STEM CELLS – LABORATORY AND CLINICAL RESEARCH

MANIPULATION OF STEM CELLS FOR DISEASE BENEFITS

STEM CELLS – LABORATORY AND CLINICAL RESEARCH

Additional books and e-books in this series can be found on Nova's website under the Series tab.

STEM CELLS – LABORATORY AND CLINICAL RESEARCH

MANIPULATION OF STEM CELLS FOR DISEASE BENEFITS

PRASAD KOKA
EDITOR

nova
Medicine & Health
New York

Library of Congress Cataloging-in-Publication Data

ISBN: 978-1-53615-468-9

Published by Nova Science Publishers, Inc. † New York

CONTENTS

PREFACE

This collection of articles deals with the benefits of different types of stem cells sources, use, manipulation, and aspects for the treatment of chronic diseases. The role of calcium channel pathway/s in the regulation of neural stem cell differentiation is quite interesting, particularly in view of the role of TRPC3 channels in cardiovascular disease as well. This leads into the cardiomyocytes vis-à-vis mesenchymal stem cells (MSCs) raising into the debate the commonalities of the evolutionary roles of the totipotent, pluripotent, or even multipotent stem cells.

The derivations of the multipotent MSCs, which are inherently conferred with immunosuppressive potential, have been discussed for their continued clinical applications through manipulations that include scaffolding and proposed targeting of cancer tissue tropism of these stem cells. Future investigations would be expected to reveal the extent of such MSC-mediated clinical applications and efficacy.

Some of the reported findings, such as that MSC differentiation into hepatocytes and the involvement of these cells with microRNA-133 in type 1 diabetes in rodents, are to be further elucidated in future studies.

Similarly as above, the role of Vitronectin in the differentiation into endoderm should be carried forward for showing wider advantages and disadvantages in terms of clinical roles.

Potential canine-derived stem cell therapies for dogs that have been suggested will be a foray into the veterinary clinics.

To what extent the stemness of dental pulp stem cells will be useful is yet another topic awaiting future lines of investigations into the clinics.

So also, PBMCs are to serve as a source for pluripotent stem cells, needs to be firmly established.

Last but not the least is that yoga and Ayurveda (ancient India pre/scripted herbal medicine) as complementary and/or alternative therapies have clearly been shown to improve the clinical conditions of spinal cord injury, type 2 diabetes, and polycystic ovarian syndrome (PCOS).

Interestingly, yoga may act in synergy with the other finding that bone marrow stromal cells provide relief from a laboratory reagent used as drug-mediated pain in spinal cord injury.

Chapter 1 - The identification and use of pharmacological agents to regulate the fate of embryonic stem cells (ESCs) and promote their differentiation into neurons has great potential in the development of novel clinical therapies. Here, the authors investigated the effect of pyrazole 3 (pyr3) on the generation of Ca^{2+} transients in mouse ESCs (mESCs), as well as on the differentiation of mESCs into neural cells. Pyr3 was originally identified as being a potent inhibitor of the transient receptor potential canonical subfamily 3 (TRPC3) channel. However, here the authors showed that pyr3 induced an increase in intracellular Ca^{2+} ($[Ca^{2+}]_i$) in a dose-dependent manner in undifferentiated mESCs. An initial, rapid increase in $[Ca^{2+}]_i$ was stimulated mainly via an influx of Ca^{2+} across the plasma membrane, whereas a subsequent longer-lasting reduced plateau phase was mediated both by Ca^{2+} influx and by Ca^{2+} release from the endoplasmic reticulum (ER) via inositol 1,4,5-trisphosphate receptors (IP_3Rs). A similar increase in $[Ca^{2+}]_i$ was recorded in mESCs following CRISPR/Cas9-mediated knock-out of *TRPC3* in the presence of the L-type Ca^{2+} channel agonist, (*S*)-(-)-Bay K 8644. A much smaller increase in $[Ca^{2+}]_i$ was recorded on addition of (*S*)-(-)-Bay K 8644 in control cells, where functional TRPC3 channels were present. Pyr3 also induced apoptosis via the disruption of the mitochondrial membrane potential ($\Delta\Psi m$) in both undifferentiated mESCs and in cells undergoing neural differentiation, and it inhibited the early stages of mESC differentiation to neural progenitors. Taken together, the authors' results suggest a novel role for TRPC3 in the regulation of $[Ca^{2+}]_i$, as well as on the survival and neural differentiation of mESCs.

Chapter 2 - The discovery, isolation, characterization and differentiation of stem cells have significantly changed the global scenario of medicinal use of these cells for diseases for which conventional drugs are of limited therapeutic potential. The presence of stem cells in virtually every multicellular organism suggests that these cells probably have a major role to play throughout the lifetime of the organism for performing specialized functions that are biologically demanded from time to time for normal development and survival. Stem cells are classified as embryonic stem cells (ESCs), induced pluripotent stem cells (iPSCs) and adult stem cells. Mesenchymal stromal cells (MSCs) are adult stem cells originally identified in mouse bone marrow, have now been discovered in many species and can be isolated from human and animal sources. Human MSCs (hMSCs) are multipotent, non-hematopoietic stromal cells which have the ability to differentiate into variety of cell types, including osteoblasts, chondrocytes, myocytes, adipocytes, cardiomyocytes, endothelial cells, hepatocytes and neural cells. These cells are identified by adherence to plastic surfaces under normal culture conditions and exhibit fibroblast-like morphology. The cultured MSCs express cell surface markers including CD29, CD44, CD49a-f, CD51, CD73, CD105, CD106, CD166, and Stro-1 and lack the expression of CD14, CD19, CD34, CD45 and HLA-DR surface molecules. Because of their immunosuppressive, anti-inflammatory properties and ability to secrete paracrine factors, hMSCs have emerged with a great potential in the field of tissue engineering and regenerative medicine and promise to be a liable source for therapeutic applications. This review article provides an overview on classification, sources and importance of mesenchymal stromal cells with an emphasis on its clinical applications. Brief updates on production technology and currently available cell therapy products have been described.

Chapter 3 - Tumor tropism of Mesenchymal Stem Cells confers them an added characteristic. Possibly, one can explore inherent anticancer potentials to deliver anti-cancer agents to the site of the tumor. It is a well-established fact that Mesenchymal Stem Cells (MSCs) are equipped with traits like multi-lineage differentiation potential, immune privilegedness and probably some affinity for tumors. The scientific community has been debating pro-cancer or anticancer nature of MSCs. It is believed that MSCs, by virtue of their reparative function, acts as a tumor-promoting entity by expressing several growth factors and helps formation of new vessels by a process called angiogenesis. However, MSCs are also reported to play an anti-cancer role by expressing molecules like TRAIL (Tumor Necrosis Factor-related Apoptosis Inducing Ligand) and DKK1 (Wnt pathway inhibitor) and many other tumor suppressor molecules. Extensive literature is available on tumor specific migration and anti-cancer nature of MSCs derived from either bone marrow or adipose tissue. The behavior of mix of MSCs derived from perinatal tissues viz. umbilical cord tissue, placenta and amniotic sac for these investigations is least explored. The advantages of utilizing perinatal tissue as a source of MSCs are obvious, which include the ease of procurement process, their abundant availability and the naive nature of cells as compared to other sources studied so far.

Chapter 4 - Tumor tropism of Mesenchymal Stem Cells confers them an added characteristic. Possibly, one can explore inherent anticancer potentials to deliver anti-cancer agents to the site of the tumor. It is a well-established fact that Mesenchymal Stem Cells (MSCs) are equipped with traits like multi-lineage differentiation potential, immune privilegedness and probably some affinity for tumors. The scientific community has been debating pro-cancer or anticancer nature of MSCs. It is believed that MSCs, by virtue of their reparative function, acts as a tumor-promoting entity by expressing several growth factors and helps formation of new vessels by a process called angiogenesis. However, MSCs are also reported to play an anti-cancer role by expressing molecules like TRAIL (Tumor Necrosis Factor-related Apoptosis Inducing Ligand) and DKK1 (Wnt pathway inhibitor) and many other tumor suppressor molecules. Extensive literature is available on tumor specific migration and anti-cancer nature of MSCs derived from either bone marrow or adipose tissue. The behavior of mix of MSCs derived from perinatal tissues viz. umbilical cord tissue, placenta and amniotic sac for these investigations is least explored. The advantages of utilizing perinatal tissue as a source of MSCs are obvious, which include the ease of procurement process, their abundant availability and the naive nature of cells as compared to other sources studied so far.

Chapter 5 - Differentiation of mesenchyal stem cells (MSCs) into biologically active hepatocytes depends on several factors. Glutathione (GSH) and antioxidant enzymes play major role in maintaining the balance between oxidative damage factors and antioxidants during the differentiation. There-fore by adding GSH modifiers to the culture media, the authors examined the impact of GSH on the process of MSC differentiation into hepatocyte-like cells. In the present study differentiation of MSCs into hepatocyte-like cells was induced using a 2-step protocol. Then production of reactive oxygen species (ROS), cellular GSH, GSH peroxidase (GPX), GSH reductase (GR) and total antioxidant capacity (TAC) were determined on days 2, 7 and 14 of differentiation onset. Besides, the experiment was carried out in cells treated with glutathione modifiers namely; buthionine sulfoximine (BSO) or N-acetylcysteine (NAC). Depletion in GSH and GPX due to BSO treatments resulted in elevation of ROS production. In contrast, ROS was substantially decreased in cells having high levels of GSH and GPX following NAC treatments. The results showed that during differentiation, the cell proliferation was affected by ROS alterations. Cell proliferation was enhanced when treated with NAC which also increased GSH, GPX and TAC. As a consequence of GSH elevation by NAC, there was a substantial increase in antioxidant activity of the cells undergoing differentiation. This data show that ROS generation and TAC status can be balanced during the process of hepatic differentiation of MSCs by inducing GSH biosynthesis using NAC in the culture media. This action is associated with improved cell proliferation and differentiation.

Chapter 6 - *Background*: Stem cells created new hope in regenerative medicine for their ability to repair damaged tissues. This present study examined the effect of bone marrow-derived mesenchymal stem cells (BM-MSCs) on miRNA-133a expression, and their relation to cardiac complications in diabetic rats. *Methods:* The current study included three groups of Wistar rats: control rats, type 1 diabetes rat model induced by streptozotocin (STZ), and diabetic rats treated with BM-MSCs. For all rats, fasting blood glucose (FBG), serum insulin as well as cardiovascular functions (heart rate, systolic blood pressure and electrocardiogram) were assessed. All rats were sacrificed after eight weeks. Specimens from cardiac and pancreatic tissues were examined to detect fluorescent labelled BM-MSCs, and their regenerative effect by hematoxylin and eosin stain. Expression of miRNA-133a was assessed in pancreatic and cardiac tissues by quantitative real time polymerase chain reaction (qRT-PCR). *Results:* This study revealed that the body weight and serum insulin levels were increased in BM-MSC treated diabetic rats, while FBG didn't reach the euglycemic level. Moreover, improvement of systolic blood pressure and corrected QT (QTc) interval was found. The expression of miR-133a was significantly increased in pancreatic and cardiac tissues of diabetic rats, and correlated with FBG. However, there was no significant difference in its expression after treatment with BM-MSCs. *Conclusion*: This study has given evidence for the first time that miR133a was expressed in pancreatic as well as cardiac tissues of diabetic rats in response to hyperglycemia. Also, BM-MSCs had the potential to improve pancreatic and cardiac functions in diabetic rats.

Chapter 7 - Current comprehension of endoderm organ development has enabled researchers to successfully direct pluripotent stem cells (PSCs) to differentiate into endodermal lineage which can give rise to cells of the lungs, liver, pancreas, stomach, and intestine. Nevertheless, variations in the differentiation efficiency have been reported mainly due the utilization of poorly defined matrices in the protocols applied. On this basis, the present study investigated the potential role of recombinant human-Vitronectin-N (VN) in inducing differentiation of human induced pluripotent stem cells (hiPSCs) into endodermal lineage. Differentiation was initiated by applying a previously established sequential step wise endodermal differentiation protocol. Expression of endodermal specific genes characteristic of each differentiation stage was investigated and analyzed by qRT-PCR and immunohistochemistry. The authors' results demonstrated a significant up-regulation of endoderm related markers characteristic of respective stages of differentiation in hiPSCs differentiated on VN coated dishes in comparison to those differentiated on routinely used feeder cells. Analysis of *PDX1* expression in differentiated cells illustrated that VN was able to further induce pancreatic progenitors as well. Altogether, the authors' results demonstrated that VN efficiently promoted endodermal differentiation of human induced pluripotent stem cells.

Chapter 8 - Previous studies have suggested that neurotransmitters may play an important role in influencing neural stem/progenitor cells (NSPCs) differentiation into oligodendrocytes (OL). Differentiated OL are known to aid in remyelination and axonal protection. In order to derive pure lineages of OL, especially for use in regenerative medicine, improved differentiation protocols are required. One potential differentiation cue is the excitatory neurotransmitter glutamate, but, its effect on NSPCs is currently unknown. Using real-time PCR, the authors examined the *in vitro* ability of glutamate, in combination of growth factors to influence the NSPCs differentiation. Glutamate (200μM) for 14-days did not induce significant changes in the gene expression profile of differentiated cultures. Moreover, the combination of growth factors (FGF2, PDGF, NT3) demonstrated no significant effect on the proportions of differentiated cell types. Although the differentiation media, containing fetal bovine serum, had an effect on appearance of neuronal lineage, the overall expression of mature cell markers continued to decrease by day-14. In contrast, Matrigel-attached cultures, demonstrated significant increase in glial markers, with possible inhibition of neuronal differentiation as observed with spontaneous attachment. Overall, these data suggest that glutamate (200μM) and combination of growth factors had no modulating effect on the gene expression profile of differentiated NSPCs culture.

Chapter 9 - This present study aims at the evaluation of different transportation, isolation, and cryopreservation conditions on the stemness properties of dental pulp stem cells (DPSCs), in an attempt to optimize those conditions to obtain high-quality cells for the needs of regenerative therapy. DPSCs were isolated from canine teeth that were placed in one of six different collection/transport solutions: phosphate buffered saline (PBS); PBS containing fetal bovine serum (FBS); Dulbecco modified Eagles' medium (DMEM); DMEM containing FBS; Hank's solution; or saline. Collected teeth were either processed after 3, 12, 24, 36, or 48 hours and using one of two different enzymes. The stemness properties of the isolated cells were evaluated in terms of proliferation, migration, and expression of stem cell markers. Moreover, DPSCs cryopreserved in one of two different cryopreservants and stored at -80°C then transferred to liquid nitrogen after either 1,12,24,48 hours or 1 week. After thawing, the cells were evaluated for viability using trypan blue test. The results indicate that dental pulp cells can be isolated from dental pulp up to 48 hours after tooth extraction, which implies that processing immediately after extraction may not be required for successful isolation. However, the stemness properties of the isolated cells were significantly affected by the transportation media and the isolation time. This study also indicates that the shorter the time elapsed between transferring the cryopreserved cells from -80°C to liquid nitrogen was, the higher the viability of the thawed cells was.

Chapter 10 - *Background:* Dental pulp stem cells (DPSCs) are considered an easily accessible source of mesenchymal stem cells holding great promise for use in tissue repair and regenerative medicine. In order for DPSCs to be used in therapeutic clinical applications, issues like safely enhancing culture expansion need to be addressed. *Objective:* In this research, the authors aimed to assess the safety of platelet-rich plasma (PRP) as a promoter of proliferation in comparison to routinely used animal derived supplements. *Methods:* The effect of PRP on the proliferation of DPSCs was assessed by MTT assay. Expression of stemness-related genes *OCT4 & INTGRIN1* was analyzed by real-time quantitative PCR. DNA sequencing was performed for *OCT4 & INTGRIN1* genes to ensure that the isolated DPSCs stem cell properties were not altered by the PRP supplemented media. *Results:* At a concentration of 1% with platelet count of 1.5 x $10^6/cm^3$, PRP was able to significantly increase the proliferation rate while maintaining the viability of DPSCs in comparison to routinely used 15% FBS. Mesenchymal stem cell surface markers expression (CD29, CD105) were not altered by PRP supplementation. Moreover, PRP in cultures significantly promoted expression of stemness markers *OCT4 & INTGRIN1* compared with 10% FBS. The results were confirmed by DNA sequencing for *OCT4 & INTGRIN1* genes where DPSCs cultured in PRP demonstrated 100% matching with the control group indicating that PRP supplementation didn't alter the nucleotide sequence of stem cell genes. *Conclusions:* Taken together, the authors' results indicate that PRP is a safe and efficient promoter of proliferation and can readily substitute traditional animal derived supplements like FBS.

Chapter 11 - Domesticated animals or companion animals are pets that share a psychological bond with their owners. Today there are some 77 million dogs in the USA.

The attitudes towards pets have changed and many pets are treated as family members. Dogs live longer lives than ever because preventive health care has become available for them by veterinarians in the health care field who devote much effort towards disease prevention, early detection, reduced invasiveness, and personalized therapies. Regular health exams and immunization programs help ensure that conditions are prevented or treated early. Millions of pets will develop diseases with close analogy to human diseases such as osteoarthritis. Pet owners will look for treatment options to help their beloved pets. Several major pet-insurance companies have recently added stem cell trans-plants to the lists of procedures for which they will pay. Stem cell therapy for dogs is a decision for the owner, and it means considering both the best interest of the dog and the owners financial possibilities. Stem cell technology is a new branch of veterinary medicine but unfortunately there is not yet much information on possible adverse side effects available. Stem cells can be harvested from a variety of adult animal tissues then be injected and induced to grow into different mature cell types.

Chapter 12 - Bone marrow stromal cells (BMSC) have been investigated in the central nervous system repair after injury. However, the effectiveness of these cells in the treatment of spinal cord injury (SCI) induced hyperalgesia, allodynia, and hypoalgesia is far from clear. In this study, the authors investigated the therapeutic effect of BMSC on formalin tonic pain and feeding behavior after thoracic complete SCI. Adult male rats underwent complete transection of the spinal cord and later at day 9 of SCI received a direct injection of pre-labeled BMSC cells around the injury site. Formalin pain behavior was studied once at the end of week 8 after SCI while feeding behavior was studied every day pre- and post-SCI. After the formalin pain study, rats were sacrificed for histological and neurochemical studies. Formalin pain behavior was decreased after SCI at week 8. This formalin pain behavior partially recovered in the BMSC transplanted rats. During the study period, feeding behavior was affected severely after SCI. However, it was improved in the BMSC group of rats. Neurochemicals such as serotonin and dopamine were affected after SCI in different brain regions which were restored partially by BMSC transplantation. Histological studies revealed the presence of pre-labeled BMSC that filled the lesion cavities in the transplanted group. Data suggest the beneficial effect of BMSC transplantation on supraspinal mediated feeding and formalin tonic pain behaviors that are associated with altered neurotransmitter levels in the SCI rats.

Chapter 13 - Induced pluripotent stem cells (iPSCs) indeed hold great potential as a basis for cell-based therapies for multiple degenerative diseases. It involves the administration of transcription factors in order to transduce multiple termin-ally differentiated cell types into pluripotent embryonic-like stem cells. These cells can overcome the issues of immune rejection, as the cells are autologous, and also eliminate any ethical issues regarding the use of human embryos. Objective: Here the authors present a onetime transfection reprogramming protocol for peripheral blood mononucleocytes (PBMNCs) Methods: PBMNCs were cultured in conditions favoring hematopoietic progenitor population. Three plasmids encoding five reprogramming factors (Oct3/4, Sox2, Klf4, L-Myc and Lin28) in addition to EBNA1, an enhancer of transfection efficiency and episomal plasmids expression were applied to reprogram the isolated cells. Results: A single transfection of this plasmid combination was sufficient to generate pluripotent markers positive iPSC colonies. Colonies resembling human ES-like cells were observed as early as 20 days after episomal plasmid neucleofection. These colonies stained positively for alkaline phosphatase. Moreover, the generated iPSCs expressed stem cell markers TRA-1-60, SSEA4, NANOG and OCT3/4 as determined by immunocytochemistry. These results demonstrated that iPSC could be effectively generated from PBMNCs using episomal plasmid vectors encoding OCT3/4, shRNA against p53, SOX2, KLF4, L-MYC and LIN28. Conclusion: Finally, it could be concluded that the method described in this research provides a promising approach for generating clinical grade induced pluripotent stem cells from highly accessible source of adult somatic cells.

Chapter 14 - *Background*: Type 2 Diabetes Mellitus (T2DM) is a metabolic condition characterized by chronic hyperglycemia. It is a highly prevalent medical problem across the globe and a leading cause of morbidity and mortality. Optimal blood glucose control is the primary goal of T2DM management. Yoga is a mind-body intervention found to be effective in various kinds of metabolic disorders including T2DM. *Aim*: This study intended to assess the impact of 3 months Integrated Yoga (IY) intervention on fasting and post-prandial blood glucose level among patients with T2DM. *Methods:* Total 251 patients with T2DM within the age range of 30-60 years (with average age; 46.04 ± 14.02 years) were enrolled in the study. Participants were divided into a yoga group (n = 137) and a control group (n = 114). Subjects in the yoga group received IY intervention consisted of Asanas, Surynamaskara, Pranayama and meditation every day for one hour/day, 6 days in a week for three months. Control group subjects followed their daily routines. Subjects on insulin therapy, with diabetic complications, uncontrolled hypertension, under steroid medication, or previous exposure to any form of yoga were excluded from the study. Fasting and post-prandial blood glucose level were assessed before and after 3 months for both the groups. *The results:* Significant decrease in both fasting and postprandial blood glucose levels was observed in IY group after 3 months compared to baseline. No improvement was seen in the control group. *Conclusion*: IY intervention helps in controlling blood glucose levels among patients with T2DM.

Chapter 15 - Type 2 Diabetes Mellitus (T2DM) is a chronic metabolic disorder and a leading cause of morbidity and mortality worldwide. Blood glucose control, prevention of DM complication and reducing the cardiovascular risk factors are the important goals of T2DM management. Having potential health benefiting effects, Yoga has become a popular alternative and complementary medicine in most of the countries around the world. There is large data evidence from RCTs for the efficacy of in various chronic problems including T2DM. In this chapter, various benefits of yoga practice in T2DM patients are discussed. The authors did a review of recent scientific studies on beneficial effects of yoga in blood glucose control, CVD risk factors and complications in T2DM. Our review found yoga as an effective intervention in reducing fasting blood sugar (FBS), postprandial blood sugar (PPBS), HbA1C and insulin resistance in T2DM. Yoga reduces cardiovascular complications in T2DM. Further, yoga improves nerve conduction velocity, cognitive function and it also improves mental health by reducing depression and stress in T2DM. This chapter concludes that yoga is a cost effective, feasible and potent intervention for optimal blood glucose control, reducing CVD risk factors, to improve cognition and mental health among patients with T2DM.

Chapter 16 - *Aim:* To study the efficacy of Yoga as a supportive therapy modality to Ayurveda treatment in improving endocrine parameters and psychopathologies in PCOS. *Methods:* The authors selected 64 women with PCOS within the age range 18 to 40 years (mean age = 29.24 years) who visited to *Ayurveda* center to seek *Ayurveda* treatment for PCOS. Subjects were randomly assigned to two groups of 32 each in *Ayurveda* group-AY and *Ayurveda* + *Yoga* group-AY + Y respectively. Women who had had; medical history of uterine fibroids, endometriosis, pelvic inflammatory disease, tubal blockage and or had exposure to yoga practices in the past 2 years were excluded from the study. All the women in AY group received cleansing therapy based on *Ayurveda* prescription which was followed by oral herbal medication intake for three months. Women in AY + Y group received 3 months of yoga intervention 1 hr daily, 5 day/week for 3 months along with *Ayurveda* treatment. The assessment of the study was for endocrine variables, ovary mass and psychological states using perceived stress scale and hospital anxiety depression invent-tory, at the baseline and after 3 months. *Results:* In the AY + Y group a significant decrease was observed for 9 variables (1) prolactin ($p = 0.003$), 2) LH ($p = 0.006$), 3) testosterone ($p = 0.003$), 4) HbA1C ($p = 0.006$), 5) AMH ($p = 0.004$), 7) T4 ($p = 0.001$), 8) TSH ($p = 0.035$), 9) right ovary mass ($p = 0.003$). In AY Group significant reduction was found for 3 variables 1) AMH ($p = 0.006$), HbA1C ($p = 0.003$), T4 ($p = 0.03$). In the between group comparison A+Y group showed significantly greater reduction in HbA1C ($p < 0.001$) and TSH ($p = 0.002$), left ($p = 0.04$) and right ($p = 0.006$) ovary mass as compared to AY group. The authors noticed significant improvement in anxiety, depression, & perceived stress in Y+A group. *Conclusion:* The present study suggests that addition of yoga intervention to the herbal medication for PCOS have additional benefits compared to only herbal treatment. This study also suggest that combination of complimentary therapies have synergetic effects in management of PCOS.

Chapter 17 - *Introduction:* Traumatic Spinal Cord Injury (TSCI) is an injury to the spinal cord that results in temporary or permanent motor, sensory, and cognitive deficits. The current conventional approach of TSCI management includes surgery, pharmacology, and physical therapy, which have some limitations and are associated with side effects. Yoga is a form of mind-body medicine found to be effective in several neurological disorders as an add-on to other therapies. *Aim:* The present study intended to see the effect of Integrated Yoga (IY) intervention as an add-on to the physiotherapy on walking index, ESR, pain and spasticity among subjects with TSCI. *Methods*: The study was conducted in a Rehabilitation Centre at Swami Vivekananda National Institute of Rehabilitation, Training and research (SVNIRTAR), Odisha. A total of 125 paraplegics within age range 18-60 years were randomly assigned to either integrated Yoga therapy + physiotherapy group (IY + PT) group (n = 62, age = 33.97 ± 10.00) or Physiotherapy (PT) group (n = 63, age = 32.84 ± 9.47). The participants in PT + IY group received one month of integrated yoga intervention consisting of yogic postures, yogic breathing techniques & chanting, and yogic relaxation practices along with physical therapy. Yoga session lasted for 75 mins per day and 6 days per week. PT group participants received only physiotherapy intervention for one month. All the participants were assessed for Erythrocyte Sedimentation Rate (ESR), Walking Index for Spinal Cord Injury II (WISCI II), Multidimensional Pain Inventory (MPI), and Modified-Modified Ashworth Scale (MMAS) at the baseline and after one month. *Results:* The authors found statically significant changes in 4 variables for IY + PT group 1) Erythrocyte Sedimentation Rate ($P < 0.001$), 2) WISCI II ($P < 0.001$) MPI-S1 ($P < 0.001$), MPI-S2 ($P = 0.003$), & MPI-S3 ($P = 0.003$), and 4) MMAS ($P < 0.001$) after one month of intervention compared to baseline. Compared to PT group, IY + PT group showed significantly better improvement in WISCI II ($P < 0.001$), MPI-S3 ($P = 0.003$), and MMAS ($P < 0.001$). *Conclusion:* The resent study suggests the usefulness of an IY intervention add on to physiotherapy in the management of patients with paraplegia.

Chapter 18 - Spinal cord injury (SCI) leads to severe disability contributing to poor quality of life. Cell-based or cell-related therapies have emerged as breakthrough therapies, both in regeneration of spinal cord and enhanced functional recovery. This review aims to discuss the therapeutic benefits of yoga in the rehabilitation of SCI in enhancing neural plasticity and emerging as an important add-on to support stem cell therapies. Conventional treatment for SCI does not bring out full recovery of loss of function. Chronic systemic inflammation prevailing years after injury is one of the obstacles in sensory and motor function improvement. Recurrence of secondary infections, risk of neural tissue death and depression disorders leading to poor quality of life are some of the factors which are barriers to recovery of SCI. Cell replacement strategies provide cells that can replace the lost function. They provide a regenerative pathway for injured adult neurons, which would then promote the regeneration of adult neurons. Transplantation of cells mostly leads to the rejection of the donor material due to a combination of humoral and cellular immune responses. Evidences how that yoga modulates immune function which is otherwise compromised by stress. It can promote neurogenesis and angiogenesis resulting from increase production of neurotrophins. Yoga as an immune modulator can thus enhance the acceptance of implanted stem cells leading to the regeneration of the spinal cord circuitry and restore function after injury. It is thus hypothesized that yoga's therapeutic benefits may prove as an approach to alleviate the barriers of cellular therapies if necessary evidences are generated.

In: Manipulation of Stem Cells for Disease Benefits
Editor: Prasad Koka
ISBN: 978-1-53615-468-9

Chapter 1

THE EFFECT OF PYRAZOLE 3 TREATMENT ON THE GENERATION OF INTRACELLULAR CA^{2+} TRANSIENTS AND MITOCHONDRIAL MEMBRANE POTENTIAL, AS WELL AS THE SURVIVAL AND NEURAL DIFFERENTIATION OF MOUSE EMBRYONIC STEM CELLS

Helen Baixia Hao[1], Sarah E. Webb[1], Jianbo Yue[2], Marc Moreau[3], Catherine Leclerc[3] and Andrew L. Miller[1,*]

[1]Division of Life Science and State Key Laboratory of Molecular Neuroscience, HKUST, Clear Water Bay, Hong Kong, PR China
[2]Department of Biomedical Sciences, City University of Hong Kong, Hong Kong, PR China
[3]Centre de Biologie du Développement, UMR-CNRS 5547, Université Toulouse III, Toulouse, France

ABSTRACT

The identification and use of pharmacological agents to regulate the fate of embryonic stem cells (ESCs) and promote their differentiation into neurons has great potential in the development of novel clinical therapies. Here, we investigated the effect of pyrazole 3 (pyr3) on the generation of Ca^{2+} transients in mouse ESCs (mESCs), as well as on the differentiation of mESCs into neural cells. Pyr3 was originally identified as being a potent inhibitor of the transient receptor potential canonical subfamily 3 (TRPC3) channel. However, here we showed that pyr3 induced an increase in intracellular Ca^{2+} ($[Ca^{2+}]_i$) in a dose-dependent manner in undifferentiated mESCs. An initial, rapid

* Corresponding Author's E-mail: almiller@ust.hk.

increase in $[Ca^{2+}]_i$ was stimulated mainly via an influx of Ca^{2+} across the plasma membrane, whereas a subsequent longer-lasting reduced plateau phase was mediated both by Ca^{2+} influx and by Ca^{2+} release from the endoplasmic reticulum (ER) via inositol 1,4,5-trisphosphate receptors (IP_3Rs). A similar increase in $[Ca^{2+}]_i$ was recorded in mESCs following CRISPR/Cas9-mediated knock-out of *TRPC3* in the presence of the L-type Ca^{2+} channel agonist, (*S*)-(-)-Bay K 8644. A much smaller increase in $[Ca^{2+}]_i$ was recorded on addition of (*S*)-(-)-Bay K 8644 in control cells, where functional TRPC3 channels were present. Pyr3 also induced apoptosis via the disruption of the mitochondrial membrane potential ($\Delta\Psi m$) in both undifferentiated mESCs and in cells undergoing neural differentiation, and it inhibited the early stages of mESC differentiation to neural progenitors. Taken together, our results suggest a novel role for TRPC3 in the regulation of $[Ca^{2+}]_i$, as well as on the survival and neural differentiation of mESCs.

Keywords: mouse embryonic stem cells, Ca^{2+} signaling, pyr3, TRPC3, CRISPR/Cas9 gene editing, apoptosis, mitochondrial membrane potential, neural differentiation

INTRODUCTION

Embryonic stem cells (ESCs) are characterized by their capacity for self-renewal and pluripotency (Evans and Kaufman, 1981; Beddington and Robertson, 1989; Thomson et al., 1998). Thus, these cells can proliferate in an unlimited manner and differentiate into the various different cell types of the three germ layers (i.e., the ectoderm, mesoderm and endoderm; Bradley et al., 1984). It is because of these unique properties that ESCs have the potential for use in the development of cell-based therapies for the treatment of various congenital, developmental and degenerative conditions including neurodegenerative diseases (Hipp and Atala, 2008; Forment et al., 2017). While the regular and successful use of ESCs in a clinical setting has many challenges still to overcome, these cells are currently very useful for disease modelling and drug discovery (Sandoe and Eggan, 2013; Marks et al., 2017).

In recent years, a considerable effort has been spent attempting to develop methods to efficiently and cost-effectively induce the differentiation of ESCs into specific types of neuron, including dopaminergic and motor neurons (Li et al., 2005; Yan et al., 2005; Kriks et al., 2011). Early methods included: Treatment of ESCs with retinoic acid (RA; Bain et al., 1995; Fraichard et al., 1995); co-culture with specific stromal cell lines such as PA6 (Kawasaki et al., 2000); or through the treatment of adherent monolayer cultures with chemically-defined medium (Ying and Smith, 2003; Ying et al., 2003). More recently, a scalable system for deriving and propagating neural stem cells from human ESCs was developed via the use of chemically-defined medium containing components derived from humans, such as serum albumin, transferrin, recombinant FGF2, and insulin (Joannides et al., 2007). However, in order to generate neurons that meet clinical application standards (Trounson and DeWitt, 2016), more detailed work needs to be conducted to characterize the properties of ESC-derived neuronal cells, as well as to increase the efficacy and promote the maturation of ESC-derived neurons. To this end, gaining a better understanding of the cellular and molecular mechanisms involved in the regulation of *in vivo* and *in vitro* neurogenesis is essential.

Ca^{2+} signaling has been reported to play an important role in neural development *in vivo* and during the neural differentiation of ESCs (Leclerc et al., 2000; Rosenberg and Spitzer, 2011; Leclerc et al., 2012; Hao et al., 2016; Toth et al., 2016). For example, Ca^{2+} transients have been implicated in the regulation of neural proliferation, migration, differentiation, and survival (Spitzer, 2006; Platel et al., 2008; Vonhoff and Keshishian, 2017). In addition, Ca^{2+} signaling has been reported to contribute to the specification of the various neuronal subtypes via the regulation of axonal guidance, dendritic growth and branching, as well as via the specification of neurotransmitter subtypes (Rosenberg and Spitzer, 2011). Moreover, during the neural differentiation of ESCs the manipulation of various Ca^{2+} channels or Ca^{2+} signaling proteins has been shown to affect cell viability, the expression of neural differentiation markers, and specification of the neural lineage, as well as the Ca^{2+} handling of the cells (Yu et al., 2008; Lin et al., 2010; Hao et al., 2014; Wei et al., 2015).

Transient receptor potential canonical subfamily 3 (TRPC3) is a Ca^{2+} permeable, non-selective cation channel. It has been reported to regulate/interact with a number of Ca^{2+} sensors, as well as other Ca^{2+} channels and receptors such as STIM1 (Yuan et al., 2007); Orai1 (Woodward et al., 2010); L-type Ca^{2+} channels (LTCCs; Gao et al., 2012); inositol 1,4,5-trisphosphate receptors (IP_3Rs; Bandyopadhyay et al., 2008) and ryanodine receptors (RyRs; Lee et al., 2006). TRPC3 channels are reported to be present in both the plasma membrane and the mitochondrial membrane of certain cell types, where they serve to regulate the influx and uptake of Ca^{2+}, respectively (Feng et al., 2013). As a result, they are reported to be associated with the regulation of a diverse range of cellular functions (Trebak et al., 2003; Putney et al., 2004). These include hypothalamic glucose detection (Chrétien et al., 2017); thrombin-induced astrocyte activation (Shirakawa et al., 2010); endothelial dysfunction and heart disease (Smedlund et al., 2012); and sinoatrial arrhythmias (Ju et al., 2015) to name just a few examples. Furthermore, TRPC3 channels have most recently been reported to be required for the survival, pluripotency and neural differentiation of mouse embryonic stem cells (mESCs; Hao et al., 2018). Thus, due to the wide range of functions, TRPC3 channels might be considered to act as a cellular signaling nexus (Groschner and Rosker, 2005; Zheng, 2013). We therefore decided to investigate the possible role played by TRPC3 during the quiescent survival of mESCs and the neural differentiation of these cells in further detail.

A variety of small molecules have been identified, which can selectively activate or block different Ca^{2+} channels, pumps, and exchangers located within the membranes of cells. They can therefore be used to regulate $[Ca^{2+}]_i$ and consequently, the associated downstream Ca^{2+}-sensitive processes within differentiating cells, including neurons (Lee, 1997; Darcy and Isaacson, 2009). One of these small molecules, pyrazole 3 (pyr3), has been reported to be a selective inhibitor of TRPC3. It was shown to inhibit TRPC3-mediated Ca^{2+} influx into DT40 B lymphocytes; attenuate activation of nuclear factor of activated T cells (NFAT); block hypertrophic growth in rat neonatal cardiomyocytes; and reduce overload-induced cardiac hypertrophy in mice (Kiyonaka et al., 2009). Since then, pyr3 has been used in a number of different studies to specifically antagonize the function of TRPC3 both *in vivo* and *in vitro* (Sabourin et al., 2012; Koenig et al., 2013; Senadheera et al., 2013; Qi et al., 2016; Oda et al., 2017). However, the TRPC3-specificity of pyr3 has also been questioned as it has been reported that in some cases where it is used at a concentration that blocks TRPC3 (i.e., ~ 0.5 μM), this drug also inhibits Orai1-mediated store-operated Ca^{2+} entry (SOCE) and mast cell activation (Schleifer et al., 2012). Thus, in this study we investigated the possible role played by TRPC3 in undifferentiated mESCs, and during their differentiation into neurons by blocking the function of TRPC3 pharmacologically with pyr3, and by knocking out its function via CRISPR/Cas9 gene editing (Hao et al., 2018).

Here, we report the effect of pyr3 on the regulation of $[Ca^{2+}]_i$ as well as on the survival and neural differentiation of mESCs. We found that the treatment of mESCs with pyr3 alone induced an immediate and rapid increase in $[Ca^{2+}]_i$, mainly due to an influx of Ca^{2+} across the plasma membrane, as well as a later secondary plateau, which was partially due to the release of Ca^{2+} from the endoplasmic reticulum (ER) via IP_3Rs. CRISPR/Cas9-mediated gene knock-out (KO) of *TRPC3* followed by exposure to (*S*)-(-)-Bay K 8644 - an LTCC agonist - suggested that functional TRPC3 might at least partially regulate $[Ca^{2+}]_i$ via an inhibitory interaction with LTCCs. We also showed that pyr3 induced apoptosis, which was stimulated via the disruption of the mitochondrial membrane potential (ΔΨm). Finally, we demonstrated that pyr3 suppressed the early neural differentiation of mESCs. Our results therefore provide new insights regarding the possible actions of pyr3 and the roles of TRPC3 on the regulation of Ca^{2+} signaling and homeostasis, as well as on cell apoptosis and differentiation, in mESCs.

RESULTS

Pyr3 Increased $[Ca^{2+}]_i$ in mESCs in a Dose-Dependent Manner

Pyr3 has previously been reported to selectively inhibit TRPC3-mediated Ca^{2+} influx in a number of cell types, including DT40 B lymphocytes, HEK293 cells, embryonic stem cell-derived cardiomyocytes, and melanoma cells (Kiyonaka et al., 2009; Qi et al., 2016; Oda et al., 2017). Initially, we measured the direct effect of exposure to 0.2 μM, 2.0 μM or 10 μM pyr3 (as well as to 0.1% DMSO as the solvent control), on the intracellular Ca^{2+} response of mESCs, which were maintained in Hank's balanced salt solution (HBSS) containing 1.26 mM Ca^{2+} (Figure 1A). Our results showed that no Ca^{2+} signals were generated in cells treated with 0.2 μM pyr3 or DMSO alone (control) (Figure 1A-1C). However, both 2 μM and 10 μM pyr3 stimulated a similar initial rapid rise in $[Ca^{2+}]_i$ (indicated by the fluorescence intensity of Fluo-4) with comparable relative peak values of 3.4 ± 0.2 at ~ 130 s (Figure 1A, 1B). At ~590 s, cells stimulated with 2 μM or 10 μM pyr3 maintained secondary plateau values of 1.3 ± 0.1 and 2.8 ± 0.2, respectively (Figure 1A, 1C). These results suggest that pyr3 alone increased $[Ca^{2+}]_i$ in a dose-dependent manner in mESCs.

Pyr3 Increased $[Ca^{2+}]_i$ by Stimulating an Influx of Ca^{2+} across the Plasma Membrane as well as a Release of Ca^{2+} from the ER via IP_3Rs

When mESCs were incubated in Ca^{2+}-free HBSS medium (+2 mM EGTA) prior to treatment with 10 μM pyr3 (Figure 1D), the initial rapid peak-rise in $[Ca^{2+}]_i$ that was observed in the Ca^{2+}-containing medium (Figure 1A) was eliminated, and the secondary slow plateau-rise was reduced by ~ 60% (Figure 1D, 1E).

mESCs were incubated in Ca^{2+}-free HBSS medium (+2 mM EGTA) and pre-treated with either 2 μM xestospongin C (an IP_3R antagonist; Miyamoto et al., 2000) or 0.1% DMSO (as the solvent control). In both cases, the addition of 10 μM pyr3 failed to induce the initial rapid peak-rise in $[Ca^{2+}]_i$ (Figure 1F), which was normally observed when Ca^{2+} was present in the extracellular medium (Figure 1A, 1D). However, xestospongin C pre-treatment also completely blocked the pyr3-induced secondary slow plateau-rise (Figure 1F, 1G). These data suggest that Ca^{2+} release from the ER via IP_3Rs contributes to the secondary slow rise in $[Ca^{2+}]_i$ induced by pyr3 and helps to maintain it at a plateau level.

Together, the data from Figure 1 suggest that in mESCs there are 2 components that result from the addition of 10 μM pyr3. The first is a rapid and instantaneous influx of Ca^{2+} across the plasma membrane; this is then followed, after a delay of ~60 seconds, by a slower release of Ca^{2+} from intracellular store(s) via IP_3Rs (Figure 1F), to help maintain the elevated plateau level. Figure 1H shows a representative fluorescent image of control mESCs loaded with fluo-4 AM.

Pyr3 Increased $[Ca^{2+}]_i$ in TRPC3 KO mESCs

In order to further explore the possible mechanism(s) behind this somewhat surprising result, we treated *TRPC3* KO mESCs (Hao et al., 2018) maintained in HBSS + Ca^{2+}, with 10 µM pyr3 (or 0.1% DMSO; Figure 2A, 2B). For controls, scrambled sequence (Scr) infected mESCs (Hao et al., 2018) were also treated with either 10 µM pyr3 or 0.1% DMSO. In the *TRPC3* KO mESCs, treatment with 10 µM pyr3 triggered a larger (i.e., by ~ 30%) initial peak increase in $[Ca^{2+}]_i$, and then maintained a higher plateau level, when compared with the Scr mESCs treated with 10 µM pyr3 (Figure 2A, 2B). This suggests that pyr3 might have an effect on mESCs, which is independent of TRPC3, but which acts via an as-yet unidentified mechanism. When *TRPC3* KO and Scr mESCs were maintained in HBSS without Ca^{2+} (plus 2 mM EGTA), and then treated with 10 µM pyr3, the initial peak was completely inhibited (Figure 2C). In addition, the *TRPC3* KO and Scr mESCs both showed similar plateau values (Figure 2C, 2D). Figure 2E and 2F show representative fluorescent images of Scr and *TRPC3* KO mESCs, respectively, when loaded with fluo-4 AM.

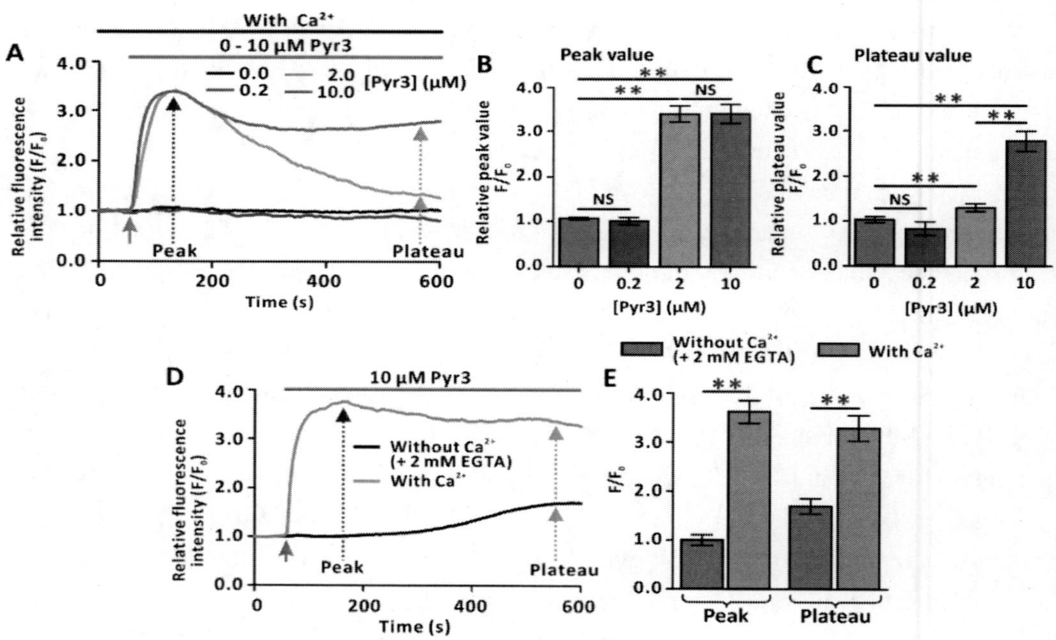

Figure 1. (Continued).

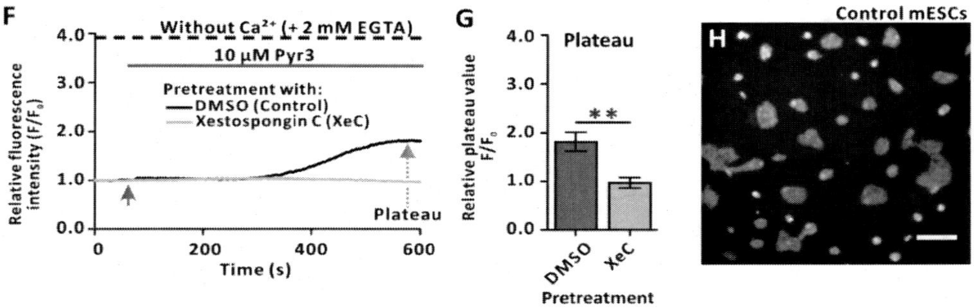

Figure 1. Pyr3 increases $[Ca^{2+}]_i$ in a dose-dependent manner by stimulating an influx of Ca^{2+} as well as a release of Ca^{2+} from the ER via IP_3Rs. (A) Line graph to show the time course of intracellular Ca^{2+} responses in control mESCs (maintained in HBSS buffer containing Ca^{2+}), following the addition (indicated by the brown arrow) of pyr3 at 0.2 μM, 2 μM or 10 μM, or 0.1% DMSO alone (as the solvent control). The peak and plateau values following the addition of pyr3 (or DMSO) are indicated by blue and orange arrows, respectively. (B,C) Quantification of the relative (B) peak and (C) plateau F/F_0 values as indicated by the blue and orange arrows, respectively in panel (A). In cases where distinct peaks and/or plateaus were not observed, these F/F_0 data were compared at the same time that the 10 μM treatment did show a peak and plateau, respectively. (D) Line graph showing the time course of Ca^{2+} responses in mESCs (maintained in HBSS buffer with/without Ca^{2+}), following the addition of 10 μM pyr3 (as indicated by the green arrow). The peak and plateau values are indicated by the blue and orange arrows, respectively. (E) Quantification of the relative peak and plateau values of F/F_0 as indicated by the blue and orange arrows, respectively in panel (D). (F) Line graph showing the time course of Ca^{2+} responses of mESCs (pretreated with 0.1% DMSO or 2 μM xestospongin C (XeC) in HBSS without Ca^{2+} and with 2 mM EGTA for 10 min), following the addition of 10 μM pyr3 (indicated by the green arrow). In both cases, the immediate early peak-rise seen in the presence of extracellular was absent. In addition, in the DMSO controls, the cells displayed a slow late rise to a much reduced plateau level (indicated by the orange arrow), whereas with XeC, this slow late rise was also inhibited. (G) Quantification of the relative plateau values of F/F_0 as indicated by the orange arrow in panel (F). In panels (B), (C), (E) and (G), the data are presented as mean ± S.E.M of n = 3 experiments, and the asterisks indicate statistically significant differences at $p < 0.01$ (**). NS indicates data that are not significantly different. (H) Representative fluorescence image of control mESCs after being loaded with fluo-4 AM. Scale bar is 100 μm.

(S)-(-)-Bay K 8644-Induced an Increase in $[Ca^{2+}]_i$ in CRISPR/Cas9-Mediated TRPC3 KO mESCs

TRPC3 KO and Scr control mESCs were treated with 10 μM (*S*)-(-)-Bay K 8644, an LTCC agonist (Figure 3A, 3B). Our results indicated that the Ca^{2+} influx mediated by LTCCs was significantly increased in the *TRPC3* KO mESCs, when compared with the Scr control cells, exhibiting significantly higher levels of $[Ca^{2+}]_i$ for both the initial peak (blue arrows) and the sustained secondary plateau of elevated Ca^{2+} (orange arrows) (Figure 3A, 3B).

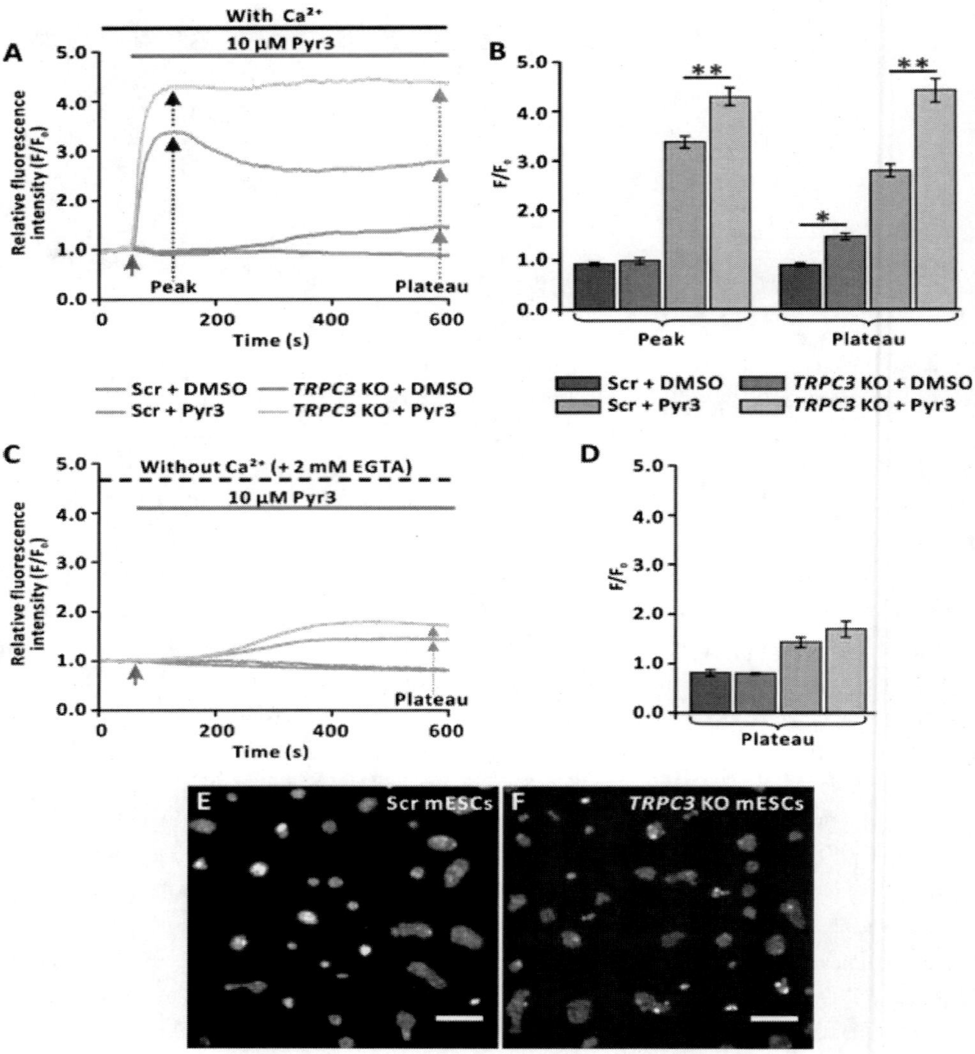

Figure 2. The pyr3-induced Ca^{2+} influx is enhanced in *TRPC3* KO mESCs. (A) Line graph showing the time course of Ca^{2+} responses in *TRPC3* KO and scrambled (Scr) mESCs (maintained in HBSS buffer with Ca^{2+}) when treated with 10 μM pyr3 or 0.1% DMSO control (indicated by the green arrow). The peak and plateau values following the addition of pyr3 (or DMSO) are indicated by blue and orange arrows, respectively. (B) Quantification of the relative peak and plateau F/F_0 values, as indicated by the blue and orange arrows, respectively in panel (A). (C) Line graph showing the time course of Ca^{2+} responses of mESCs in HBSS buffer minus Ca^{2+} (and plus 2 mM EGTA), following the addition of 10 μM pyr3 (indicated by the green arrow). The immediate early peak-rise seen in the presence of extracellular is absent and cells display only a slow late rise to a much reduced plateau level. The plateau value is indicated by the orange arrows. (D) Quantification of the relative resting values of F/F_0 as indicated by the orange arrows in panel (C). In panels (B) and (D), the data are presented as mean ± S.E.M of n = 3 experiments, and the asterisks indicate statistically significant differences at $p < 0.05$ (*) and $p < 0.01$ (**). (E,F) Representative fluorescence images of (E) Scr and (F) *TRPC3* KO mESCs after being loaded with fluo-4 AM. Scale bars are 100 μm.

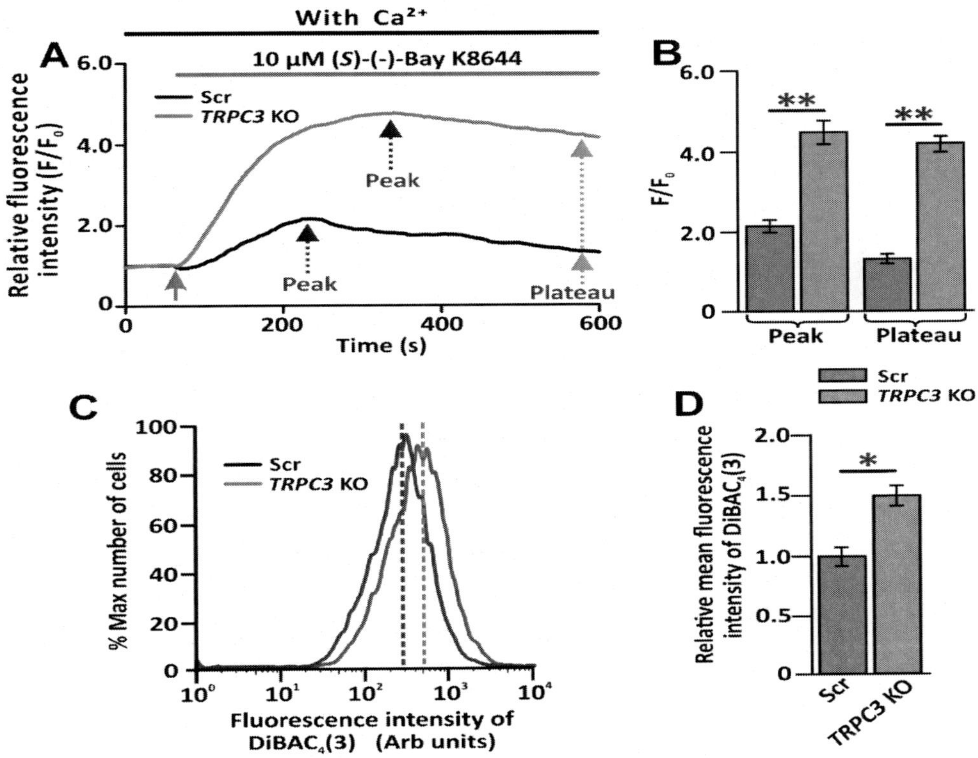

Figure 3. In the presence of (*S*)-(-)-Bay K 8644, the LTCC-mediated Ca^{2+} influx and the plasma membrane potential is greater in the *TRPC3* KO mESCs than in the Scr controls. (A) Line graph showing the time course of Ca^{2+} responses in *TRPC3* KO and Scr mESCs when treated with 10 µM (*S*)-(-)-Bay K 8644 (indicated by the pink arrow). The peak and plateau levels are indicated by blue and orange arrows, respectively. (B) Quantification of the peak and plateau values of F/F_0 as indicated by the blue and orange arrows, respectively in panel (A). (C) Flow cytometry analysis following $DiBAC_4(3)$ staining of *TRPC3* KO and Scr mESCs to compare the membrane potentials. (D) Quantification of the relative mean fluorescence intensity of $DiBAC_4(3)$ in panel (C). The mean value of fluorescence intensity in the *TRPC3* KO cells was normalized to the mean fluorescence intensity value of the Scr controls. In panels (B) and (D), the data are presented as mean ± S.E.M of n = 3 experiments, and the asterisks indicate statistically significant differences at $p < 0.05$ (*) and $p < 0.01$ (**).

As the activation and inactivation of LTCCs are dependent, respectively on the depolarization and hyperpolarization of the plasma membrane potential (Striessnig et al., 2014), the membrane potential in both the *TRPC3* KO and Scr mESCs was compared using the dye $DiBAC_4(3)$ (Figure 3C, 3D). As shown in Figure 3D, the *TRPC3* KO mESCs exhibited a ~ 50% higher membrane potential than the Scr cells. These results suggest that in mESCs where functional TRPC3 was knocked-out, treatment with 10 µM (*S*)-(-)-Bay K8644 resulted in an influx of Ca^{2+} via LTCC. However, when functional TRPC3 was present (i.e., in the case of the Scr control mESCs), it appeared to play an inhibitory role with regards to the regulation of Ca^{2+} influx through LTCC on the addition of 10 µM (*S*)-(-)-Bay K8644 (Figure 3A, 3B).

Pyr3 Induced Apoptosis and a Disruption of the Mitochondrial Membrane Potential (ΔΨm) in Undifferentiated mESCs

As Ca^{2+} homeostasis is crucial for cell viability (Orrenius et al., 2015), we investigated the effect of pyr3 on the viability of mESCs using several different assays (Figure 4A-4C). The MTT assay provides a measure of the metabolic activity of cells and in this way it can be used to provide an indication of the level of cell viability. The assay involves NAD(P)H-dependent oxidoreductase enzymes in cells reducing the yellow-colored MTT reagent to purple-colored formazan.

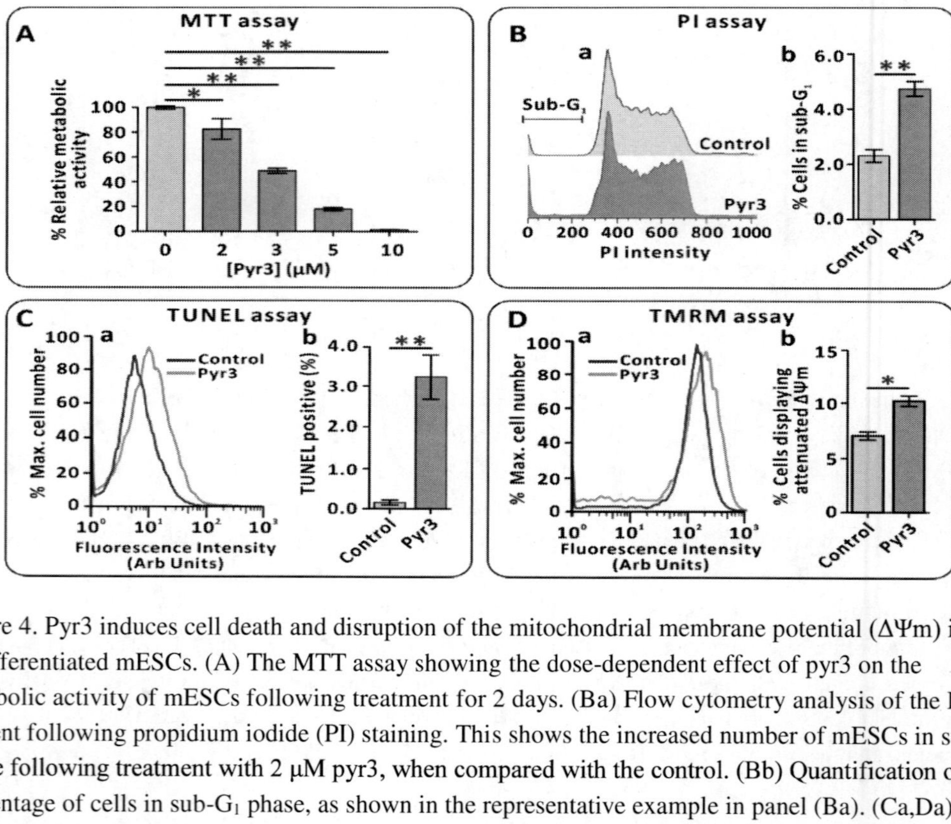

Figure 4. Pyr3 induces cell death and disruption of the mitochondrial membrane potential (ΔΨm) in undifferentiated mESCs. (A) The MTT assay showing the dose-dependent effect of pyr3 on the metabolic activity of mESCs following treatment for 2 days. (Ba) Flow cytometry analysis of the DNA content following propidium iodide (PI) staining. This shows the increased number of mESCs in sub-G_1 phase following treatment with 2 µM pyr3, when compared with the control. (Bb) Quantification of the percentage of cells in sub-G_1 phase, as shown in the representative example in panel (Ba). (Ca,Da) Flow cytometry analysis following: (Ca) TUNEL and (Da) TMRM staining in mESCs in the presence or absence of 2 µM pyr3, to show the distribution of mESCs undergoing cell death and with a disrupted ΔΨm, respectively. (Cb,Db) Quantification of the percentage of: (Cb) TUNEL-positive cells, and (Db) cells displaying an attenuated ΔΨm in panels (Ca) and (Da), respectively. In panels (A) and (Bb-Db), the data are presented as the mean ± S.E.M of n = 3 experiments, and the asterisks indicate statistically significant differences at $p < 0.05$ (*) and $p < 0.01$ (**).

Our data showed that pyr3 affected the metabolic activity of mESCs in a dose-dependent manner such that the percentage of relative metabolic activity was 82.6% ± 8.3%, 48.9% ± 2.0%, 18.0% ± 1.3% and 1.7% ± 0.1% following 2-day treatment with 2 µM, 3 µM, 5 µM or 10 µM pyr3, respectively, when compared with the untreated controls (Figure 4A). In addition, analysis of the cell cycle profile via propidium iodide (PI) staining, showed that 2 μM pyr3 increased the percentage of cells in sub-G_1 phase (indicating dead cells), when compared with the control group with no pyr3 (Figure 4B).

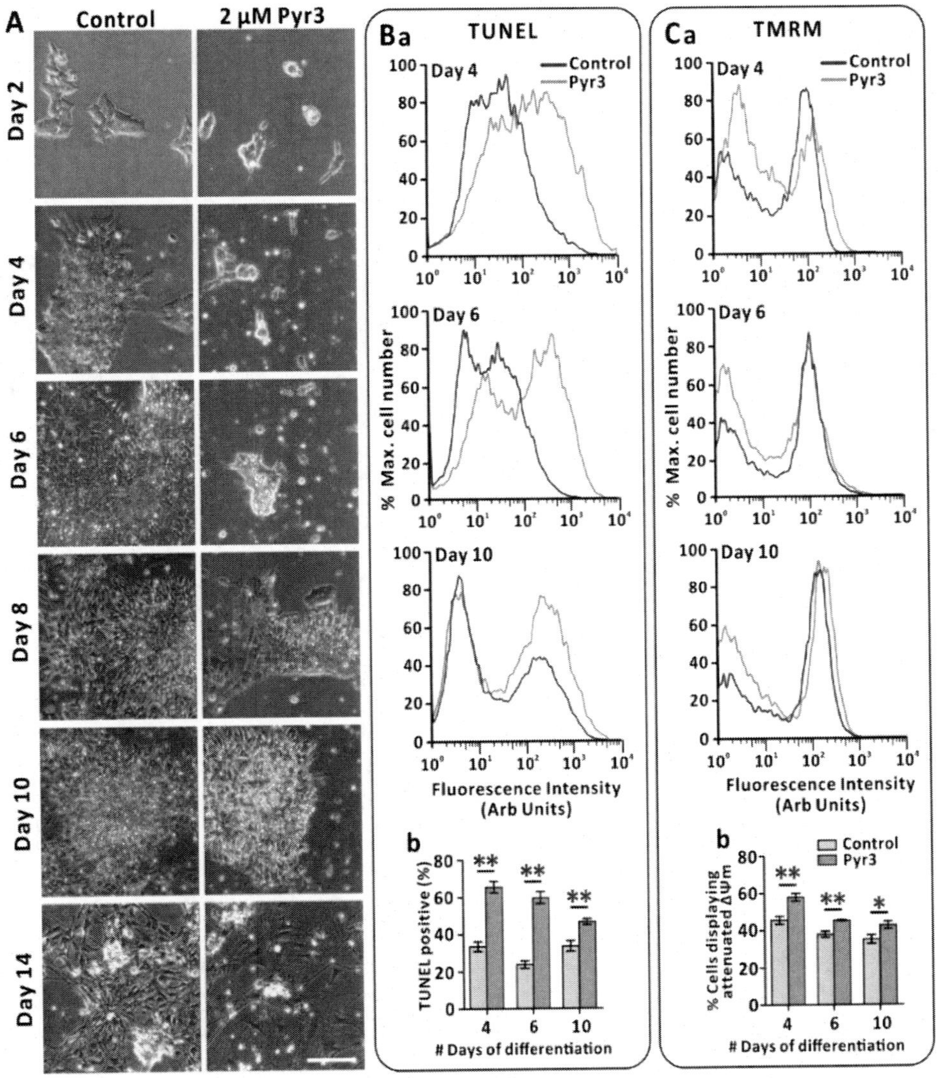

Figure 5. Pyr3 induces cell death and disruption of the mitochondrial membrane potential (ΔΨm) during neural differentiation of mESCs. (A) Bright-field images showing the morphology of mESCs in the presence or absence of 2 μM pyr3 at day 2 to day 14 following the initiation of neural differentiation. Scale bar, 100 μm. (Ba,Ca) Flow cytometry analysis following: (Ba) TUNEL and (Ca) TMRM staining in mESCs in the presence or absence of 2 μM pyr3 at differentiation days 4, 6 and 10, to show the distribution of cells undergoing cell death and with a disrupted ΔΨm, respectively. (Bb,Cb) Quantification of the percentage of: (Bb) TUNEL positive cells, and (Cb) cells displaying an attenuated ΔΨm in panels (Ba) and (Ca), respectively. In panels (Bb) and (Cb) the data are presented as the mean ± S.E.M of n = 3 experiments, and the asterisks indicate statistically significant differences at $p < 0.05$ (*) and $p < 0.01$ (**).

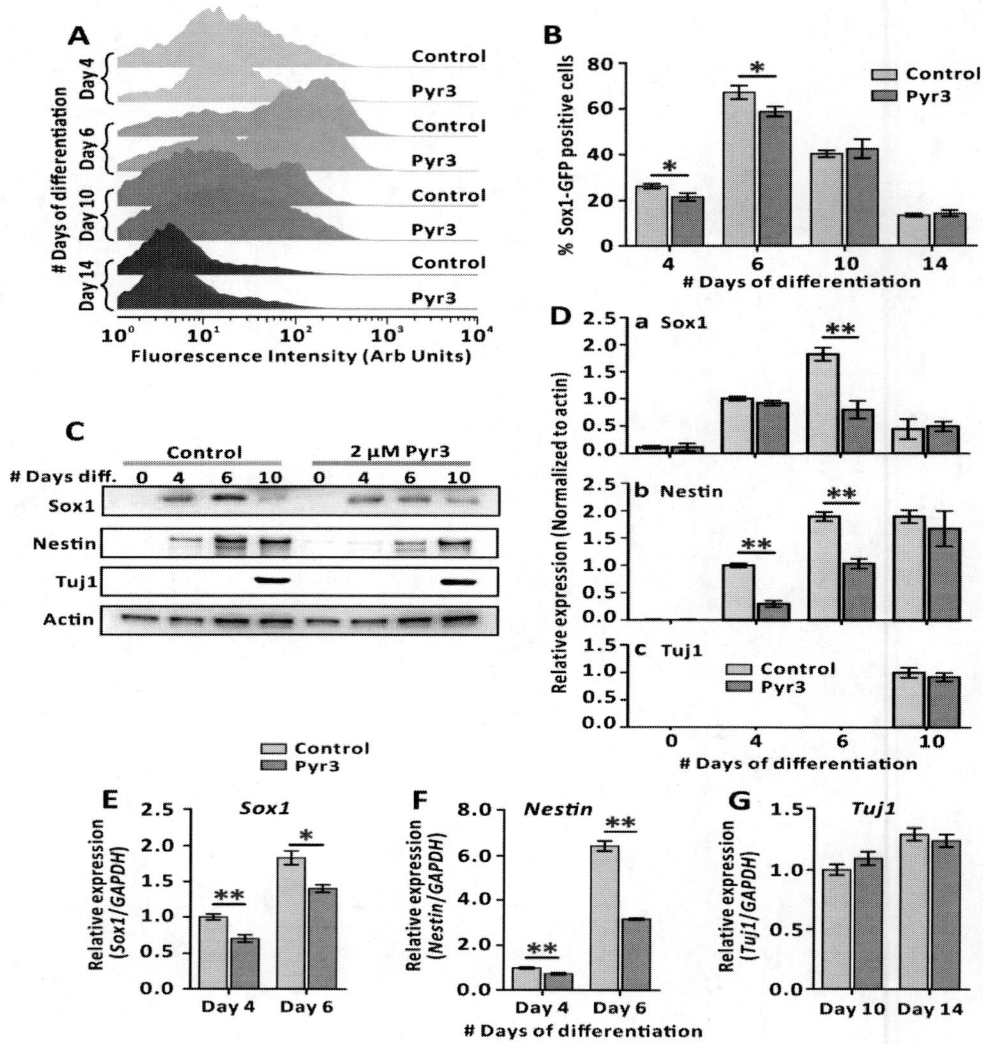

Figure 6. Pyr3 represses the early differentiation of mESCs into neural progenitors but it has little effect on the later differentiation of progenitors into neurons. (A) Flow cytometry analysis showing the numbers of Sox1-GFP-expressing cells incubated in the presence or absence of 2 μM pyr3 at day 4 to 14 of neural differentiation. (B) Bar graph showing the percentage of Sox1-GFP-expressing cells, derived from panel (A). (C) Western blot analysis showing the expression of Sox1 and Nestin (neural progenitor markers); and Tuj1 (a neuronal marker) in cells cultured in the presence or absence of 2 μM pyr3, at day 0 to 10 of neural differentiation. Actin was used as the internal control. (D) Quantification of the Western blot band intensities of (Da) Sox1, (Db) Nestin and (Dc) Tuj1; the band intensities were all first normalized to that of actin (internal control), after which they were normalized to the values at day 4 (for Sox1 or Nestin), or day 10 (for Tuj1). (E-G) *q*RT-PCR analysis showing the expression of (E) *Sox1*, (F) *Nestin* and (G) *Tuj1* in cells incubated in the presence or absence of 2 μM pyr3, at the indicated days of neural differentiation. *GAPDH* was used as the internal control. In panels (B), (D) and (E-G), the data are presented as mean ± S.E.M of n = 3 experiments and the asterisks indicate statistically significant differences at $p < 0.05$ (*) and $p < 0.01$ (**).

In order to confirm that pyr3 induced cell death, terminal deoxynucleotidyl transferase (TdT) dUTP Nick-End labeling (TUNEL) was applied to detect DNA fragmentation in mESCs with or without 2 μM pyr3 treatment (Figure 4C). This assay detects DNA degradation (an important event in cell death), without differentiating between the various mechanisms of cell death, i.e., apoptosis, necrosis or autosis (Fink and Cookson, 2005; Lopilly Park et al., 2012). We showed that the percentage of non-viable cells was increased by ~ 3% in mESCs treated with pyr3.

To investigate if the increased cell death observed might be due to apoptosis, we examined the effect of pyr3 on the ΔΨm as mitochondrial dysfunction is known to be an early indicator of apoptosis. Thus, untreated or pyr3-treated mESCs were labeled with tetramethylrhodamine methyl ester, (TMRM; Figure 4D). Our data showed that there was a higher percentage of mESCs (i.e., 10.2% ± 0.5%) displaying an attenuated ΔΨm following treatment with 2 μM pyr3, when compared with that in control cells (i.e., 7.0% ± 0.4%). Together, these data suggest that pyr3 treatment induces a higher level of cell death via apoptosis in mESCs, and an early step in this process is the disruption of the ΔΨm. Notably, 2 μM pyr3 did not affect the pluripotency of mESCs, as detected both by alkaline phosphatase (AP) staining and *q*RT-PCR analysis (Figure 8).

Pyr3 also Induced Cell Death and a Disruption of ΔΨm during the Neural Differentiation of mESCs

It has been reported that as mESCs undergo differentiation, then certain properties of the cells, such as the electrical parameters, cell size and nucleus-to-cytoplasm ratio, undergo change (Zhou et al., 2016). Thus, we investigated the effect of pyr3 on cell death and ΔΨm when mESCs undergo neural differentiation (Figure 5). Live cell imaging showed that starting at day 4 of neural differentiation, some cell death was apparent whether in the presence or absence of pyr3 (Figure 5A, 5B). Pyr3 treatment appeared to induce a higher level of cell death than the DMSO controls, such that on day 4, day 6 and day 10 of neural differentiation, the percentage of pyr3-treated cells undergoing cell death was 65.4%, 59.5% and 46.5%, respectively, when compared with 33.7%, 23.9% and 33.7%, respectively, in the DMSO-treated control group (Figure 5Ba, 5Bb). In addition, in the presence of 2 μM pyr3, significantly more cells exhibited an attenuated ΔΨm (Figure 5C). For example, on day 4, ~ 12% more cells exhibited an attenuated ΔΨm in the pyr3 treated group when compared with the control group; and on day 6 and day 10, ~ 8% more of the pyr3-treated cells exhibited an attenuated ΔΨm, when compared with the controls (Figure 5Ca, 5Cb). These data suggest that pyr3 might induce apoptosis via the disruption of ΔΨm during the neural differentiation of mESCs.

Pyr3 Repressed the Early Differentiation of mESCs into Neural Progenitors but had Little Effect on the Later Differentiation of Progenitors into Neurons

As pyr3 induced cell death and compromised the ΔΨm during day 4 to day 10 of neural differentiation (Figure 5), its effect on the neural differentiation process itself was also investigated (Figure 6). FACS analysis showed that in DMSO-treated control cells, the percentage of Sox1-GFP-positive cells (i.e., neural progenitor cells) increased from 26.3% ± 1.0% at day 4 to a peak of 67.1% ± 3.0% at day 6. This was followed by a decrease in the percentage of Sox1-GFP-positive cells at day 10 (40.2% ± 1.5%) and at day 14 (13.5% ± 0.8%; Figure 6B). When cells were treated with pyr3, the percentage of Sox1-GFP-positive cells followed a similar trend. However, when comparing the pyr3 and DMSO data together, there were significantly fewer Sox1-GFP-positive cells during early neural differentiation (i.e., on day 4 and day 6) following pyr3 treatment, whereas there were no significant differences during later neural differentiation (i.e., at day 10 and day 14; Figure 6B). Western blot analysis also showed that following pyr3 treatment, the expression of Sox1 and Nestin (both neural progenitor markers) were decreased early on (i.e., at day 4 and/or day 6) when compared with the controls, but at day 10 the level of expression in the pyr3-treated cells and controls was similar (Figure 6C, 6Da, 6Db). Tuj1 (a neuronal marker) was not expressed in mESCs at day 4 and day 6. In addition, at day 10, when Tuj1 was expressed in cells, there was no observed difference in the level of expression when comparing the pyr3-treated cells and the DMSO-treated controls (Figure 6C, 6Dc). Consistent with this, *q*RT-PCR showed a similar pattern of *Sox1*, *Nestin* and *Tuj1* expression during the neural differentiation of mESCs in the presence or absence of pyr3 (Figure 6E-6G). These results indicate that pyr3 might inhibit the early differentiation of mESCs into neural progenitors, whereas it has little effect on the later events when the neural progenitors differentiate into neurons.

Discussion

Pyrazole (pyr) compounds were originally designed as a class of immunosuppressants analogous to cyclosporine A, and they were initially shown to inhibit cytokine production in Jurkat T cells (Djuric et al., 2000). Pyr3 was first identified as being a TRPC3 antagonist via its ability to bind directly to TRPC3 as well being able to inhibit its channel activity (Kiyonaka et al., 2009). Although pyr3 has been widely used to inhibit the activity of the TRPC3 channel (Shirakawa et al., 2010; Kim et al., 2012; Dragoni et al., 2013), it is also known to inhibit the Orai1-mediated Ca^{2+} entry and current (Schleifer et al., 2012). Here, we showed that a rapid increase in $[Ca^{2+}]_i$ was induced in a dose-dependent manner when pyr3 was added to mESCs in the presence of extracellular Ca^{2+} (Figure 1A, 1B). A similar increase in $[Ca^{2+}]_i$ has also been reported in acute lymphoblastic leukemia cells following treatment with pyr3 (Abdoul-Azize et al., 2016). The concentration of pyr3 that we used might be considered to be quite high. For example, it has been reported that pyr3 inhibits Ca^{2+} influx in YFP-TRPC3-transfected HEK293 cells and thapsigargin-depleted RBL-2H3 cells with an IC_{50} value of ~ 0.54 μM (Schleifer et al., 2012). Moreover, it has also been reported that pyr3 at 0.3 μM to 1 μM inhibits TRPC3-mediated Ca^{2+} influx in DT40 B lymphocytes, rat uterine artery, and ESC-derived cardiomyocytes (Kiyonaka et al., 2009; Senadheera et al.; 2013; Qi et al., 2016). However, pyr3 has also been used at 10 μM, and at this concentration it was shown to inhibit the TRPC3-mediated Ca^{2+} influx in atrial and ventricular myocytes from chick embryos, and in human coronary artery smooth muscle and human microvascular endothelial cells (Sabourin et al., 2012; Koenig et al., 2013). We used pyr3 at 0.2 μM, 2 μM and 10 μM to investigate its effect on the $[Ca^{2+}]_i$ and it only increased the intracellular Ca^{2+} in mESCs at 2 μM and 10 μM (Figure 1A-1C). In early experiments we also used pyr3 at 1 μM and it had no obvious effect on the $[Ca^{2+}]_i$ or cell viability (data not shown). Since 10 μM pyr3 showed the most pronounced effect in our initial experiments, we continued to use this concentration to investigate the source of Ca^{2+} (i.e., Ca^{2+} influx or release of Ca^{2+} from internal stores; Figure 1D-1G), and to test the effect of this drug on the $[Ca^{2+}]_i$ in *TRPC3* KO cells (Figure 2).

Following our initial observations, we found that the initial rapid peak-increase in $[Ca^{2+}]_i$ induced by pyr3 was due mainly to Ca^{2+} influx across the plasma membrane from the extracellular Ca^{2+} store, whereas the later, smaller plateau-rise above resting level included a component that was due to Ca^{2+} release from the ER via IP_3Rs (Figure 1F). This was demonstrated in part because Ca^{2+}-free HBSS (plus 2 mM EGTA) totally eliminated the initial rapid peak-rise, as well as ~ 70% of the plateau amplitude of the Ca^{2+} response (Figure 1D, 1E). Furthermore, pretreatment with 10 μM xestospongin C (an IP_3R antagonist) completely blocked the pyr3-induced generation and maintenance of the secondary plateau (Figure 1F, 1G). Such pyr3-induced Ca^{2+} release from the ER has also been reported in human leukemia cell lines (Abdoul-Azize et al., 2016). These results suggest a novel function of pyr3 in mESCs with regards to the regulation of intracellular Ca^{2+} transients, by stimulating both Ca^{2+} influx across the plasma membrane and Ca^{2+} release from the ER. TRPC3 channels have also been reported to be localized to the membrane of mitochondria isolated from adult rat liver and brain, where they help regulate mitochondrial Ca^{2+} uptake (Feng et al., 2013). It has previously been reported that TRPC3 is expressed in undifferentiated mESCs as well as in cells undergoing differentiation (both neural progenitor cells and neuron-like cells), with a significant amount of expression being observed in the cytosol of these cells (Hao et al., 2018). However, it was not clear from these data if TRPC3 was expressed in the mitochondria. Thus, the pyr3-induced slow plateau-rise in $[Ca^{2+}]_i$ might be due in part to the release of Ca^{2+} from the ER via IP_3Rs, and in part due to the inhibition of TRPC3-mediated Ca^{2+} uptake into the mitochondria.

Emerging data suggest that in many cell types Ca^{2+} entry into cells results from the coordinated regulation and interaction between a variety of different Ca^{2+}-permeable ion channels and receptors. For example, it has been reported that there are regulatory interactions between TRPC3 and LTCCs in isolated neonatal rat ventricular myocytes (Gao et al., 2012). Thus, in order to investigate the somewhat surprising finding that pyr3 treatment stimulated an increase in Ca^{2+} influx across the plasma membrane in further detail, we proceeded to knock-out *TRPC3* in mESCs via CRISPR/Cas9-mediated gene editing. This allowed us to explore whether functional TRPC3 channels in control cells might in some way help regulate Ca^{2+} entry across the plasma membrane via an alternative membrane-bound Ca^{2+} channel.

We decided, therefore, to focus on exploring possible interactions between TRPC3 and LTCCs in order to investigate the rapid rise in $[Ca^{2+}]_i$ recorded when TRPC3 function was attenuated. We showed that on exposure to the LTCC agonist (*S*)-(-)-Bay K 8644, there was an immediate and significant increase in $[Ca^{2+}]_i$ in *TRPC3* KO mESCs, whereas this was not the case in Scr control mESCs (Figure 3A-3C). A possible explanation for this effect might be that TRPC3, as well as functioning as a non-specific plasma membrane cation channel, might also act to regulate alternative Ca^{2+} entry pathways across the plasma membrane, including that via LTCCs. When this regulatory function is removed, either via genetic (CRISPR/Cas9-based gene editing) or pharmacological (pyr3) means, Ca^{2+} might then enter cells via LTCCs, resulting in a rapid increase in $[Ca^{2+}]_i$. The entry of Ca^{2+} across the plasma membrane might in turn directly stimulate the release of additional Ca^{2+} into the cytoplasm from the ER via Ca^{2+}-sensitive IP_3Rs (Joseph et al., 2005), and in the case of pyr3 treatment, also by direct stimulation of IP_3Rs in the ER (Bandyopadhyay et al., 2008; Abdoul-Azize et al., 2016). Our xestospongin C experiments support the proposition that this secondary release is via IP_3Rs (Figure 2C).

When viewed in isolation, the response elicited by pyr3 treatment alone might be explained by suggesting that pyr3 is interacting directly with an alternate Ca^{2+} channel or release mechanism, to elicit the instantaneous and rapid rise in $[Ca^{2+}]$ observed, and that the inhibition of TRPC3 function plays little-to-no role in the Ca^{2+} rise observed following pyr3 treatment. However, the observation that CRISPR/Cas9-mediated KO of *TRPC3* removes what appears to be a regulator function of TRPC3 with respect to the activity of LTCCs, suggests that functional TRPC3, although normally viewed as a Ca^{2+} influx channel in its own right, might also play a role in regulating the influx of Ca^{2+} through LTCCs (Gao et al., 2012). We provide a summary of the data shown in Figures 1-3, as well as our developing hypothesis for the effect of pyr3 on the generation of intracellular Ca^{2+} transients in mESCs (see Figure 7).

Our new data provide additional evidence regarding the complexity of Ca^{2+} signaling within cells, and the difficulties associated with measuring and understanding it. The complex nature of Ca^{2+} signaling is due in part to the various internal and external Ca^{2+}

stores available to provide a supply of Ca^{2+} to generate specific signals. It is also due to the Ca^{2+} sensing elements that monitor and regulate the [Ca^{2+}] within each store, and the channels/receptors that mediate the release of Ca^{2+} from the individual stores into both localized and global cytosolic domains (Berridge et al., 2003; Pinto et al., 2015). Furthermore, investigating intracellular Ca^{2+} signaling via the use of agonists and antagonists can often be difficult due to the non-specific nature of the agents used to probe the functions of the channels, receptors and sentinel complexes involved in generating and monitoring a signal. This may indeed be the case with regards to investigating the action of pyr3, as it appears to have an effect on Ca^{2+} entering the cell across the plasma membrane via more than one channel type; as well as on the release of Ca^{2+} from the ER; and perhaps even the uptake of Ca^{2+} by mitochondria.

Ca^{2+} has long been known to play an important role in regulating apoptosis by disturbing the function of mitochondria (Orrenius et al., 2015). Persistent or excess cytoplasmic [Ca^{2+}] leads to apoptosis via the overloading of mitochondrial [Ca^{2+}] and the loss of $\Delta\Psi m$ (Pinton et al., 2008). Here, we report that pyr3 treatment induced a higher level of cell death, which we suggest is in part due to apoptosis due to the increased disruption of the $\Delta\Psi m$ in both undifferentiated mESCs and neural differentiating cells (Figures 4 and 5). In our PI, TUNEL and TMRM experiments, pyr3 was used at 2 μM (Figure 4B-4D).

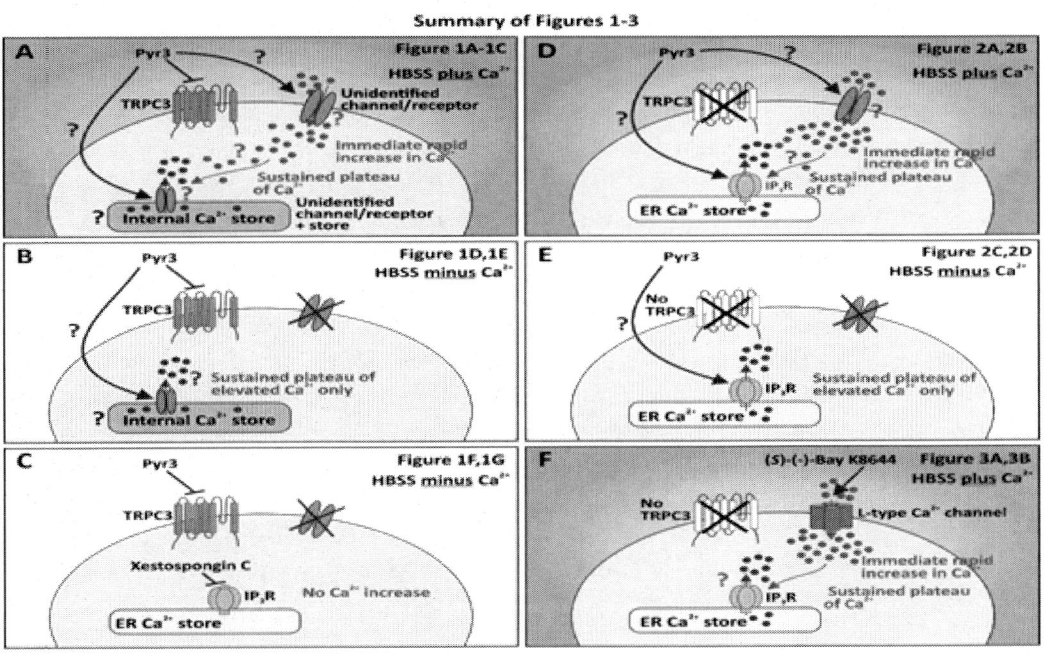

Figure 7. (Continued).

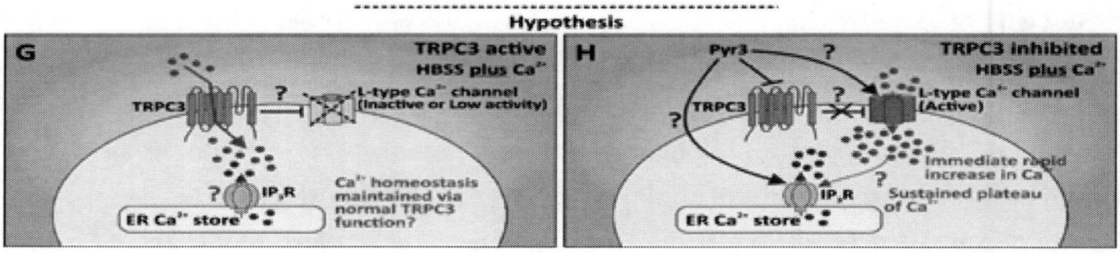

Figure 7. Schematics to summarise the data shown in Figures 1-3, and illustrate our developing hypothesis regarding the effect of pyr3 on the generation of intracellular Ca^{2+} transients in mESCs. Summary of data from Figures 1–3: (A) Treatment of mESCs (maintained in HBSS containing Ca^{2+}) with pyr3 show an immediate rapid increase and a later sustained plateau of Ca^{2+}. The identity of the plasma membrane channel/receptor responsible for the immediate rapid rise in $[Ca^{2+}]_i$, and the identity of the Ca^{2+} store and channel/receptor responsible for the subsequent release to help maintain the later sustained peak, are not known. (B) Treatment of mESCs (maintained in HBSS minus Ca^{2+}) with pyr3 results in only the later sustained plateau of elevated Ca^{2+}. This suggests that the Ca^{2+} contributing to the sustained plateau is due to release from intracellular stores, and that the immediate rapid Ca^{2+} increase observed in the Ca^{2+}-containing medium is due to the influx of extracellular Ca^{2+} across the plasma membrane. It also suggests that pyr3 alone might in some way stimulate the release of Ca^{2+} from an internal store. (C) Treatment of mESCs (maintained in HBSS minus Ca^{2+}) with pyr3 following pre-treatment with xestospongin C, results in no Ca^{2+} response. This suggests that Ca^{2+} release from the ER via IP_3Rs might be responsible for generating the later sustained plateau of Ca^{2+} observed in the earlier experiments. (D) Treatment of *TRPC3* KO mESCs (maintained in HBSS containing Ca^{2+}) with pyr3 still show an immediate rapid increase and a later sustained plateau of Ca^{2+}, suggesting that pyr3 might directly/indirectly stimulate the influx of extracellular Ca^{2+} via a channel/receptor other than TRPC3, as well as the release of Ca^{2+} from the ER via IP_3Rs. (E) Treatment of *TRPC3* KO mESCs (maintained in HBSS minus Ca^{2+}) with pyr3 result only in the late sustained plateau of elevated Ca^{2+}, suggesting once again that pyr3 might directly/indirectly stimulate the release of Ca^{2+} from the ER via IP_3Rs without requiring an influx of extracellular Ca^{2+}. (F) Treatment of *TRPC3* KO mESCs (maintained in HBSS containing Ca^{2+}) with (*S*)-(-)-Bay K8644 show an immediate rapid increase and a later sustained plateau of Ca^{2+}, suggesting that L-type Ca^{2+} channels might play a role in the influx of extracellular Ca^{2+} into these cells. Hypothesis: (G) We suggest that normally, when TRPC3 is functional, then this channel is sufficient to maintain the normal Ca^{2+} homeostasis in mESCs and in some, as yet unknown manner, exerts a negative regulatory influence on L-type Ca^{2+} channels. (H) When TRPC3 activity is inhibited with pyr3, however, the inhibitory regulation is removed, and L-type Ca^{2+} channels can be activated. This results in Ca^{2+} entering the cell from the extracellular medium resulting in the immediate Ca^{2+} rapid response. This increase in $[Ca^{2+}]_i$ might in turn help stimulate release of Ca^{2+} from the ER via IP_3Rs. It is still not known by which mechanism functional TRPC3 can act to negatively regulate Ca^{2+} entry via L-type Ca^{2+} channels, and if pyr3 can directly activate L-type Ca^{2+} channels and/or IP_3Rs. The question marks in the schematics indicate cell processes that are still not confirmed.

This is because when mESCs were treated with 5 μM or 10 μM pyr3, there was excessive cell death within ~12 hours, which meant that at these concentrations it was not possible to collect enough cells for experimentation. In addition, we suggest that at 2 μM, pyr3 might have also stimulated necrosis in a proportion of the cells. This is because in the MTT assay the 2 μM pyr3-treated cells exhibited a ~ 17% reduction in metabolic activity (i.e., overall cell viability) when compared with the DMSO controls. In contrast, the TUNEL and TMRM assays indicated that 2 μM pyr3 stimulated only a ~ 3% increase in cells exhibiting DNA fragmentation and in those with attenuated ΔΨm, indicating a ~ 3% increase in apoptosis. Thus, the additional ~ 14% reduction in cell viability observed in the MTT assay with 2 μM pyr3 might be due to necrosis. Methods are available to differentiate between apoptosis and necrosis (Krusko et al., 2008) but this was beyond the remit of our current study. Regarding the PI assay, the cell cycle histograms did not show a typical G_1, S, G_2/M pattern (Figure 4B). We suggest that this might be because mESCs have a high rate of cell division, which means that the percentage of cells in S-phase is very high, and thus the proportion in the G_2/M phase is negligible. Our mESC cell cycle profile data are supported by those published previously when a very high S phase and a small G_2/M phase peak were also observed (Tsubouchi et al., 2013). Without BrDu and PI double staining, it is difficult to specifically quantify the G_0/G_1, S and G_2/M phases with a fitted model. In our experiments, however, we simply used the PI staining assay to quantify the percentage of cells in the sub-G_1 phase in order to monitor the level of cell death. The robust Ca^{2+} peak and the sustained plateau of elevated $[Ca^{2+}]_i$ induced by pyr3 might contribute to apoptosis via compromising the ΔΨm. However, further studies are needed to verify this hypothesis. Interestingly, it has been shown that pyr3 synergistically potentiates the effect of dexamethasone on inducing apoptosis and inhibiting normal mitochondrial function (i.e., both ΔΨm and reactive oxygen species production) in acute lymphoblastic leukemia cells (Abdoul-Azize et al., 2016). In addition, we recently showed that apoptosis was induced, and the mitochondrial membrane potential was disrupted in both un-differentiated mESCs and in cells undergoing neural differentiation following *TRPC3* KO (Hao et al., 2018).

Notably, in this new study, cells treated with pyr3 during neural differentiation showed a higher level of cell death and a more disrupted ΔΨm (Figure 5), than did undifferentiated mESCs (Figure 4). Similar results were obtained when *TRPC3* was knocked-out (Hao et al., 2018), and we suggest that this might be due to differences in the Ca^{2+} handling properties of pluripotent ESCs, and that of neural differentiating cells. For example, it has been shown that treatment of pluripotent ESCs with agonists of the RyR (i.e., caffeine or a low concentration of ryanodine) or LTCCs did not elicit obvious Ca^{2+} transients (Yanagida et al., 2004). However, during neural differentiation of embryonic P19 carcinoma stem cells (CSCs) and adult murine bone-marrow mesenchymal stem cells (MSCs), caffeine induced an increased $[Ca^{2+}]_i$ response (Resende et al., 2010). In addition, the dynamic expression of genes encoding Ca^{2+} channels, pumps and/or Ca^{2+} related proteins, including *RyR2*, *STIM1*, *Orai1*, *TPC2* and *CD38* were also identified during the neural differentiation of mESCs (Yu et al., 2008; Zhang et al., 2013; Hao et al., 2014; Wei et al., 2015; Hao et al., 2018). Manipulation of several of these Ca^{2+} channel genes, such as *STIM1* knock-down, or *CD38* or

TPC2 over-expression resulted in increased apoptosis in cells undergoing neural differentiation, but not in undifferentiated mESCs. Together with these previous studies, our new results suggest that mESCs might be more sensitive to changes in $[Ca^{2+}]_i$ during neural differentiation than when they are in an undifferentiated state.

Here, we showed that pyr3 only repressed the early differentiation of mESCs into neural progenitors (Figure 6). This is not surprising, as the neural differentiation of ESCs is known to be a highly dynamic process, which can be separated into three stages: Neural induction, the differentiation into neural progenitors, and the neuro-glial switch (Leclerc et al., 2012). In addition, RNA sequencing data have revealed the occurrence of a wide spectrum of gene transcription and splicing dynamics at each successive stage of neural differentiation of human ESCs (Wu et al., 2010). Furthermore, it has been suggested in a number of reports that Ca^{2+} signaling and apoptosis can play a role in the neural or cardiac differentiation of mESCs and on embryo development (Fuchs and Steller, 2011; Zhong et al., 2014; Tang et al., 2016). Here, we demonstrated that pyr3 induced dramatic apoptosis on days 4 to 10 of neural differentiation. Thus, together with its effect on $[Ca^{2+}]_i$, the apoptosis induced by pyr3 might also contribute to the impairment of neural progenitor differentiation from mESCs.

In summary, we demonstrated that pyr3 induced an immediate and rapid peak-increase in $[Ca^{2+}]_i$ via Ca^{2+} influx across the plasma membrane, as well as a later, secondary plateau of elevated Ca^{2+}, due to a combination of Ca^{2+} entry across the plasma membrane and Ca^{2+} release from the ER via IP_3Rs. Our results also showed that pyr3 induced apoptosis and disrupted $\Delta\Psi m$ in mESCs. Further-more, it also suppressed early, rather than later, neural differentiation of mESCs. These results provide a novel view of the role of pyr3 and TRPC3 in regulating $[Ca^{2+}]_i$, as well as in apoptosis and neural differentiation.

Materials and Methods

Cell Culture

The Sox1-GFP 46C mESC line, which expresses GFP knocked-in in the *sox1* locus, was kindly provided by Prof. Austin Smith (Ying et al., 2003). Undifferentiated Sox1-GFP 46C mESCs were maintained in Millipore ESGRO Complete PLUS Clonal Grade medium on 0.1% gelatin-coated plates, and were passaged every 2 days.

The neural differentiation of mESCs was induced according to established protocols (Ying et al., 2003; Ying and Smith, 2003), where undifferentiated cells were plated in N2B27 medium (Hao et al., 2014) on 0.1% gelatin-coated plates and the medium was renewed every 2 days for 2 weeks.

Ca^{2+} Measurements

Cells were cultured in a 24-well plate in ESGRO medium for 24 hr. They were then incubated with 2 μM fluo-4 AM in Hank's balanced salt solution (HBSS) at room temperature for 30 min, after which they were washed with HBSS 3 times and incubated in HBSS (containing its usual 1.26 mM Ca^{2+}) at room temperature for 15 min to allow time for de-esterification of the dye. Images were acquired every 5 s with a Nikon Epi-fluorescence Live Cell Imaging System using a 20x/0.45 NA Plan Fluor Dry objective lens. One minute after the start of data acquisition, the cells were treated with 0.2 μM, 2 μM or 10 μM pyr3, or with 0.1% DMSO as the solvent control. In another series of experiments, mESCs were treated with 10 μM pyr3 or 0.1% DMSO, while being incubated in HBSS minus Ca^{2+} plus 2 mM EGTA (to chelate any Ca^{2+} contamination from the other components of HBSS). Cells were washed 3 times with Ca^{2+}-free HBSS just prior to the start of data acquisition. In another series of experiments, mESCs were pretreated with 0.1% DMSO or 2 μM xestospongin C, for 10 min before adding 10 μM pyr3. Pyr3 and xestospongin C were from obtained from Tocris Bioscience (UK). Stock solutions of pyr3 and xestospongin C were prepared in 0.1% DMSO. The data were analyzed with Image J. (NIH, http://imagej.nih.gov/ij/).

TRPC3 Knock-Out with CRISPR/Cas9

TRPC3 knock-out mESCs were prepared using CRISPR/Cas9, as previously described (Hao et al., 2018).

MTT Assay (for Assessing the Metabolic Activity of Cells)

Cells were plated in a 96-well plate at a density of 5,000 cells/well and cultured for 2 days with 2 μM, 3 μM, 5 μM, or 10 μM pyr3, or with DMSO alone. MTT solution (20 μl of 5 mg/ml) was added to the cells in culture at 37°C for 4 hr. These cells were then solubilized with DMSO and the amount of light generated was quantified in a Multiskan FC plate reader (Abs = 570 nm; Thermo Scientific).

Propidium Iodide (PI) Analysis

Cell fixation and PI staining were performed as described previously (Hao et al., 2014). Cells were analyzed using a FACS Aria II system (BD Bioscience) and the data were analyzed with the FlowJo software (FlowJo LLC).

Flow Cytometry Analysis of Sox1-GFP Expression, Cell Viability, and Mitochondrial Membrane Potential (ΔΨm)

Sox1-GFP expression: Cells were fixed every other day from day 2 to day 14 with phosphate buffered saline (PBS) containing 4% paraform-aldehyde at room temperature for 20 min. They were then washed once and stored in PBS at 4°C prior to FACS analysis, as described above.

Table 1. Sequences of the primers used for RNA isolation and quantitative RT-PCR

Gene name	Direction	Primer sequences (5'-3')
Nanog	Forward	CCAGGTTCCTTCCTTCTTCC
	Reverse	GGTGAGATGGCTCAGTGGAT
Oct4	Forward	AAGCCCTCCCTACAGCAGAT
	Reverse	CTGGGAAAGGTGTCCCTGTA
Nestin	Forward	AGATCGCTCAGATCCTGGAA
	Reverse	GAGTTCTCAGCCTCCAGCAG
Sox1	Forward	AGGAACACCCGGATTACAAGT
	Reverse	CGCTCATGTAGCCCTGAGAG
Tuj1	Forward	AGTCAGCATGAGGGAGATCG
	Reverse	GCTGATGACCTCCCAGAACT
GAPDH	Forward	CGTCCCGTAGACAAAATGGT
	Reverse	TTGATGGCAACAATCTCCAC

Cell Death

Cells were dissociated on days 0, 4, 6, or 10 of neural differentiation and washed once with PBS. The TUNEL assay was then performed with an *in situ* cell death detection kit (Roche). Cells were fixed with 4% paraformaldehyde at room temperature for 1 hr and washed once with PBS. After permeabilization, cells were stained with terminal deoxynucle-otidyl transferase (TdT) reaction mixture at 37°C for 1 hr in the dark. Cells were washed twice with PBS before FACS analysis.

ΔΨm

Cells were dissociated on days 0, 4, 6, or 10 of neural differentiation and washed once with PBS. They were then incubated with 250 nM TMRM (Thermo Fisher Scientific) in HBSS buffer at 37°C for 30 min and washed twice before FACS analysis. Following FACS analysis, the data were analyzed with the FlowJo software.

Live Cell Imaging

Bright-field images of mESCs undergoing neural differentiation were acquired on days 2, 4, 6, 8, 10 and 14 with a Nikon Epi-fluorescence Live Cell Imaging System using a 20x/0.45 NA Plan Fluor Dry objective lens.

Western Blot Analysis

Western blot analysis was performed (Hao et al., 2014). The primary antibodies used to probe the poly-vinylidene fluoride (PVDF) membrane (Millipore) were nestin (NES, Aves; used at a dilution of 1:1,000); SOX1 (MAB3369, R&D; used at a dilution of 1:1,000); Tuj1 (MAB1195, R&D; used at a dilution of 1:2,000) and actin (A2066, Sigma-Aldrich Co. Ltd; used at a dilution of 1:5,000). The appropriate HRP-conjugated chick (sc- 2428), mouse (sc-2005) or rabbit (sc-2004)-secondary antibodies (Santa Cruz Biotechnology) were used at a dilution of 1:5,000.

RNA Isolation and Quantitative RT-PCR (qRT-PCR)

The total RNA of mESCs and of neural differentiating cells at days 4, 6 and 10 was extracted with TRIzol reagent (Thermo Fisher Scientific). Reverse transcription was performed with a High-capacity cDNA Reverse Transcription kit (Thermo Fisher Scientific), and *q*RT-PCR was performed with the primers listed in Table 1 using SYBR Green I Master mix and a LightCycler 480 system (both from Roche). The relative level of gene expression was normalized to the expression of *GAPDH* with the LightCycler 480 software.

Statistical Analysis

Data were presented as mean ± SEM. and statistical analyses were conducted with the Student's *t*-test, such that $p < 0.05$ was considered to be significant.

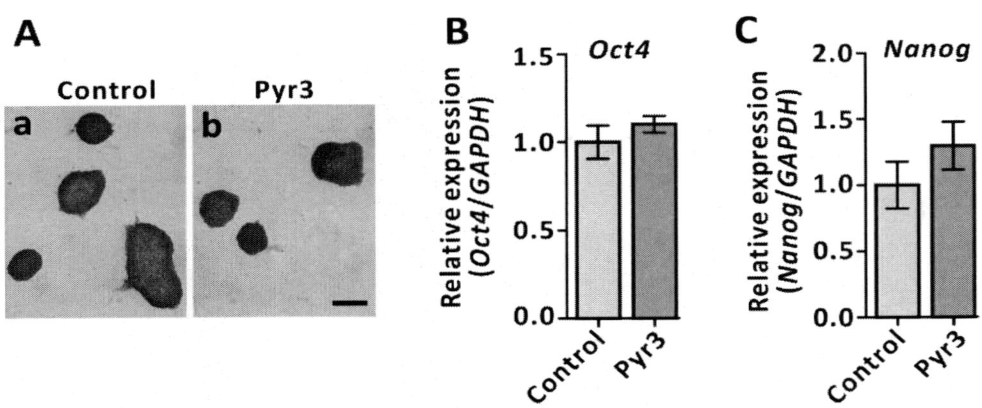

Figure 8. Pyr3 has a negligible effect on the pluripotency of mESCs. (A) Alkaline phosphatase (AP) staining of mESCs cultured for 4 days in the presence or absence of 2 μM pyr3. Scale bar, 100 μm. (B, C) *q*RT-PCR analysis of: (B) *Oct4* and (C) *Nanog* in mESCs in the presence or absence of 2 μM pyr3. *GAPDH* was used as the internal control.

Acknowledgments

We thank Prof. Austin Smith (Cambridge Stem Cell Institute, Cambridge, UK), for kindly providing us with the 46C cells. We also thank Prof. Klaus Groschner (Medical University of Graz, Austria) for his advice regarding the pyr3 data obtained, and Ms. Mandy Chan (HKUST, Hong Kong) for her technical support. This work was funded by the Hong Kong Research Grants Council (RGC) General Research Fund awards 16101714 and 16100115, and the ANR/RGC joint research scheme award A-HKUST601/13. We also acknowledge funding support from the Hong Kong Innovation and Technology Commission (ITCPD/17-9).

Supplemental Information

Materials and Methods

Alkaline Phosphatase (AP) Staining

mESCs were cultured in ESGRO medium for 4 days, after which they were fixed for 2 min, and then incubated with the AP Detection kit staining solution (Millipore) for 15 min at room temperature in the dark. The cells were washed with PBS and visualized with a Zeiss Axioskop upright microscope using a 20x/0.45 NA Plan Fluor Dry objective lens.

References

Abdoul-Azize, S., Buquet, C., Vannier, J. P. & Dubus, I. (2016). Pyr3, a TRPC3 channel blocker, potentiates dexamethasone sensitivity and apoptosis in acute lymphoblastic leukemia cells by disturbing Ca^{2+} signaling, mitochondrial membrane potential changes and reactive oxygen species production. *Eur. J. Pharmacol.*, *784*, 90–98.

Bain, G., Kitchens, D., Yao, M., Huettner, J. E. & Gottlieb, D. I. (1995). Embryonic stem cells express neuronal properties *in vitro*. *Dev. Biol.*, *168*, 342–357.

Bandyopadhyay, B. C., Ong, H. L., Lockwich, T. P., Liu, X., Paria, B. C., Sing, B. B. & Ambudkar, I. S. (2008). TRPC3 controls agonist-stimulated intracellular Ca^{2+} release by mediating the interaction between inositol 1,4,5-trisphosphate receptor and RACK1. *J. Biol. Chem.*, *283*, 32821-32830.

Beddington, R. S. & Robertson, E. J. (1989). An assessment of the developmental potential of embryonic stem cells in the midgestation mouse embryo. *Development*, *105*, 733–737.

Berridge, M. J., Bootman, M. D. & Roderick, H. L. (2003). Calcium signaling: Dynamics, homeostasis and remodeling. *Nat. Rev. Mol. Cell Biol.*, *4*, 517-529.

Bradley, A., Evans, M., Kaufman, M. H. & Robertson, E. (1984). Formation of germ-line chimaeras from embryo-derived teratocarcinoma cell lines. *Nature*, *309*, 255–256.

Chrétien, C., Fenech, C., Liénard, F., Grall, S., Chevalier, C., Chaudy, S., Brenachot, X., Berges, R., Louche, K., Stark, R., et al. (2017). Transient receptor potential canonical 3 (TRPC3) channels are required for hypothalamic glucose detection and energy homeostasis. *Diabetes*, *66*, 314-324.

Darcy, D. P. & Isaacson, J. S. (2009). L-type calcium channels govern calcium signaling in migrating newborn neurons in the postnatal olfactory bulb. *J. Neurosci.*, *29*, 2510–2518.

Djuric, S. W., BaMaung, N. Y., Basha, A., Liu, H., Luly, J. R., Madar, D. J., Sciotti, R. J., Tu, N. P., Wagenaar, F. L., Wiedeman, P. E., et al., (2000). 3,5-Bis (trifluoromethyl) pyrazoles: A novel class of NFAT transcription factor regulator. *J. Med. Chem.*, *43*, 2975–2981.

Dragoni, S., Laforenza, U., Bonetti, E., Lodola, F., Bottino, C., Guerra, G., Borghesi, A., Stronati, M., Rosti, V., Tanzi, F., et al., (2013). Canonical transient receptor potential 3 channel triggers vascular endothelial growth factor-induced intracellular Ca^{2+} oscillations in endothelial progenitor cells isolated from umbilical cord blood. *Stem Cells Dev.*, *22*, 2561–2580.

Evans, M. J. & Kaufman, M. H. (1981). Establishment in culture of pluripotential cells from mouse embryos. *Nature*, *292*, 154–156.

Forment, J. V., Herzog, M., Coates, J., Konopka, T., Gapp, B. V., Nijman, S. M., Adams, D. J., Keane, T. M. & Jackson, S. P. (2017). Genome-wide genetic screening with chemically mutagenized haploid embryonic stem cells. *Nat. Chem. Biol.*, *13*, 12–14.

Fraichard, A., Chassande, O., Bilbaut, G., Dehay, C., Savatier, P. & Samarut, J. (1995). *In vitro* differentiation of embryonic stem cells into glial cells and functional neurons. *J. Cell Sci.*, *108*, 3181–3188.

Feng, S., Li, H., Tai, Y., Huang, J., Su, Y., Abramowitz, J, Zhu, M. X., Birnbaumer, L. & Wang, Y. (2013). Canonical transient receptor potential 3 channels regulate mitochondrial calcium uptake. *Proc. Natl. Acad. Sci. USA*, *110*, 11011-11016.

Fink, S. L. & Cookson, B. T. (2005). Apoptosis, pyroptosis, and necrosis: Mechanistic description of dead and dying eukaryotic cells. *Infec. Immun.*, *73*, 1907-1916.

Fuchs, Y. & Steller, H. (2011). Programmed cell death in animal development and disease. *Cell*, *147*, 742–758.

Gao, H., Wang, F., Wang, W., Makarewich, C. A., Zhang, H., Kubo, H., Berretta, R. M., Barr, L. A., Molkentin, J. D. & Houser, S. R. (2012). Ca^{2+} influx through L-type Ca^{2+} channels and transient receptor potential channels activate pathological hypertrophy signaling. *J. Mol. Cell Cardiol.*, *53*, 657-667.

Groschner, K. & Rosker, C. (2005). TRPC3: A versatile transducer molecule that serves integration and diversification of cellular signals. *Naunyn-Schmiedeberg's Arch. Pharmacol.*, *371*, 251-256.

Hao, B., Lu, Y., Wang, Q., Guo, W., Cheung, K. H. & Yue, J. (2014). Role of STIM1 in survival and neural differentiation of mouse embryonic stem cells independent of Orai1-mediated Ca^{2+} entry. *Stem Cell Res.*, *12*, 452–466.

Hao, B., Webb, S. E., Miller, A. L. & Yue, J. (2016). The role of Ca^{2+} signaling on the self-renewal and neural differentiation of embryonic stem cells (ESCs). *Cell Calcium*, *59*, 67–74.

Hao, B., Webb, S. E., Yue, J., Moreau, M., Leclerc, C. & Miller, A. L. (2018). TRPC3 is required for the survival, pluripotency and neural differentiation of mouse embryonic stem cells. *China Sci. Life Sci.*, *61*, 253-265.

Hipp, J. & Atala, A. (2008). Sources of stem cells for regenerative medicine. *Stem Cell Rev.*, *4*, 3–11.

Joannides, A. J., Fiore-Hériché, C., Battersby, A. A., Athauda-Arachchi, P., Bouhon, I. A., Williams, L., Westmore, K., Kemp, P. J., Compston, A., Allen, N. D., et al., (2007). A scaleable and defined system for generating neural stem cells from human embryonic stem cells. *Stem Cells*, *25*, 731–737.

Joseph, S. K., Brownell, S. & Khan, M. T. (2005). Calcium regulation of inositol 1,4,5-trisphosphate receptors. *Cell Calcium*, *38*, 539-546.

Ju, Y. K., Lee, B. H., Trajanovska, S., Hao, G., Allen, D. G., Lei, M. & Cannell, M. B. (2015). The involvement of TRPC3 channels in sinoatrial arrhythmias. *Front. Physiol.* doi:10.3389/fphys.2015.00086.

Kawasaki, H., Mizuseki, K., Nishikawa, S., Kaneko, S., Kuwana, Y., Nakanishi, S., Nishikawa, S. I. & Sasai, Y. (2000). Induction of midbrain dopaminergic neurons from ES cells by stromal cell-derived inducing activity. *Neuron*, *28*, 31–40.

Kim, D. S., Ryu, H. J., Kim, J. E. & Kang, T. C. (2012). The reverse roles of transient receptor potential canonical channel-3 and -6 in neuronal death following pilocarpine-induced status epilepticus. *Cell. Mol. Neurobiol.*, *33*, 99–109.

Kiyonaka, S., Kato, K., Nishida, M., Mio, K., Numaga, T., Sawaguchi, Y., Yoshida, T., Wakamori, M., Mori, E., Numata, T., et al., (2009). Selective and direct inhibition of TRPC3 channels underlies biological activities of a pyrazole compound. *Proc. Natl. Acad. Sci. USA*, *106*, 5400–5405.

Koenig, S., Schernthaner, M., Maechler, H., Kappe, C. O., Glasnov, T. N., Hoefler, G., Braune, M., Wittchow, E. & Groschner, K. (2013). A TRPC3 blocker, ethyl-1-(4-(2,3,3-Trichloroacrylamide)Phenyl)-5-(Trifluoromethyl)-1H-Pyrazole-4-Carboxylate (Pyr3), prevents stent-induced arterial remodeling. *J. Pharmacol. Exp. Ther.*, *344*, 33–40.

Kriks, S., Shim, J. W., Piao, J., Ganat, Y. M., Wakeman, D. R., Xie, Z., Carrillo-Reid, L., Auyeung, G., Antonacci, C., Buch, A., et al. (2011). Dopamine neurons derived from human ES cells efficiently engraft in animal models of Parkinson's disease. *Nature*, *480*, 547–551.

Krysko, D. V., Vanden Berghe, T., Parthoens, E., D'Herde, K. & Vandenabeele, P. (2008). Methods for distinguishing apoptotic from necrotic cells and measuring their clearance. *Meth. Enzymol.*, *442*, 307-341.

Leclerc, C., Webb, S. E., Daguzan, C., Moreau, M. & Miller, A. L. (2000). Imaging patterns of calcium transients during neural induction in *Xenopus laevis* embryos. *J. Cell Sci.*, *113*, 3519-3529.

Leclerc, C., Moreau, M. & Néant, I. (2012). The calcium: An early signal that initiates the formation of the nervous system during embryogenesis. *Front. Mol. Neurosci.*, *5*, *3*. doi: 10.3389/fnmol.2012.00064.

Lee, H. C. (1997). Mechanisms of calcium signaling by cyclic ADP-ribose and NAADP. *Physiol. Rev.*, *77*, 1133–1164.

Lee, E. H., Cherednichenko, G., Pessah, I. N. & Allen, P. D. (2006). Functional coupling between TRPC3 and RyR1 regulates the expression of key triadic proteins. *J. Biol. Chem.*, *281*, 10042-10048.

Li, X. J., Du, Z. W., Zarnowska, E. D., Pankratz, M., Hansen, L. O., Pearce, R. A. & Zhang, S. C. (2005). Specification of motoneurons from human embryonic stem cells. *Nat. Biotechnol.*, *23*, 215–221.

Lin, H. H., Bell, E., Uwanogho, D., Perfect, L. W., Noristani, H., Bates, T. J. D., Snetkov, V., Price, J. & Sun, Y. M. (2010). Neuronatin promotes neural lineage in ESCs via Ca^{2+} signaling. *Stem Cells*, *28*, 1950–1960.

Lopilly Park, H. Y., Kim, J. H. & Park, C. K. (2012). Activation of autophagy induces retinal ganglion cell death in a chronic hypertensive glaucoma model. *Cell Death Dis.*, *3*, e290; doi:10,1038/cddis.2012.26.

Marks, P. W., Witten, C. M. & Califf, R. M. (2017). Clarifying stem-cell therapy's benefits and risks. *N. Engl. J. Med.*, *376*, 1007-1009.

Miyamoto, S., Izumi, M., Hori, M., Kobayashi, M., Ozaki, H. & Karaki, H. (2000). Xestospongin C, a selective and membrane-permeable inhibitor of IP_3 receptor, attenuates the positive inotropic effect of α-adrenergic stimulation in guinea-pig papillary muscle. *Br. J. Pharmacol.*, *130*, 650-654.

Oda, K., Umemura, M., Nakakaji, R., Tanaka, R., Sato, I., Nagasako, A., Oyamada, C., Baljinnyam, E., Katsumata, M., Xie, L. H., et al. (2017). Transient receptor potential cation 3 channel regulates melanoma proliferation and migration. *J. Physiol. Sci.*, *67*, 497-505.

Orrenius, S., Gogvadze, V. & Zhivotovsky, B. (2015). Calcium and mitochondria in the regulation of cell death. *Biochem. Biophys. Res. Commun.*, *460*, 72–81.

Pinto, M. C. X., Tonelli, F. M. P., Viera, A. L. G., Kihara, A. H., Ulrich, H. & Resende, R. R. (2015). Studying complex systems: Calcium oscillations as attractor of cell differentiation. *Integr. Biol.*, *8*, 130-148.

Pinton, P., Giorgi, C., Siviero, R., Zecchini, E. & Rizzuto, R. (2008). Calcium and apoptosis: ER-mitochondria Ca^{2+} transfer in the control of apoptosis. *Oncogene*, *27*, 6407–6418.

Platel, J. C., Dave, K. A. & Bordey, A. (2008). Control of neuroblast production and migration by converging GABA and glutamate signals in the postnatal forebrain. *J. Physiol.*, *586*, 3739–3743.

Putney, J. W., Trebak, M., Vazquez, G., Wedel, B. & Bird, G. S. (2004). Signalling mechanisms for TRPC3 channels. *Novartis Found. Symp.*, *258*, 123-133.

Qi, Z., Wong, C. K., Suen, C. H., Wang, J., Long, C., Sauer, H., Yao, X. & Tsang, S. Y. (2016). TRPC3 regulates the automaticity of embryonic stem cell-derived cardiomyocytes. *Int. J. Cardiol.*, *203*, 169–181.

Resende, R. R., da Costa, J. L., Kihara, A. H., Adhikari, A. & Lorençon, E. (2010). Intracellular Ca^{2+} regulation during neuronal differentiation of murine embryonal carcinoma and mesenchymal stem cells. *Stem Cells Dev.*, *19*, 379–394.

Rosenberg, S. S. & Spitzer, N. C. (2011). Calcium signaling in neuronal development. *Cold Spring Harb. Perspect. Biol.*, *3*, a004259.

Sabourin, J., Antigny, F., Robin, E., Frieden, M. & Raddatz, E. (2012). Activation of transient receptor potential canonical 3 (TRPC3)-mediated Ca^{2+} entry by A1 adenosine receptor in cardiomyocytes disturbs atrioventricular conduction. *J. Biol. Chem.*, *287*, 26688–26701.

Sandoe, J. & Eggan, K. (2013). Opportunities and challenges of pluripotent stem cell neurodegenerative disease models. *Nat. Neurosci.*, *16*, 780–789.

Schleifer, H., Doleschal, B., Lichtenegger, M., Oppenrieder, R., Derler, I., Frischauf, I., Glasnov, T., Kappe, C., Romanin, C. & Groschner, K. (2012). Novel pyrazole compounds for pharmacological discrimination between receptor-operated and store-operated Ca^{2+} entry pathways. *Br. J. Pharmacol.*, *167*, 1712–1722.

Senadheera, S., Bertrand, P. P., Grayson, T. H., Leader, L., Tare, M., Murphy, T. V. & Sandow, S. L. (2013). Enhanced contractility in pregnancy is associated with augmented TRPC3, L-type, and T-type voltage-dependent calcium channel function in rat uterine radial artery. *Am. J. Physiol. Regul. Integr. Comp. Physiol.*, *305*, R917–R926.

Shirakawa, H., Sakimota, S., Nakao, K., Sugishita, A., Konno, M., Iida, S., Kusano, A., Hashimoto, E., Nakagawa, T. & Kaneko, S. (2010). Transient receptor potential canonical 3 (TRPC3) mediates thrombin-induced astrocyte activation and upregulates its own expression in cortical astrocytes. *J. Neurosci.*, *30*, 13116-13129.

Smedlund, K., Bah, M. & Vazquez, G. (2012). On the role of endothelial TRPC3 channels in endothelial dysfunction and cardiovascular disease. *Cardio. Hematol. Agents Med. Chem.*, *10*, 265-274.

Spitzer, N. C. (2006). Electrical activity in early neuronal development. *Nature*, *444*, 707–712.

Streissnig, J., Pinggera, A., Kaur, G., Bock, G. & Tuluc, P. (2014). L-type Ca^{2+} channels in heart and brain. *WIREs Membr. Transp. Signal*, *3*, 15-38.

Tang, Y., Hong, Y. Z., Bai, H. J., Wu, Q., Chen, C. D., Lang, J. Y., Boheler, K. R. & Yang, H. T. (2016). Plant homeo domain finger protein 8 regulates mesodermal and cardiac differentiation of embryonic stem cells through mediating the histone demethylation of pmaip1. *Stem Cells*, *34*, 1527–1540.

Thomson, J. A., Itskovitz-Eldor, J., Shapiro, S. S., Waknitz, M. A., Swiergiel, J. J., Marshall, V. S. & Jones, J. M. (1998). Embryonic stem cell lines derived from human blastocysts. *Science*, *282*, 1145–1147.

Toth, A. B., Shum, A. K. & Prakriya, M. (2016). Regulation of neurogenesis by calcium signaling. *Cell Calcium*, *59*, 124–134.

Trebak, M., Bird, G. St. J., McKay, R. R., Birnbaumer, L. & Putney, J. W. Jr. (2003). Signaling mechanism for receptor-activated canonical transient receptor potential 3 (TRPC3) channels. *J Biol Chem.*, *278*, 16244–16252.

Trounson, A. & DeWitt, N. D. (2016). Pluripotent stem cells progressing to the clinic. *Nat. Rev. Mol. Cell Biol.*, *17*, 194–200.

Tsubouchi, T., Soza-Ried, J., Brown, K., Piccolo, F. M., Cantone, I., Landeira, D., Bagci, H., Hochegger, H., Merkenschlager, M. & Fisher, A. G. (2013). DNA synthesis is required for reprogramming mediated by stem cell fusion. *Cell*, *152*, 873–883.

Vonhoff, F. & Keshishian, H. (2017). *In vivo* calcium signaling during synaptic refinement at the *Drosophila* neuromuscular junction. *J. Neurosci.*, *37*, 5511-5526.

Wei, W., Lu, Y., Hao, B., Zhang, K., Wang, Q., Miller, A. L., Zhang, L. R., Zhang, L. H. & Yue, J. (2015). CD38 is required for neural differentiation of mouse embryonic stem cells by modulating reactive oxygen species. *Stem Cells*, *33*, 2664–2673.

Woodard, G. E., Lopez. J. J., Jardin, I., Salido, G. M. & Rosado, J. A. (2010). TRPC3 regulates agonist-stimulated Ca^{2+} mobilization by mediating the interaction between type I inositol 1,4,5-trisphosphate receptor, RACK1, and Orai1. *J. Biol. Chem.*, *285*, 8045-8053.

Wu, J. Q., Habegger, L., Noisa, P., Szekely, A., Qiu, C., Hutchison, S., Raha, D., Egholm, M., Lin, H., Weissman, S., et al., (2010). Dynamic transcriptomes during neural differentiation of human embryonic stem cells revealed by short, long, and paired-end sequencing. *Proc. Natl. Acad. Sci. USA*, *107*, 5254–5259.

Yan, Y., Yang, D., Zarnowska, E. D., Du, Z., Werbel, B., Valliere, C., Pearce, R. A., Thomson, J. A. & Zhang, S. C. (2005). Directed differentiation of dopaminergic neuronal subtypes from human embryonic stem cells. *Stem Cells*, *23*, 781–790.

Yanagida, E., Shoji, S., Hirayama, Y., Yoshikawa, F., Otsu, K., Uematsu, H., Hiraoka, M., Furuichi, T. & Kawano, S. (2004). Functional expression of Ca^{2+} signaling pathways in mouse embryonic stem cells. *Cell Calcium*, *36*, 135–146.

Ying, Q. L. & Smith, A. G. (2003). Defined conditions for neural commitment and differentiation. *Methods Enzymol.*, *365*, 327–341.

Ying, Q. L., Stavridis, M., Griffiths, D., Li, M. & Smith, A. (2003). Conversion of embryonic stem cells into neuro-ectodermal precursors in adherent monoculture. *Nat. Biotechnol.*, *21*, 183–186.

Yu, H. M., Wen, J., Wang, R., Shen, W. H., Duan, S. & Yang, H. T. (2008). Critical role of type 2 ryanodine receptor in mediating activity-dependent neurogenesis from embryonic stem cells. *Cell Calcium*, *43*, 417–431.

Yuan, J. P., Zeng, W., Huang, G. N., Worley, P. F. & Muallem, S. (2007). STIM1 heteromultimizers TRPC channels to determine their function as store-operated channels. *Nature Cell Biol.*, *9*, 636-645.

Zhang, Z. H., Lu, Y. Y. & Yue, J. (2013). Two pore channel 2 differentially modulates neural differentiation of mouse embryonic stem cells. *PLoS ONE*, *8*, e66077.

Zheng, J. (2013). Molecular mechanism of TRP channels. *Compr. Physiol.*, *3*, 221-242.

Zhong, J. X., Zhou, L., Li, Z., Wang, Y. & Gui, J. F. (2014). Zebrafish Noxa promotes mitosis in early embryonic development and regulates apoptosis in subsequent embryogenesis. *Cell Death Differ.*, *21*, 1013–1024.

Zhou, Y., Basu, S., Laue, E. & Seshia, A. A. (2016). Single cell studies of mouse embryonic stem cell (mESC) differentiation by electrical impedance measurements in a microfluidic device. *Biosens. Bioelectron.*, *81*, 249–258.

In: Manipulation of Stem Cells for Disease Benefits
Editor: Prasad Koka
ISBN: 978-1-53615-468-9

Chapter 2

Mesenchymal Stromal Cells: Basics, Classification, and Clinical Applications

***Sanjay Gottipamula*[1,*], *Samatha Bhat*[1,*], *Udaykumar*[1] *and Raviraja N. Seetharam*[1,2,†]**
[1]Stempeutics Research Pvt. Ltd, Manipal, India
[2]Shirdi Sai Baba Cancer Hospital, Manipal, India

Abstract

The discovery, isolation, characterization and differentiation of stem cells have significantly changed the global scenario of medicinal use of these cells for diseases for which conventional drugs are of limited therapeutic potential. The presence of stem cells in virtually every multicellular organism suggests that these cells probably have a major role to play throughout the lifetime of the organism for performing specialized functions that are biologically demanded from time to time for normal development and survival. Stem cells are classified as embryonic stem cells (ESCs), induced pluripotent stem cells (iPSCs) and adult stem cells. Mesenchymal stromal cells (MSCs) are adult stem cells originally identified in mouse bone marrow, have now been discovered in many species and can be isolated from human and animal sources. Human MSCs (hMSCs) are multipotent, non-hematopoietic stromal cells which have the ability to differentiate into variety of cell types, including osteoblasts, chondrocytes, myocytes, adipocytes, cardiomyocytes, endothelial cells, hepatocytes and neural cells. These cells are identified by adherence to plastic surfaces under normal culture conditions and exhibit fibroblast-like morphology. The cultured MSCs express cell surface markers including CD29, CD44, CD49a-f, CD51, CD73, CD105, CD106, CD166, and Stro-1 and lack the expression of CD14, CD19, CD34, CD45 and HLA-DR surface molecules. Because of their immunosuppressive, anti-inflammatory properties and ability to secrete paracrine

* These authors equally contributed to this work.
† Corresponding Author's E-mail: raviraja.ns@stempeutics.com.

factors, hMSCs have emerged with a great potential in the field of tissue engineering and regenerative medicine and promise to be a liable source for therapeutic applications. This review article provides an overview on classification, sources and importance of mesenchymal stromal cells with an emphasis on its clinical applications. Brief updates on production technology and currently available cell therapy products have been described.

Keywords: mesenchymal stromal cells, sources, clinical applications, cell therapy products

INTRODUCTION

Mesenchymal stromal cells (MSCs) are multipotent, heterogeneous subset of stromal cell population that can be isolated from various sources of adult tissues that have the ability to differentiate into several types of specialized cells related to, but not including blood cells. These stem cells give rise to cells that forms specialized connective tissues, as well as that support the formation of blood. Mesenchymal stromal cells have therapeutic potential in the treatment of Osteoarthritis (OA) [1], Critical Limb Ischemia (CLI) [2], Liver Cirrhosis (LC) [3], Chronic Obstructive Pulmonary Disease (COPD) [4], Diabetes Mellitus (DM) [5], Acute Myocardial Infarction, Cerebral Stroke (CS) [6], Parkinson Disease (PD) [7], spinal cord injuries [8] etc. MSCs are non- hematopoietic clonogenic cells capable of providing safe and reliable way to repair, restore, maintain or replace the damaged cells and help in retaining functional properties. They are also capable of self-renewal and differentiation into multiple tissues [9]. *In vivo* administration of MSCs has peripheral tolerance and migrates to injured site, where they can inhibit the release of pro-inflammatory cytokines and enhance the survival of damaged tissues [10]. Overall, the MSCs hold great promise for regenerative medicine as they are not only involved in regeneration of tissue, but also in prognostics and diagnostics use.

MSCs can be classified into different types broadly based on source, immune response and cell shape/size.

CLASSIFICATION OF MSCS BASED ON SOURCE

MSCs can be derived from various different sources. These MSCs can be found in nearly all tissues and are mostly located in perivascular niches. Based on the source, MSCs are classified as bone marrow derived MSCs, adipose derived MSCs, cord blood derived MSCs, Wharton's Jelly MSCs, placental derived MSCs, amniotic fluid derived MSCs, synovial MSCs, dental pulp MSCs, peripheral blood derived MSCs (PB-MSCs), MSCs derived from embryonic stem cells, bronchoalveolar lavage (BAL) fluid, atrium tissue from heart, spleen tissue and perirenal fat tissue.

Bone-Marrow-Derived MSCs

Bone marrow derived mesenchymal stem cells (BM-MSCs) first described by Friedenstein et al., (1976) are still the most widely studied cell type and often designated as the gold standard [11]. Bone marrow aspiration (BMA) is an invasive and painful procedure for healthy volunteer donors. The commonly used procedure for the generation of mononuclear cells (MNCs) from bone marrow is density gradient centrifugation [12] and then MSCs are isolated from MNCs during culture process. While isolating MSCs from bone marrow, some hematopoietic cells also adhere to the plastic surface but these cells are washed away during sub-culturing leaving only adherent fibroblast like cells. Recently an alternate method to isolate BM-MSCs using novel marrow filter device is identified, which is less time consuming and avoids the risk of external contamination [13]. MSCs isolated from bone marrow are generally cultured in Dulbecco's modified Eagle's media (DMEM)/DMEM-F12 supplemented with 10% fetal bovine serum (FBS). The expression of specific set of cell surface CD markers is one of the important characteristics of hMSCs. BM-MSCs are positive for CD73, CD90, CD105, STRO-1 and negative for CD14, CD34, CD45, HLA-DR [13-16]. The morphological characteristics of MSCs may slightly differ based on the source, for example BM-MSCs are morphologically larger than adipose tissue derived MSCs (AT-MSCs) [17]. The mean population doubling time (PDT) of BM-MSCs is about 49 h up to passage 7 and it increases thereafter [18]. Peng et al., (2008) described the PDT of 61.2 h in BM-MSCs and 45.2 in AT-MSCs based on logarithmic growth phase [17]. Kern et al., (2006) found the sign of cell senescence in BM-MSCs at passage 7, whereas AT-MSCs showed the same at passage 8 onwards [18]. There have been extensive preclinical studies using MSCs wherein most of these are performed in mice, rats and monkey models. BM-MSCs can be easily isolated, expanded and harvested, abundantly available in bone marrow (BM), differentiates into chondrogenic and osteogenic lineages at a higher rate than adipose tissue-derived MSCs [19]. In the human system, BM-MSCs are most frequently used in multiple clinical trials for various disease indications. Treatment with BM-MSCs can improve type 2 diabetes, liver fibrosis and arthritis via its immunoregulatory functions and hematopoietic stem cell support [20]. Kastrinaki et al., (2008) reported the use of autologous BM-MSCs in rheumatoid arthritis which may have important implications for the repair of tissue injury [21]. Wehbe et al., (2016) showed normalization of the fasting glucose and the glycosylated hemoglobin after infusion of autologous BM-MSCs into patients with type 2 diabetes mellitus [22]. Autologous transplantation of BM-MSCs showed improved liver function as reported by Mohamadnejad et al., (2007) and Kharaziha et al., (2009) [23, 24]. The immunosuppressive and anti-inflammatory property of BM-MSCs is mediated by the secretion of soluble factors such as IL-6, M-CSF, IL-10, TGF-β, HGF and PGE2 which in turn regulates T-cell proliferation [25, 26]. BM-MSCs suppress DC function, regulate

T and B cell activity and prevent the development of acute graft versus host disease (GVHD) [27]. Additionally, they increase T reg cells, modulate immune response via inducing the generation of T reg *in vitro* [25]. The immune-suppressive effect of BM-MSCs is favourable for organ transplantation. MSCs have been used in clinical trials as immunosuppressants (20), but the long term safety of the administration of MSCs needs to be proven prior to their clinical applications.

Adipose-Derived MSCs

Adipose tissue derived MSCs (AT-MSCs), also called as adipose-derived stem cells (ASCs) are usually isolated from the stromal vascular fraction (SVF) of homogenized adipose tissue material generated during liposuction, lipoplasty, or lipectomy procedures by enzymatic digestion with collagenase followed by centrifugation and washing [28] and also by membrane filtration method. MSCs isolated from adipose tissue are cultured in DMEM/DMEM-Low glucose (LG) supplemented with 10% FBS [29-32]. AT-MSCs may in fact be vascular stem cells (VSC), as these cells differentiate into smooth muscle and endothelial cells that are assembled into newly formed blood vessels during angiogenesis and neovasculogenesis. Schaffler et al., (2007) defined the surface marker set for AT-MSCs as positive for CD9, CD29, CD44, CD54, CD73 (SH3), CD90, CD105 (SH2), CD106, CD146, CD166 and HLA-I expression, and negative for CD14, CD31, CD34, CD45, CD133, CD144, HLA-DR, STRO-1 and HLA-II expression [33]. STRO-1 is reported positive in dental and bone marrow whereas negative in human AT-MSCs [29]. AT-MSCs have shown higher proliferation capacity than BM-MSCs [18]. AT-MSCs have PDT in the range of 45-61 h depending on the origin of ASCs from various region of the body [17, 18]; Chondrogenic differentiation of AT-MSCs (ASCs) has been observed at enhanced levels under hypoxic conditions where osteogenesis is inhibited. In contrast, enhanced osteogenic differentiation of AT-MSCs (ASCs) can be induced under normoxia [34, 35].

Cord-Blood-Derived MSCs

The umbilical cord blood (UCB) collected immediately after the birth can be used as a rich source of stem cells. UCB derived stem cells are rejected less often by the host tissue, possibly because they do not possess cell-surface molecules that can be recognized and attacked by the host's immune system. Cord blood derived MSCs (CB-MSCs) were first described by Erices et al., in 2000 [36] and were isolated using Ficoll gradient centrifugation method [37]. An average of 40-45% of the processed cord blood samples have colony forming efficiency of 1-11% and visible morphological features appear within 7-21 days [37]. These CB-MSCs were characterized by higher proliferation and differentiation potential with longer telomeres. There is no significant variation in phenotypic marker expression while compared to BM-MSCs. CB-MSCs do not elicit tumorigenicity after subcutaneous injection in immune-deficient nude mice, and its gene expression profile showed expression of POU5F1, OCT4, Nanog, SOX2 which are also markers of embryonic stem cells [38].

Wharton's-Jelly-Derived MSCs

Wharton's jelly MSCs (WJ-MSCs) can be described as an amenable, plentiful, and inexpensive source of multipotent MSCs with promising potential for use in regenerative medicine applications. Fresh human umbilical cords can be obtained after full-term births after undergoing proper standardization process for processing the cord [39]. The clean and non-contaminated tissues should be used for processing of umbilical cords [40]. Explants culture and enzymatic digestion are two basic methods to isolate MSCs from the human umbilical cord. In explants culture, based on the mesenchymal migratory capabilities which are also called "plate and wait" where the cord segments are simply plated in the medium and the MSCs are obtained by waiting for them to migrate out [41]. The explants culture protocol is simple, reliable and less labor-intensive, leading to pure and viable cultures, when dealing with a large number of samples received simultaneously [42]. In enzymatic digestion, the cord tissue pieces are digested in an enzyme solution to release the cells. With this method, the number of cells isolated from the umbilical cord is fixed and known while compared with explants culture. But over digestion of tissue may result in diminished cellular viability and altered cellular function [42-46]. MSCs isolated from Wharton's jelly are cultured in DMEM supplemented with 10% FBS. WJ-MSCs are positive for CD73, CD90, and CD105 and negative for CD14, CD34, CD45, CD79, HLA-DR [47-49]. WJ-MSCs' stemness and immune properties appear to be more robustly expressed and are more comparable with fetal than adult-derived MSCs. Other advantageous features include ease of sourcing, *in vitro* expandability up to 80 or more population doublings, differentiation abilities, immune-evasion, and immune-regulation capacities [50, 51]. WJ-MSCs possess the typical extra-embryonic perinatal MSCs properties. Generally WJ-MSCs are very similar to the properties of placenta-derived MSCs (PD-MSCs) and cord blood-derived MSCs (UCB-MSCs) [51]. Clinical application of WJ-MSCs includes improvement in cardiac function, when co-cultured with fetal MSCs [52].

Placental-Derived MSCs

The human PD-MSCs can be isolated from the cotyledons present towards the maternal side of the placenta. PD-MSCs are isolated by enzymatic digestion method and are generally cultured in DMEM-LG supplemented with 10% FBS. MSCs derived from placenta are positive for CD29, CD73, CD90, CD105, and CD146 and negative for CD34, CD45 [53]. The unique properties of multipotent PD-MSCs can be described as an amenable, widely available without ethical concerns and without compromising cell cycle pattern, apoptosis and pluripotency associated endogenous gene expression pattern even after culturing up to 25-30 passages [54]. PD-MSCs exhibit low or no immunogenicity as the placenta acts as an immunological barrier between the fetus and the maternal immune system [55, 56]. Further, placenta synthesizes various hormones, enzymes, neurotransmitters, and cytokines [57, 58]. PD-MSCs may secrete active factors that facilitate the repair of bone defects.

Amniotic-Fluid-Derived MSCs

The human amniotic fluid derived MSCs (AF-MSCs) were first reported in 2003 by Prusa et al., (2003) as OCT-4 positive cells, a marker of pluripotent stem cells [59]. Subsequently there were several reports on the use of AF-MSCs for further characterization [60-63]. Both amniotic membrane and AF contains sub-population of MSCs and these AF are usually obtained during amniocentesis and express all the MSC characteristics that are determined by International Society for Cellular Therapy (ISCT). Second trimester AF are considered to be rich source of multipotent MSCs. These AF-MSCs are reported to possess increased *in vitro* proliferation potential of about 250 population doublings with a doubling time of 1.6 days [64]. Besides, it shows increased multipotency with long telomeric lengths and these cells can be placed in between ESCs and post-natal cell sourcing material like WJ, UB etc. The procedure for the isolation of MSCs from amniotic fluid is density gradient centrifugation. AF-MSCs are also isolated by enzymatic digestion method and are generally cultured in α-Minimal Essential Medium (α-MEM)/DMEM-F12 with 10% FBS. AF-MSCs are positive for CD29, CD44, CD90, CD105, CD, SH2, SH3, HLA-DR and negative for CD10, CD14, CD34, HLA-DR [65-67]. Miranda S et al., (2011) reported that AF-MSCs could be expanded *in vitro* culture conditions with population doublings of 54.95 ± 3.17 and accumulated cell number of about 1.0×10^{22} and 9.7×10^{23} with no visible chromosomal alterations and retain their tri-lineage differentiation capacity during their life span [68]. These MSCs exhibit embryonic intra cellular markers like Nanog and Sox2 throughout their life span. Recently, AF-MSCs are considered the most valuable tools to induce liver repair and function by cell transplantation as they can release many factors in curing liver related diseases [69]. CD44+/CD105 sorted MSCs from AF are tested in mouse model for premature ovarian failure and has shown long term *in vivo* survival and proliferation [70].

MSCs isolated from fetal parts like placenta, umbilical cord and umbilical cord blood have advantage of wide availability, no ethical concern, low/no oncogenicity, high expandability and low risk of bacterial/viral contamination [71-73]. ESCs have highest proliferation and potency and then it decreases gradually from prenatal cell source like AF-MSCs and post-natal cell source like WJ-MSCs, adult tissue like AT-MSCs, and then BM-MSCs and lastly the peripheral blood derived MSCs [74-76].

Synovial MSCs

Synovium also has considerable regeneration capability seen during its reappearances following surgical synovectomy [77]. Synovial MSCs are isolated by Ficoll density gradient method and are generally cultured in α-MEM supplemented with 10% FBS. Synovial MSCs are positive for CD44, CD90, CD105, CD147 and STRO-1 and negative for CD31, CD34, CD45, and CD106 [78]. Synovial Fluid-MSCs (SF-MSCs) from intraarticular ligament injury patients have 100 times more MSCs than healthy donors. SF-MSCs are more in OA than other arthropathies suggesting its possible role in arthritis pathophysiology [78]. Hence understanding the characteristics of SF-MSCs in diseased OA patients will help to develop strategy for OA treatment. SF-MSCs exhibit potential role in ligament regeneration and these SF-MSCs consistently show higher differentiation potential during *in vitro* chondrogenesis compared to BM-MSCs [79]. Further, strategies are developed to pre-condition the MSCs with 10 ng/ml of TGF-β1 resulted in higher proteoglycan expression. This is of high importance in tissue engineering application of MSCs in chondral defects [80].

Dental-Pulp-Derived MSCs

The dental pulp is the center part of the tooth consisting of small mass of living connective tissue, blood vessels, nerves and stem cells. The search for easily accessible MSCs has originated the investigations in dental tissue cells. The first type of MSC like cells were isolated from human dental pulp by enzymatic digestion method and termed as post-natal dental pulp stem cells (DPSCs) [81]. MSCs derived from dental tissues are generally cultured in α-MEM supplemented with 10% FBS or FCS and these cells are positive for CD29, CD44, CD90,CD105 and show negative expression of CD14, CD34, CD45 [82-84]. Recently, MSC characteristics were identified in cells derived from dental pulp, stem cells from human exfoliated deciduous teeth (SHEDs), periodontal ligament stem cells, dental follicle precursor cells and apical papilla of dental tissue [85]. Besides,

DPSCs possess all mesenchymal characteristics like differentiation, phenotypic marker expression, immune-privilege properties and have characteristics of ectomesenchyme (due to its interaction with neural crest), express a few embryonic markers and possess higher neurogenic potential [82]. DPSCs are highly proliferative as compared to BM-MSCs and ASCs and transcriptome profiling of DPSCs revealed an inherent propensity towards the neuro-ectoderm lineage [86]. DPSCs are a source of neurotrophic factors like nerve growth factor (NGF), brain derived neurotrophic factor (BDNF), glial derived neurotrophic factor (GDNF), CXCL12 etc. [87, 88]. The neuroprotective effect of DPSCs can be used to cure the central nervous disorders such as spinal cord injury, Alzheimer' disease and Parkinson disease, as it promote the *in vivo* survival of trigeminal and sympathetic ganglia [87, 89].

Peripheral-Blood-Derived MSCs (PB-MSCs)

PB-MSCs are one of the easily accessible sources and form the alternative to painful cell sourcing of BM-MSCs. MSCs isolated from peripheral blood shows all basic MSCs characteristics and can be compared with their BM-MSCs. PB-MSCs are isolated from peripheral blood by Ficoll-Paque density-gradient separation method and are generally cultured in α-MEM supplemented with 10% newborn calf serum (NBCS). PB-MSCs are positive for CD44, CD90, CD105, HLA-ABC and show negative expression of CD45, CD133 (90). PB-MSCs and BM-MSCs demonstrated similar tri-lineage differentiation, and similar phenotypic marker expression. Moreover, qualitative and quantitative test of chondrogenic potential showed similar s-GAG levels in both cultures [91]. Comparison of UC-MSCs and PB-MSCs exhibited similar morphology, proliferation capacity and multilineage differentiation potential; differences were only in the clonogenic efficiency and the immune-phenotype [92]. These results also demonstrate that the PB-MSCs are good alternative source for cellular therapies.

MSCs Derived from Embryonic Stem Cells

Search for alternative source that provides consistency, robustness and enable large scale manufacturing to produce downstream progenitor cells by MSCs has led to ESCs as a source for MSCs [93]. Potential of manufacturing cell therapy products sufficient to repeat treatments in multiple patients eliminating the variability and improving the cell quality can be achieved by MSCs derived from ESCs. The use of ESC derived MSCs enables cost-effective production system. Several researchers have developed methods for differentiating MSCs from ESCs [94-96]. These hESC-MSCs are very similar to BM-MSCs in morphology, function, biology and even in the gene expression profile [97].

Recently; MSCs were even derived from human induced pluripotent stem cells (hiPSCs), confirmed the MSCs characteristics *in vitro* and showed *in vivo* bone formation in mice [98]. MSCs are even derived from lung [99], heart [100].

Table 1. Summary of different sources of MSCs, method of isolation, expansion media with serum supplements, cell surface markers and the references

Sl No	Source	Method of Isolation	Media	Serum Supplement	Cell Surface Markers		References
					Positive	Negative	
1	Bone marrow	Ficoll density gradient method Novel marrow filter device	DMEM DMEM-F12A/DMEM	FBS	CD73, CD90, CD105, STRO-1	CD14, CD34, CD45, HLA-DR	[12-16]
2	Adipose tissue	Digestion method Membrane filtration method	DMEM DMEM-LG	FBS FCS	CD73, CD90, CD29, CD44, CD71, CD105, CD13, CD166	CD14, CD31, CD34, CD45, STRO-1	[29-32]
3	Amniotic fluid and membrane	Density gradient method Digestion method	α-MEM DMEM/F12	FBS	CD29, CD44, CD90, CD105, CD, SH2, SH3, HLA-DR	CD10, CD14,CD34, HLA-DR	[65-67]
4	Dental tissues	Digestion method	α-MEM MEM	FCS FBS	CD29, CD44, CD90, CD105	CD14, CD34, CD45	[82-84]
5	Endometrium	Digestion method	DMEM-F12	FCS	CD73, CD90, CD105, CD146	CD34, CD45	[104]
6	Limb bud	Digestion method	DMEM-LG	FBS	CD13, CD29,CD90, CD105, CD106	CD3, CD4, CD14, CD15, CD34, CD45, HLA-DR	[105]
7	Peripheral blood	Ficoll density gradient	α-MEM	NBCS	CD44, CD90, CD105, HLA-ABC	CD45, CD133	[90]
8	Placenta and fetal membrane	Digestion method	DMEM-LG	FBS	CD29, CD73, CD90, CD105	CD34, CD45	[53]
9	Salivary gland	Digestion method (Ringer solution)	DMEM	FCS	CD13, CD29, CD44, CD90, STRO-1	CD34, CD45	[106]
10	Skin and foreskin	Digestion method	DMEM-HG DMEM DMEM-F12	FBS	CD44, CD73, CD90, CD105, CD166, SSEA-4, Vimentin	CD34, CD45, HLA-DR	[107, 108]
11	Sub amniotic umbilical cord lining membrane	Digestion method	DMEM-HG DMEM CMRL1660	FBS	CD29, CD44, CD73, CD90, CD105	CD34, CD45	[31, 109, 110]

Table 1 (Continued)

Sl No	Source	Method of Isolation	Media	Serum Supplement	Cell Surface Markers		References
12	Synovial fluid	Ficoll density gradient method	α-MEM	FBS	CD44, CD90, CD105, CD147, STRO-1	CD31, CD34, CD45, CD106	[78]
13	Wharton's jelly	Explants culture Enzymatic digestion method	DMEM	FBS	CD73, CD90, CD105	CD14, CD34, CD45, CD79, HLA-DR	[47, 48]
14	Bronchoalveolar lavage (BAL) fluid	Filtration and Centrifugation at 1,000 g for 5 minutes	DMEM HG	FBS	CD73, CD90, CD105	CD14, CD34,CD45, HLA-DR	[101]
15	Atrium tissue from heart	Digestion with collagenase type IV	α-MEM	FBS	CD90, CD105, CD166, and HLA class I	CD34, CD45, HLA class II, CD80, and CD86	[102]
16	Spleen tissue	Digestion with collagenase type IV	α-MEM	FBS	CD90, CD105, CD166, and HLA class I	CD34, CD45, HLA class II, CD80, and CD86	[102]
17	Perirenal fat tissue	Digestion with collagenase type IV followed by centrifugation at 1,200 g for 10 min	α-MEM	FBS	CD90, CD105, CD166, and HLA class I	CD34, CD45, HLA class II, CD80, and CD86	[102]

Source: [103], modified.

MSCs Derived from Bronchoalveolar Lavage (BAL) Fluid, Atrium Tissue from Heart, Spleen Tissue and Perirenal Fat Tissue

Mesenchymal cell populations are even derived from human lung allografts. BAL fluid is initially filtered through sterile gauze to remove cellular debris and mucus. Cells are pelleted by centrifugation at 1,000g for 5 minutes and maintained in medium consisting of high-glucose DMEM supplemented with 10% FBS. MSCs from BAL fluid express cell-surface proteins, CD73, CD90, and CD105, commonly found on mesenchymal stem cells (MSCs) and are negative for hematopoietic lineage markers CD14, CD34, and CD45. BAL-derived MSCs exhibits several characteristics typical of BM- MSCs. Moreover, these cells possess multipotent differentiation capacity and give rise to adipocytes, chondrocytes, and osteocytes. Report by Lama et al., (2007) is the first one to demonstrate the presence of lung tissue–specific MSCs in the human adult lung. They also observed survival of these cells for more than a decade in transplanted lung allografts [101]. Hoogduijn et al., (2007) reported the isolation and characterization of MSCs from human heart, spleen, and perirenal adipose tissue. MSCs from these tissues were similar to those derived from bone marrow and expressed cell-surface markers CD90, CD105, CD166, and HLA class I, were negative for CD34, CD45, HLA class II, CD80, and CD86 expression, and were able to differentiate into osteogenic and adipogenic lineages. In addition, these cells inhibited the proliferative response of allogeneic peripheral blood mono-nuclear cells (PBMCs) after stimulation with phytohemagglutinin (PHA). MSCs from atrium, spleen and perirenal fat tissue was isolated using collagenase IV digestion method and then cultured in α-MEM supplemented with 10% FBS [102].

Table 1 represents the list of different sources of MSCs of human origin, their cell surface markers, method of isolation, expansion media with serum supplements and the references summarized by Ullah et al., (2015) [103] (modified).

Classification of MSCs Based on Immune Response

MSCs have been reported to be hypoimmunogenic which facilitates the transplantation of MSCs across the major histocompatibility barriers favoring its potential therapeutic applications. Waterman et al., (2010) classified two homogenously acting phenotypes as proinflammatory MSC1 and anti-inflammatory MSC2 based on MSC polarization of toll-like receptor (TLR) signaling [49]. MSC1 are TLR4-primed MSCs which elaborate pro-inflammatory mediators whereas MSC2 are TLR3 primed MSCs having immunosuppressive properties. MSCs are sensors of inflammatory microenvironment able to switch over between these two phenotypes depending on their interaction with components of the innate and/or adaptive immune system. As a consequence of inflammatory response, molecules associated with tissue injury are recognized by the TLRs which activate phagocytosis and release of inflammatory mediators. TLR activation not only stimulates phagocytic cells but also stromal cells including MSCs, thus creating inflammatory microenvironment.

The proinflammatory MSC1 phenotype aids in establishing an early inflammatory response, while the anti-inflammatory MSC2 phenotype aids at later stages to suppress inflammatory T-cell responses, the property that has been exploited for therapeutic use. Further studies performed by the same group showed that MSC1 does not support *in vitro* tumor cell growth whereas MSC2 favor tumor cell growth [111, 112]. MSC2 respond to proinflammatory cytokines such as tumor necrosis factor alpha (TNF-α) and interferon gamma (IFN-γ) leading to the release of soluble factors including indoleamine 2,3-dioxygenase (IDO), prostaglandin E2 (PGE2), nitric oxide (NO), transforming growth factor beta (TGF-β) which in turn suppress T-cell proliferation. [113]. Low levels of TNF-α and IFN-γ may stimulate MSCs to adopt a proinflammatory phenotype (MSC1) which enhances T cell proliferation by secreting chemokines such as MIP-1α and MIP-1β, RANTES, CXCL9, and CXCL10. These chemokines bind to receptors present on T cells decreasing the level of immune -suppressive mediators (IDO, NO). The balance between these two MSC phenotypes may serve as host defense mechanism and promotes tissue repair [111]. MSCs express low level of major histocompatibility complex (MHC) class I molecules with minimal or no expression for MHC class II molecules and co-stimulatory molecules CD40, CD40 ligand, CD80 and CD86. MSCs when stimulated with proinflammatory cytokine induce the expression of MHC class II but cannot vary the expression of costimulatory molecules. MHC class II in the absence of costimulatory molecules cannot activate alloreactive T cells thus leading to immunosuppression [114]. MSCs from different sources exhibit distinct surface marker expression according to the tissue from which they were obtained. The expression of these surface markers effectively contributes to the MSC-mediated inhibition of T-cell proliferation. For example, the surface marker CD90 is involved in controlling the production of molecules involved in immunosuppression. The absence of this marker may lead to the loss of immunosuppressive potential of MSCs. Likewise, CD271, CD39, CD73 and VCAM-1 positive MSCs possess immunomodulatory functions [115]. Clinical benefit of cell based therapy prevails even if 0.1 to 1% of infused cells reach target sites. These benefits are due to local immune modulation by these cells rather than differentiation or replacement of damaged target tissue [116, 117].

Classification of MSCs Based on Shape and Size

MSCs derived from various cell sources have heterologous cell population and within the same source, MSCs tends to generate various sub-populations. Mets and Verdonk (1981) classified MSCs based on cell shape into rapidly proliferating smaller spindle-shaped cells as type-I MSCs and very slow proliferating, large and flat cells as type-II MSCs [118]. Similarly, Colter et al., (2000) have identified, defined and classified MSC subpopulations [119] based on rapidly proliferating small cyclic self-renewal cells as recycling stem (RS) cells. The RS cells grow very rapidly at low seeding densities of 1.5 or 3.0 cells/cm^2 to produce single cell derived colonies. The cultures exhibited lag phase (5 days), log phase (5 days) and stationary phase. The stationary phase cultures included major proportion of large and moderately granular cells and a minor population of small and agranular cells. These major populations of large cells at stationary phase are called mature MSCs or mMSCs and minor population of small granular cells are called as RS-1. These RS-1 cells during lag phase give rise to a new population of small and densely granular cells (RS-2 cells) which decreased in number during late log phase and regenerated the pool of RS-1 cells found in stationary cultures. The cells retained their ability to generate single-cell derived colonies during repeated reseeding at low seeding density. Colter et al., (2001) extended their previous observation to demonstrate a third type of cells that are rapidly self-renewing extremely small, round cells as RS cells [120] characterized by their extremely small size, rapid rate of replication and enhanced potential for multilineage differentiation. RS enriched MSCs have a higher potential and express a distinct surface epitopes which can be used to distinguish the small cells from the large cells. Sekiya et al., (2002), further classified the RS based MSCs into thin spindle shaped cells as RS-1A, little wider spindle shaped cells as RS-1B and still wider spindle shaped cells as RS-1C [121]. A time dependent transition of early progenitors of RS1A to RS1B and RS1C was observed after seeding cells at density of 1 to 1000 cells/cm^2. Taken together, these studies evaluated the distinct morphological subpopulations of MSCs as rapidly self-renewing cells (RS cells), elongated, fibroblastic-like, spindle-shaped cells (SS cells) and slowly replicating, large, cuboidal or flattened cells (FC cells). Moreover, these different subpopulations displayed discrete intrinsic qualities wherein small RS cells showed the highest multipotentiality and wider, spindle-shaped cells showed the greatest potential to differentiate into cartilage. The larger MSCs were more matured cells that were differentiated in part, into osteoblastic precursors. These observations suggest that the heterogeneity of MSC cultures is due to different mesenchymal progenitors and the RS cells constitute the earliest precursors [122]. Morphological properties of cells depend on cytoskeleton organization, cell adhesion and signaling pathways [123]. Furthermore, Florian et al., correlated these sub-population of MSCs with the expression pattern of the three MSC surface markers CD73, CD90 and CD105. The percentage of RS cells was positively correlated with the percentage of cells positive for all three MSC surface markers. However, the percentage of flattened cells was inversely correlated with the percentage of cells positive for all three surface markers since these cells likely downregulated CD73 and was prone for differentiation [124]. Recent studies reported downregulation of CD73 in MSC after adipogenic and osteogenic induction and that the subpopulation of FC cells represented an early osteogenic progenitor [125]. Hence the deeper knowledge about MSC subpopulations during culturing is of key importance. It may not be appropriate to use single sourced MSCs to treat various target diseases. MSCs from various sources and types possess distinct and unique gene and molecular signatures which propels them to specific lineage propensity, besides qualifying basic MSCs characteristics. Therefore careful attention is needed in choosing appropriate MSC source for specific disease indications.

LARGE SCALE PRODUCTION OF MSCs

As the number of clinical applications of MSCs is increasing, the cell therapy companies are interestingly looking towards robust, scalable production and expansion process to cater their clinical as well as commercial needs while adhering to GMP compliances. Currently, multilayer vessels such as CellSTACKS are used for the production and expansion of MSCs. However, these processes are not fully closed system requiring class A biosafety cabinet. To adhere to GMP compliance, use of closed automated system is essential which allows large surface area to volume, automated culturing and harvesting and automated control of various parameters required for MSC expansion [126]. Various designs of bioreactors such as Multi plate bioreactors, Micro carrier based systems, Roller bottles, Hollow fiber bioreactors, packed bed bioreactors, Wave bioreactors are now available which assist in improving these criteria (Figure 1). The translation of concept driven process to commercial scale production of therapeutic MSCs is based on various factors like characterization of cells, feeding strategy and control of critical quality variables in the manufacturing process.

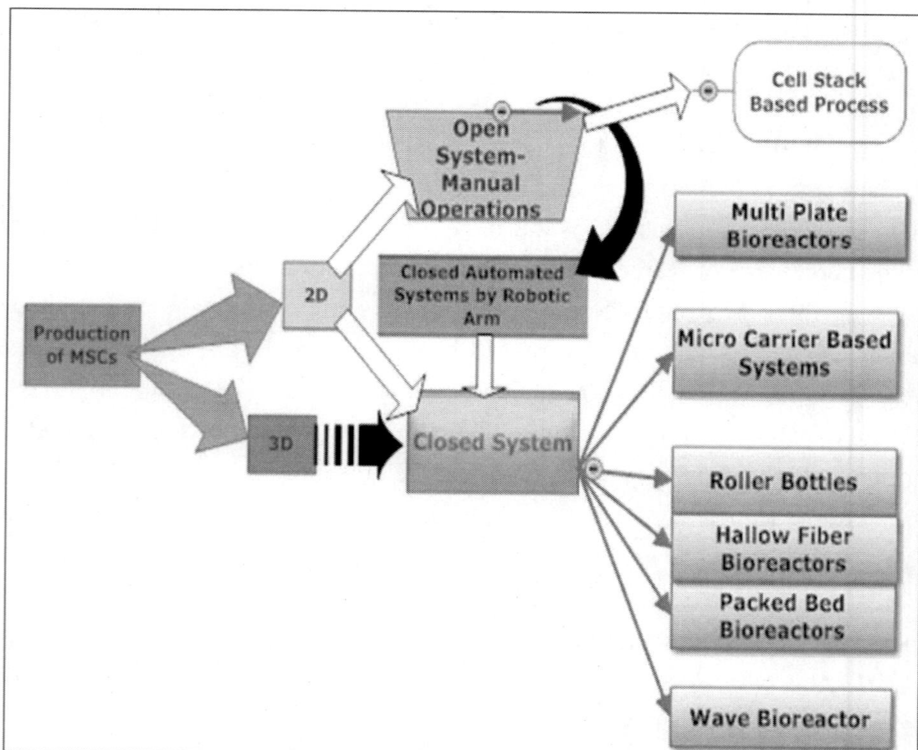

Figure 1. Diagrammatic overview of various scale-up methods for the bioprocessing of mesenchymal stromal cells. Transition from open system of manual operations to closed controlled system of automation is observed through robotics.

BASED ON THE SIZE OF THE PRODUCTION BATCH, THE PRODUCTION SYSTEM IS CLASSIFIED

Lab Scale

Laboratory or bench-top scale processing capacity is up to few lakhs to few millions of cells for characterization or testing purpose. The culture system used in this lab-scale is cell culture flask, where the optimization of media, feeding strategy and identifying the crucial process parameters are usually carried out at this stage. The cells produced in lab-scale are mostly used for characterization and to determine the growth kinetics patterns. Most of the process variables will be defined and tested.

Pilot Scale

Pilot scale is a small scale production that is larger than lab-scale used for product and process characterization purpose. Pilot scale batches simulate exact production batches and are used for optimization, troubleshooting and for process development activities. Once the MSC process conditions, variables (feeding regime) and media optimization are defined, the process is transferred to pilot scale production in GMP suite. A number of pilot scale batches will be tested again to confirm the process specifications and critical quality parameters and it can then be fine-tuned to derive the process quality specifications. Usually pilot scale batches are used for pre-clinical safety studies, master cell bank preparations, working cell bank preparations, validation studies and phase-I clinical trials.

Large Scale

The large scale manufacturing of MSCs usually happens in cGMP production suites, where initial technology transfer batches will be conducted to again check the process efficacy after change in scale of manufacturing. Multiples of CellSTACK-10 or Cell STACK-40 will be used and cells produced will be tested to confirm the QC release specifications. The cells produced will be used for validation studies, stability studies, pre-clinical efficacy studies, Phase-II/III clinical trials and commercial purpose.

Based on the Type of Culture System, the Production System Is Classified

2D Surface Based Systems

When MSCs are grown on flat plastic surfaces either on small dishes or on large surface area plates such as CellSTACKS or on flat plate bioreactors, it is called 2D culture system. Typical 2D culture dishes and plates are pre-treated for better cell attachment and growth of MSCs. Some of the 2D surface based systems are multi-plate stacks, multi-plate reactors, and roller bottle based systems.

3D Suspension

There are several 3D based systems available to culture the MSCs in closed loop and to enhance scalability of production operations. At present there are various options available for scale-up of adherent cell populations to cater clinical trials as well as to cater market demands.

Microcarrier in Stirred Tank Bioreactors (Microcarrier Beads)

Stem cell based therapies requires scaling up the culture process for culturing of cells in large quantities. Stirred tank bioreactors facilitate growth of MSCs while meeting the requirement. Microcarriers are tiny spheres or particles (typically 90–300 μm in diameter) used for culturing adherent cells in stirred-tank bioreactors. The geometry of microcarriers provides investigators with an ability to increase the amount of surface area in a given volume (cm^2/mL) of medium. Increase in the ratio of surface area to volume improves product consistency and decreases cost. Mobius® 3L Bioreactor (Merck) and Xcellerex (GE Healthcare) are some of the examples for microcarrier beads

Single Cell Suspension in Stirred Tank Bioreactor

Stirred tank bioreactors are relatively simple vessels that have a centrally located impeller agitating the contents of the vessel which provides relatively uniform conditions throughout the medium. The impeller speed is controlled by either a magnetic field generated by a stirrer placed under it or a top-driven motor. A large number of cells can be expanded in one vessel, thereby avoiding vessel-to-vessel variability and minimizing costs related to labor and consumables. In addition, computer based online monitoring is possible which allows tight control of process parameters such as pH, temperature, oxygen concentration [127]. Examples for stirred tank bioreactors are PADReactor (Pall Life Sciences) and MiniBio (Applikon Biotechnology).

Hollow Fiber Bioreactor

A Hollow fiber bioreactor is a 3D cell culturing system based on hollow fibers, which are small, semi-permeable capillary membranes arranged in parallel array with a typical molecular weight cut- off (MWCO) range of 10-30 kDa. It is a robust, functionally closed, automated system designed to reproducibly grow both adherent and suspension cells [128]. The best example is Quantum® Cell Expansion System - Terumo BCT.

3D Scaffold-Based Technology

3D scaffolds are the most common stem cell culture method. Stem cells form structures called "scaffold" through a variety of methods when seeded in 3D scaffolds, and under the proper conditions, the cells undergo proliferation, differentiation, and secretion of specific ECM molecules, which can form additional scaffold and promote cell adhesion and proliferation *in vivo*. The ideal scaffold should be 3D, porous with an open pore network, biocompatible, biodegradable, and mechanically amenable to proper cell growth [129]. Example for 3D scaffold based bioreactor is iCELLis® bioreactor, from ATMI.

Packed-Bed Bioreactor (Nonwoven Microfibers)

Packed-bed bioreactor is an automated closed system suitable for large-scale MSCs expansion. The packed bed bioreactor is designed to decouple the oxygen transport from the bulk nutrient supply from the medium flow operates efficiently at a lower perfusion rate, resulting in lower shear stress acting on the cells. It provides a continuous and connected surface area with no need for mixing [130]. Medorex fixed bed bioreactor is one of the examples for packed bed bioreactor.

These 3D bioreactors provide efficient growth micro-environment for the cells and increase the greater possibility of proliferation and differentiation.

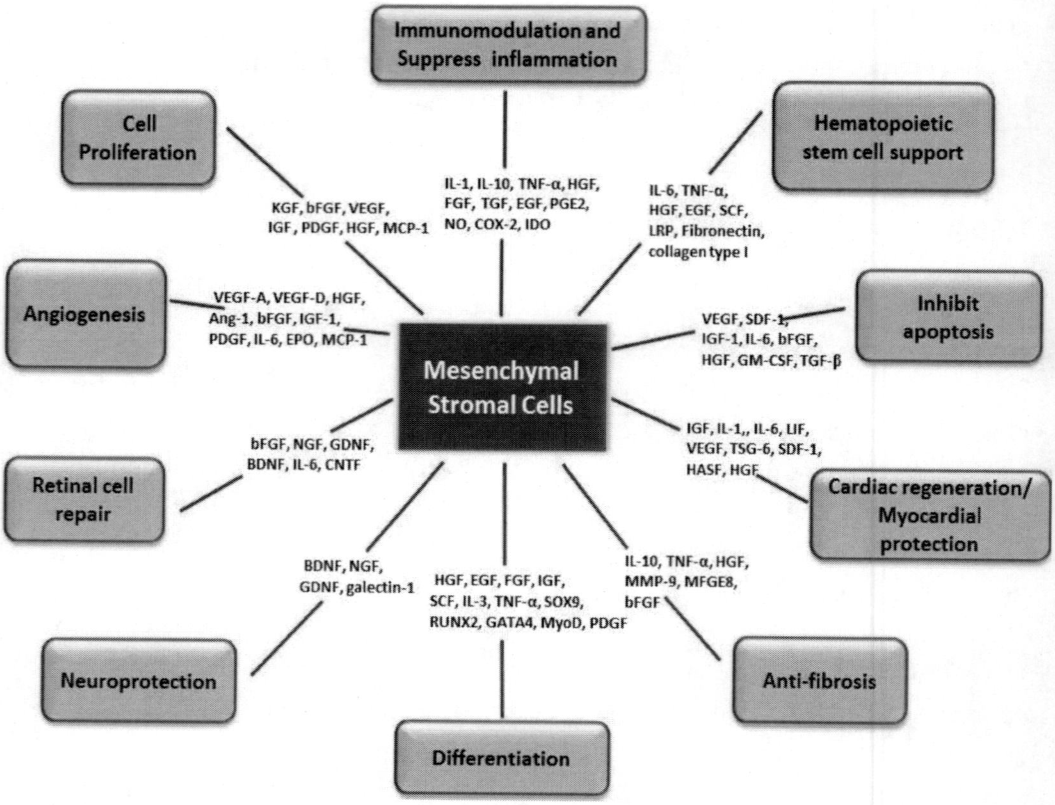

Abbreviations: Angiopoietin (Ang), basic fibroblast growth factor (bFGF), brain derived neurotrophic factor (BDNF), ciliary neurotrophic factor (CNTF), Cyclooxygenase-2 (COX-2), erythropoietin (EPO), GATA binding protein 4 (GATA4), glial cell line-neurotrophic factor (GDNF), granulocyte macrophage-colony stimulating factor (GM-CSF), Hypoxia And Akt Induced Stem Cell Factor (HASF), heme oxygenase (HO), hepatocyte growth factor (HGF), human leucocyte antigen (HLA), indoleamine 2,3-dioxygenase (IDO), insulin growth factor (IGF), interleukin (IL), keratinocyte growth factor (KGF), leukemia inhibitory factor (LIF), human cathelicidin (LL37), Low density lipoprotein receptor-related protein (LRP), monocyte chemoattractant protein (MCP), Milk Fat Globule-EGF Factor 8 (MFGE8), matrix metalloproteinase (MMP), myogenic differentiation (MyoD), nerve growth factor (NGF), nitric oxide (NO), platelet derived growth factor (PDGF), prostaglandin (PGE), placental growth factor (PIGF), runt related transcription factor 2 (RUNX2), stem cell factor (SCF), stromal cell-derived factor (SDF), SRY (Sex-Determining Region Y)-box (SOX), tissue inhibitor of metalloproteinase (TIMP), transforming growth factor (TGF), tumor necrosis factor (TNF), thrombopoietin (TPO), TNF- α -stimulated gene/protein (TSG), vascular endothelial growth factor (VEGF). Source: (173), modified.

Figure 2. Schematic diagram showing the biological properties of MSCs associated with their therapeutic effects. Several different paracrine/secreted factors released by MSCs may exert different functions via different types of molecules depending on specific signaling events. These factors influence the surrounding microenvironment leading to various therapeutic effects.

POTENTIAL CLINICAL APPLICATIONS OF MSCS IN REGENERATIVE MEDICINE

Mesenchymal stromal cells are self-renewal, multipotent progenitor cells with the ability to differentiate into different cell types of mesodermal origin. Clinical applications of MSC are mainly attributed to their important four biological properties- the ability to home to sites of inflammation following tissue injury when injected intravenously; to differentiate into various cell types; to secrete multiple bioactive molecules capable of stimulating recovery of injured cells and inhibiting inflammation and to perform immunomodulatory functions [131]. Various distinct paracrine factors such as cytokines, chemokines and growth factors released by MSCs mediates cross-talk between different cells influencing the surrounding micro-environment leading to various therapeutic effects [132-134].

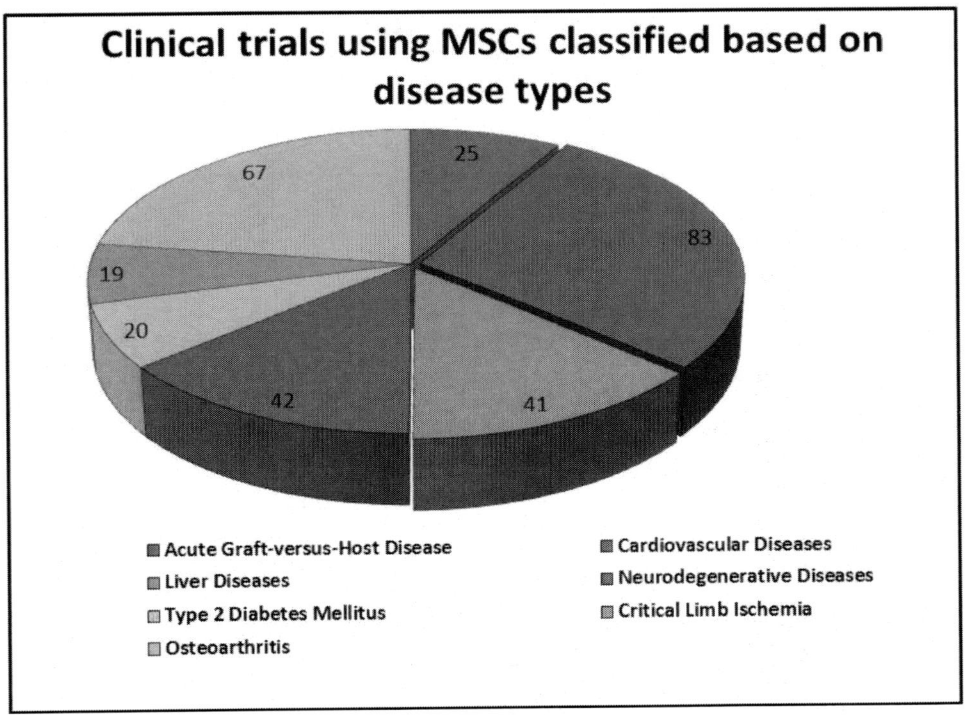

Figure 3. Clinical trials using MSCs categorized based on disease types. Numerous clinical trials have been registered (https://clinicaltrials.gov/) evaluating the use of MSCs in disease indications such as graft versus host disease, cardiovascular disease, osteoarthritis, critical limb ischemia, type 2 diabetes, liver and neurodegenerative diseases.

MSCs and osteoblasts form the stromal fraction in bone marrow and control proliferation and differentiation of stem cells. MSCs produce various molecules regulating hematopoiesis and form an integral part of the hematopoietic stem cell (HSC) niche [135]. The soluble factors secreted by MSCs may act directly by activating the intracellular mechanisms of injured cells, or indirectly by inducing the neighboring cells to secrete functionally active molecules thus aiding in tissue regeneration. During tissue injury, MSCs inhibit fibrotic remodeling and apoptosis, promote angiogenesis, stimulate endogenous stem cell proliferation and suppress immune responses/inflammation (Figure 2). These unique properties of MSCs have made them an attractive therapeutic tool for the treatment of various diseases. At the time of writing, more than 660 clinical trials are ongoing/completed according to ClinicalTrials.gov (https://clinicaltrials.gov/) evaluating the use of MSCs for treatment of various diseases; of which more than 300 clinical trials have been registered elucidating the role of MSCs in cardiovascular disease, graft versus host disease, osteoarthritis, critical limb ischemia, type 2 diabetes, liver and neurodegenerative diseases (Figure 3). These studies aim to explicate the safety and efficacy of MSCs for its use in clinical settings [136].

MSCs Infusion for the Treatment of Acute Graft-versus-Host Disease

Graft versus host disease (GvHD) is a condition that might occur after an allogeneic transplant and is associated with high mortality. Although corticosteroids are used as the initial treatment for GvHD, they are effective only in some patients. Potential treatment option for acute GvHD (aGvHD) consists of BM-MSC infusion of HLA-unrelated, or related donor. MSCs have the capability of homing and engrafting into inflammation sites exerting its functional effects on local tissues. The immunomodulatory and anti-inflammatory properties of MSCs serve as an attractive therapeutic approach for the treatment of GvHD [137]. Numerous studies reported the use of allogeneic MSCs for treatment of severe GvHD wherein the higher response rate after MSC infusion was observed suggesting the beneficial effect of MSC therapy [138-140]. The clinical efficacy in aGvHD was first observed in a 9-year-old boy with steroid-resistant grade IV aGvHD [141, 142], wherein the patient who was not responding to other therapies showed a complete response after receiving MSCs. Following this, MSCs have been studied extensively for this particular disease condition. Prochymal (Osiris Therapeutics Inc., Columbia, MD, USA) is an FDA approved, commercialized allogenic stem cell therapy product derived from bone marrow of healthy donors used in the treatment of steroid-refractory aGvHD in pediatric patients [138].

MSCs for Cardiovascular Repair

MSC therapy is gaining interest for cardio-vascular repair due to its regenerative and immune-modulatory properties. Several pre-clinical studies have shown improvement in cardiac repair after the administration of MSCs. Few clinical trials using MSCs for treatment of cardiovascular diseases have provided promising results wherein the patients with acute myocardial infarction receiving the autologous MSCs showed improvement in cardiac function with-out any serious adverse effects. Currently MSCs have been used to treat patients with myocardial infarction. The use of allogeneic MSCs derived from bone marrow and placenta for cardiovascular therapy has also been reported. Allogeneic MSCs are demonstrated to be safe and effective in phase I and II clinical trials for cardiovascular diseases [143]. Several bio-active molecules secreted by MSCs, promote myocardial tissue growth through endogenous activation of angiogenesis, immunomodulation, neurogeneration and proliferation of cardio-myocytes [144]. The administration of Prochymal, the commercial MSC therapy product in myocardial infarction patients resulted in significant clinical improvements [141].

MSCs to Treat Liver Diseases

MSCs have been used to treat hepatic fibrosis, liver cirrhosis and other acute liver diseases. Liver transplantation is the only option for the patients with advanced stages which has disadvantages such as lack of donors, complications during surgery and rejection. Recently, the therapeutic potential of MSCs for the treatment of liver diseases has been explored. More than 40 clinical trials using MSCs derived from umbilical cord tissue, bone marrow and adipose tissue for the treatment of liver diseases has been registered in ClinicalTrials.gov (https://clinicaltrials.gov/). BM-MSCs have the ability to differentiate into hepatocyte like cells *in vitro* under suitable conditions and stimulate liver regeneration. BM-MSCs are involved in immunomodulation and anti-inflammation wherein they exert a suppressive effect on T and B lymphocytes and natural killer cells (NKs). In addition, they secrete wide variety of growth factors which exert paracrine effects including anti-apoptosis, anti-fibrosis and stimulate the repopulation of endogenous cells in necrotized tissue [145-147]. Numerous reports showed that both autologous and allogeneic MSC injection was found to be safe and revealed the improvement in liver function in human clinical trials [136, 148-152].

Potential of MSCs to Treat Neurodegenerative Diseases

The ability of MSCs to transdifferentiate into neural cells under specific conditions and their neuroprotective and immunomodulatory properties have made them an attractive therapeutic tool for neurodegenerative diseases such as Alzheimer's disease (AD), Parkinson's disease (PD), Amyotrophic Lateral Sclerosis (ALS), Huntington's disease (HD) and Multiple Sclerosis (MS). MSCs are delivered via intracerebral or intrathecal injection. MSCs produce neurotrophic and growth factors that induce regeneration of damaged tissue stimulate endogenous neuronal growth, decrease apoptosis, reduce levels of free radicals, encourage synaptic connection from damaged neurons and regulate inflammation, primarily through paracrine actions upon transplantation into brain [153]. Clinical trials are currently ongoing involving MSCs for treating MS, ALS, traumatic brain injuries, spinal cord injuries and stroke [154]. Mazzini et al., conducted human clinical trial wherein autologous MSCs were implanted into the central nervous system of ALS patients and decrease in motor neuron death was assessed. Transplant-related toxicities were not observed and slowing of the decline in muscular strength was seen [155]. The immunomodulatory and neuroregenerative properties of MSCs in treatment of MS are also examined [156].

MSCs to Treat Type 2 Diabetes Mellitus

Type 2 diabetes mellitus (T2DM) is characterized by relative insulin deficiency and insulin resistance and the condition cannot be reversed with existing therapies. The use of MSCs for the treatment of diabetes has been extensively researched where several reports have demonstrated its beneficial effect in glycemic control which has been translated into clinical settings. MSCs promote the restoration of pancreatic islet beta cells, inhibit apoptosis of pancreatic islet beta cells and decrease insulin resistance of peripheral tissues by the secretion of paracrine factors or the deposition of extracellular matrix thus providing a suitable microenvironment for insulin producing cells (IPCs) [157-159]. MSCs have the potential to differentiate into IPCs by which MSCs ameliorate hyperglycemia in T2DM [160, 161]. More than 20 clinical trials in T2DM patients have been registered in http://www.clinicaltrials.gov. evaluating the clinical effects of MSC treatment in the management of T2DM. However, the survival of engrafted MSCs and the duration of its function *in vivo*, optimal dosage, long lasting effect of multiple injections has to be further evaluated before MSC transplantation becomes routine therapy for T2DM [162].

Therapeutic Potential of MSCs in the Treatment of Critical Limb Ischemia

Critical limb ischemia (CLI) represents the advanced stage of peripheral arterial obstructive disease (PAOD) with a severe obstruction of the arteries with reduced blood flow to the extremities and is characterized by severe rest pain and/or even tissue loss. Treatment strategies include pharmacologic therapy and invasive procedures; however 25% of patients still progress to limb amputations every year [163]. In the last decade, cell based therapies have been explored as an alternative option for the treatment of CLI. Preclinical studies have suggested that MSCs enhance neo-vascularization in ischemic limbs [164]. Bone marrow derived mesenchymal stromal cells induce angiogenesis and immunomodulatory environment *in situ* and may ameliorate the consequences of CLI. Recently, Gupta et al., (2013) conducted randomized double-blind placebo-controlled phase I/II study to assess the safety and efficacy of allogeneic BM-MSCs in patients with critical limb ischemia and reported that MSCs were safe when injected at a dose of 2 million cells/kg body weight and showed improvements in the rest pain [165]. Similar studies have been reported that confirmed the beneficial role of cell therapy in reducing the rate of amputations, improving distal perfusion, increasing walking distance, reducing pain and improving overall ischemic symptoms in patients with CLI and their quality of life [166-168].

MSCs to Treat Osteoarthritis

Osteoarthritis (OA) is a common and devastating chronic degenerative disease of the joints and has a significant impact on the quality of life. The prevalence of OA further increases with an aging population. Current treatment strategies aim at controlling the symptoms rather than disease modification. Joint replacement often poses significant complications. Growing interest in the area of regenerative medicine has seen efforts to explore the potential of mesenchymal stem cell therapy in the management of osteoarthritis. Fourteen clinical trials addressing OA with MSCs have been registered in ClinicalTrials.gov. Both pre-clinical and clinical studies using MSCs showed the beneficial effect for OA wherein reduction in pain and functional improvement was observed [169]. MSCs are capable of differentiating into musculoskeletal tissues, secrete bioactive molecules that stimulate angiogenesis and tissue repair, and reduce the response of T cells and inflammation. Recently, Gupta et al., (2016) have shown that the low dose intra-articular injection of BM-MSCs was safe in patients with OA [170]. Numerous clinical trials have reported that OA can be treated efficiently using autologous or allogenic MSCs through implantation, micro fracture or intra-articular injections [171]. However, determining the ideal MSC source, processing, and delivery vehicle are further challenges that must be addressed to optimize stem cell based therapy for OA.

Overview of Cell Therapy Products

Currently, there are a significant number of cell based clinical trials approved by many national and international regulatory bodies that are on-going and many of them are registered in clinicalTrials.gov. The fast growing cell therapy industry is integrated with many public companies and private partnerships for product launch and services.

Table 2. List of regulatory approved cell therapy products, source from which they are derived and their clinical applications

1997	**Carticel**	**Genzyme**	**Auto-Chon**	**Articular cartilage**	**USFDA**
1998	Apligraf	Oganogenisis	Allo-Keratino + Scaffold	Diabetic foot ulcers	USFDA
2008	ReliNethra	Reliance Life Science	limbal stem cells	Eye diseases	Not known
2009	Chondro Celect	TiGenix	Auto-Chondrocytes	Cartilage defects	EMEA
2009	Osteocel Plus	NuVasive	Allo-BM-MSCs	Orthopedics	USFDA
2010	CardioRel	Reliance Life Science	Auto- BM MSC	Post-acute myocardial infarction	Not known
2010	Provenge	Dendreon	Auto-Dendritic cells	Prostate cancer	USFDA
2010	Gintuit	Organogenisis	Auto-Dendritic cells	Prostate cancer	USFDA
2011	Grafix	Osiris Therapeutics	Allo-placenta matrix + MSC + other cells	Wounds, soft tissue defects	USFDA
2011	HeartiCell Gram-AMI	FCB-PharmiCell	Auto- BM-MSCs	Post-acute myocardial infarctions	KFDA
2012	Prochymal	Osiris Therapeutics	Allo-BM-MSCs	GVHD	Canada
2012	La Viv	Fibrocell Science inc	Auto-fibroblast	Severe nasolabial fold wrinkles	USFDA
2012	Cartistem	Medipost	Allo-MSCs from UCB	Traumatic OA	KFDA
2012	Cupistem	Anterogen	Auto-fat derived stem cells	Anal fistula in Crohns Disease	KFDA
2012	Ducord	Duke university	Allo- HPC cord blood	GVHD	USFDA
2013	Allocord	SSM cardinal	Allo- HPC cord blood	GVHD	USFDA
2013	Hemacord	New York Blood Center	Allo- HPC cord blood	GVHD	USFDA
2013	HiQCell	Regeneus	adipose SVF	Osteoarthriitis, tendonitis	TGA medical practitioner exemption
2013	OvationOS	Osiris Therapeutics	Allo-bone matrix + MSC + osteoblasts	Bone defects/ orthopedics	USFDA
2013	Trinity ELITE	Orthofix	Bone matrix with MSC and osteoprogenitors	Orthopedics	USFDA
2014	map3	RTI Surgical	Bone matrix with MAPC	Orthopedics	USFDA
2015	Holoclar	Chiesi Farmaceutici S.p.A.	limbal stem cells	Eye diseases	EMEA
Not known	Trinity Evolution	Orthofix	Allo- bone matrix with MSC	Orthopedics	USFDA
Not known	AlloStem	AlloSource	Allo- bone matrix with MSC	Orthopedics	USFDA
2016	TEMCELL® HS Inj	Mesoblast	Allo- stem cell product	Acute GVHD	Japanese Government regulatory approval
2017	Stempeucel CLI	Stempeutics Research Pvt Ltd	Allo-BM-MSCs	Critical Limb Ischemia- due to Buerger's disease	DCGI

Abbreviations: Allo- Allogeneic; Auto- Autologous; BM-MSCs- Bone marrow mesenchymal stromal cells; Chon- Chondrocytes; Diab – Diabetic; EMEA – European medical agency; GvHD – Graft versus host disease; HPC - *hematopoietic progenitor cell*; Keratino – keratinocytes; OA- *Osteoarthritis* (OA); UCB- Umbilical cord blood; KFDA – Korean federal drug administration; USFDA – United states federal drug administration.

These primarily depend on the level of investments in these sectors and the growth may slow slightly, but it may still outpace the majority of the economy largely revolving pharmaceuticals, biotechnology and medical device manufacturing companies. Many of the cell therapy industry already are aiming to create new blockbuster treatments and some cell therapy companies have already launched the product (Table 2) in the market and creating a way and market edge in cell therapy space. These translational researches towards cell therapy products create clarity on guidelines, review process and streamline the product approval requirement to market. The outcome of the cell therapy products bring critical factors in evaluating the process and improves the timely approval of regulatory bodies for the use of these cell based products for clinical trials.

Table 3. Table represents the major on-going clinical trials in regenerative medicine

1	**Lxmyelocel-T**	**Aastrom**	**Fast track approval**
2	Prochymal	Osiris	Phase-III
3	ADH001	Shire	Phase-III
4	Cx601	TiGenix	Phase-III
5	MPC	Mesoblast	Phase-III
6	StemEx	Gamida Cell	Phase-II/III
7	Liftegrast	Shire	Phase-III
8	PLX Cell	Pluristem	Phase-III
9	Lenti-D	Bluebirdbio	Phase-III
10	Chondrogen (OA)	Osiris	Phase-II
11	Multistem	Athersys	Phase-III
12	Enbuctrial RC	Medistem	Phase-II
13	AMR-001	Amorcyte	Phase-II
14	RGN-259	Regenex	Phase-III
15	Renew	Baxter International	Phase-III
16	TB4	Regenex	Phase-II
17	Stempeucel OA	Stempeutics Research Pvt Ltd	Phase-III
18	NT-501	Neurotech Pharmaceuticals	Fast track approval
19	Neocart	Histogenics	Phase-III
20	DeNovo ET	ISTO Technologies	Phase-III
21	MyoCell	Bioheart	Phase-III
22	HP802	Healthpoint Biotherapeutics	Phase-III
23	StemEx	Gamida Cell and Teva Pharmaceutical	Fast track approval
24	LaViv	Fibrocell Science	Phase-III

Overview of cell based clinical trials help us to understand the opportunities and challenges for successful therapeutic applications. Moreover, the outcomes of a large number of cell based clinical-trial outcomes for treatments are not documented in peer-reviewed journals. Unfortunately rationale for the clinical applications has lagged behind laboratory observations [172]. Well-designed clinical trials will be critical for determining whether MSCs can be effective in treating disease indications. Currently there are various clinical trials on regenerative medicine with various approaches to succeed in clinical trial end points. Table 3 represents the major on-going clinical trials in regenerative medicine. In these studies, several initiatives were implemented to accelerate our understanding to bring safe and efficacious development of regenerative medicinal product.

CONCLUSION

The efforts to bring the regenerative medicinal product are being undertaken with many types of stem cells from various sources and with distinct approaches. Most of the efforts from researchers to define, refine and characterize various types of stem cells in cell therapy industry field have occurred in the past last two decades. The anti-inflammatory and immunomodulatory properties of MSCs are remarkable to form the basis for cell based therapy. Major findings revealed that the mesenchymal stromal cells were of high promise to bring translational research to commercialization as potent cell therapy drug much faster than other cell types. Numerous studies have shown several strategies involving the use of MSCs from various sources for different disease indications, some of them currently being tested clinically. Although modest clinical success has been achieved in some areas, the field is still in its infancy stage. Further studies are required to determine the distribution and mechanism of action of MSCs *in vivo* to optimize their use for personalized regenerative medicine approach. Clinical studies carried out so far have not reported critical adverse effects of MSCs on disease conditions, hence MSC based cellular therapy can be considered safe. However, more clinical data is still essential to ensure immunogenicity; long term safety and efficacy of MSCs, the suitable source and dosage of cells to be infused before the MSC based therapy become the standard therapy for unmet medical needs of certain diseases. We hope that eventually safe and effective therapy with MSCs emerges and revolutionize the treatment strategies of patients with serious diseases.

ACKNOWLEDGMENTS

Support for this work from Stempeutics Research Pvt. Ltd. is greatly acknowledged.

CONFLICT OF INTEREST

The authors declare no conflicts of interest.

ETHICAL COMPLIANCE

The authors have stated all possible conflicts of interest within this work. The authors have stated all sources of funding for this work. If this work involved human participants, informed consent was received from each individual. If this work involved human participants, it was conducted in accordance with the 1964 Declaration of Helsinki. If this work involved experiments with humans or animals, it was conducted in accordance with the related institutions' research ethics guidelines.

REFERENCES

[1] Burke J, Hunter M, Kolhe R, Isales C, Hamrick M, Fulzele S. Therapeutic potential of mesenchymal stem cell based therapy for osteoarthritis. *Clin Transl Med.* 2016 Dec; 5(1):27.

[2] Han KH, Kim AK, Kim DI. Therapeutic Potential of Human Mesenchymal Stem Cells for Treating Ischemic Limb Diseases. *Int J Stem Cells.* 201; 9(2):163-8.

[3] Dai LJ, Li HY, Guan LX, Ritchie G, Zhou JX. The therapeutic potential of bone marrow-derived mesenchymal stem cells on hepatic cirrhosis. *Stem Cell Res.* 2009 Jan; 2(1):16-25.

[4] D'Agostino B, Sullo N, Siniscalco D, De Angelis A, Rossi F. Mesenchymal stem cell therapy for the treatment of chronic obstructive pulmonary disease. *Expert Opin Biol Ther.* 2010 May; 10(5):681-7.

[5] El-Badawy A, El-Badri N. Clinical Efficacy of Stem Cell Therapy for Diabetes Mellitus: A Meta-Analysis. *PLoS One.* 2016; 11(4):e0151938.

[6] Wang L, Ji H, Zhou J, Xie J, Zhong Z, Li M, et al. Therapeutic potential of umbilical cord mesenchymal stromal cells transplantation for cerebral palsy: a case report. *Case Rep Transplant.* 2013; 2013:146347.

[7] Inden MYD, Hijioka M, Kitamura Y. Therapeutic Effects of Mesenchymal Stem Cells for Parkinson's Disease. *Ann Neurodegener Dis.* 2016; 1(1):1002.

[8] Qu J, Zhang H. Roles of Mesenchymal Stem Cells in Spinal Cord Injury. *Stem Cells Int.* 2017; 2017:5251313.

[9] Gerson SL. Mesenchymal stem cells: no longer second class marrow citizens. *Nat Med.* 1999 Mar; 5(3):262-4.

[10] Uccelli A, Moretta L, Pistoia V. Mesenchymal stem cells in health and disease. *Nat Rev Immunol.* 2008 Sep; 8(9):726-36.

[11] Friedenstein AJ, Gorskaja JF, Kulagina NN. Fibroblast precursors in normal and irradiated mouse hemato-poietic organs. *Exp Hematol.* 1976 Sep; 4(5):267-74.

[12] Pittenger MF, Mackay AM, Beck SC, Jaiswal RK, Douglas R, Mosca JD, et al. Multilineage potential of adult human mesenchymal stem cells. *Science.* 1999 Apr 02; 284(5411):143-7.

[13] Otsuru S, Hofmann TJ, Olson TS, Dominici M, Horwitz EM. Improved isolation and expansion of bone marrow mesenchymal stromal cells using a novel marrow filter device. *Cytotherapy.* 2013 Feb; 15(2):146-53.

[14] Gronthos S, Graves SE, Ohta S, Simmons PJ. The STRO-1+ fraction of adult human bone marrow contains the osteogenic precursors. *Blood.* 1994 Dec 15; 84(12):4164-73.

[15] Mamidi MK, Nathan KG, Singh G, Thrichelvam ST, Mohd Yusof NA, Fakharuzi NA, et al. Comparative cellular and molecular analyses of pooled bone marrow multipotent mesenchymal stromal cells during continuous passaging and after successive cryo-preservation. *J Cell Biochem.* 2012 Oct; 113(10): 3153-64.

[16] Stewart K, Walsh S, Screen J, Jefferiss CM, Chainey J, Jordan GR, et al. Further characterization of cells expressing STRO-1 in cultures of adult human bone marrow stromal cells. *J Bone Miner Res.* 1999; 14(8): 1345-56.

[17] Peng L, Jia Z, Yin X, Zhang X, Liu Y, Chen P, et al. Comparative analysis of mesenchymal stem cells from bone marrow, cartilage, and adipose tissue. *Stem Cells Dev*. 2008 Aug; 17(4):761-73.

[18] Kern S, Eichler H, Stoeve J, Kluter H, Bieback K. Comparative analysis of mesenchymal stem cells from bone marrow, umbilical cord blood, or adipose tissue. *Stem Cells*. 2006 May; 24(5):1294-301.

[19] Gimble JM, Katz AJ, Bunnell BA. Adipose-derived stem cells for regenerative medicine. *Circ Res.* 2007 May 11; 100(9):1249-60.

[20] Ikehara MLaS. Immunomodulatory Properties and Therapeutic Application of Bone Marrow Derived-Mesenchymal Stem Cells. *Journal of Bone Marrow Researc*h. 2013; 1(4).

[21] Kastrinaki MC, Sidiropoulos P, Roche S, Ringe J, Lehmann S, Kritikos H, et al. Functional, molecular and proteomic characterisation of bone marrow mesenchymal stem cells in rheumatoid arthritis. *Ann Rheum Dis.* 2008 Jun; 67(6):741-9.

[22] Wehbe T, Chahine NA, Sissi S, Abou-Joaude I, Chalhoub L. Bone marrow derived stem cell therapy for type 2 diabetes mellitus. *Stem Cell Investig*. 2017; 3:87.

[23] Kharaziha P, Hellstrom PM, Noorinayer B, Farzaneh F, Aghajani K, Jafari F, et al. Improvement of liver function in liver cirrhosis patients after autologous mesenchymal stem cell injection: a phase I-II clinical trial. *Eur J Gastroenterol Hepatol*. 2009; 21(10):1199-205.

[24] Mohamadnejad M, Alimoghaddam K, Mohyeddin-Bonab M, Bagheri M, Bashtar M, Ghanaati H, et al. Phase 1 trial of autologous bone marrow mesenchymal stem cell transplantation in patients with decompensated liver cirrhosis. *Arch Iran Med.* 2007 Oct; 10(4):459- 66.

[25] Aggarwal S, Pittenger MF. Human mesenchymal stem cells modulate allogeneic immune cell responses. *Blood.* 2005 Feb 15; 105(4):1815-22.

[26] Ramasamy R, Fazekasova H, Lam EW, Soeiro I, Lombardi G, Dazzi F. Mesenchymal stem cells inhibit dendritic cell differentiation and function by preventing entry into the cell cycle. *Transplantation.* 2007 Jan 15; 83(1):71-6.

[27] Zhang B, Liu R, Shi D, Liu X, Chen Y, Dou X, et al. Mesenchymal stem cells induce mature dendritic cells into a novel Jagged-2-dependent regulatory dendritic cell population. *Blood*. 2009 Jan 1; 113(1):46-57.

[28] Kuhbier JW, Weyand B, Radtke C, Vogt PM, Kasper C, Reimers K. Isolation, characterization, differentiation, and application of adipose-derived stem cells. *Adv Biochem Eng Biotechnol*. 2010; 123:55-105.

[29] Gronthos S, Franklin DM, Leddy HA, Robey PG, Storms RW, Gimble JM. Surface protein character-ization of human adipose tissue-derived stromal cells. *J Cell Physiol*. 2001 Oct; 189(1):54-63.

[30] Pendleton C, Li Q, Chesler DA, Yuan K, Guerrero-Cazares H, Quinones-Hinojosa A. Mesenchymal stem cells derived from adipose tissue vs bone marrow: *in vitro* comparison of their tropism towards gliomas. *PLoS One*. 2013; 8(3):e58198.

[31] Wagner W, Wein F, Seckinger A, Frankhauser M, Wirkner U, Krause U, et al. Comparative characteristics of mesenchymal stem cells from human bone marrow, adipose tissue, and umbilical cord blood. *Exp Hematol*. 2005 Nov; 33(11):1402-16.

[32] Zhang X, Hirai M, Cantero S, Ciubotariu R, Dobrila L, Hirsh A, et al. Isolation and characterization of mesenchymal stem cells from human umbilical cord blood: reevaluation of critical factors for successful isolation and high ability to proliferate and differentiate to chondrocytes as compared to mesenchymal stem cells from bone marrow and adipose tissue. *J Cell Biochem*. 2011 Apr; 112(4):1206-18.

[33] Schaffler A, Buchler C. Concise review: adipose tissue-derived stromal cells--basic and clinical implications for novel cell-based therapies. *Stem Cells*. 2007; 25(4):818-27.

[34] Malladi P, Xu Y, Chiou M, Giaccia AJ, Longaker MT. Effect of reduced oxygen tension on chondrogenesis and osteogenesis in adipose-derived mesenchymal cells. *Am J Physiol Cell Physiol*. 2006 Apr; 290(4):C1139-46.

[35] Markway BD, Tan GK, Brooke G, Hudson JE, Cooper-White JJ, Doran MR. Enhanced chondrogenic differentiation of human bone marrow-derived mesen-chymal stem cells in low oxygen environment micro-pellet cultures. *Cell Transplant*. 2009; 19(1):29-42.

[36] Erices A, Conget P, Minguell JJ. Mesenchymal progenitor cells in human umbilical cord blood. *Br J Haematol*. 2000 Apr; 109(1):235-42.

[37] Kogler G, Sensken S, Airey JA, Trapp T, Muschen M, Feldhahn N, et al. A new human somatic stem cell from placental cord blood with intrinsic pluripotent differentiation potential. *J Exp Med*. 2004; 19; 200(2): 123-35.

[38] Jeltsch KS, Radke TF, Laufs S, Giordano FA, Allgayer H, Wenz F, et al. Unrestricted somatic stem cells: interaction with CD^{34+} cells *in vitro* and *in vivo*, expression of homing genes and exclusion of tumorigenic potential. *Cytotherapy*. 2010; 13(3):357-65.

[39] Peng J, Wang Y, Zhang L, Zhao B, Zhao Z, Chen J, et al. Human umbilical cord Wharton's jelly-derived mesenchymal stem cells differentiate into a Schwann-cell phenotype and promote neurite outgrowth *in vitro*. *Brain Res Bull*. 2011 Feb 28; 84(3):235-43.

[40] Zhao Z, Wang Y, Peng J, Ren Z, Zhang L, Guo Q, et al. Improvement in nerve regeneration through a de-cellularized nerve graft by supplementation with bone marrow stromal cells in fibrin. *Cell Transplant*. 2012 Jan; 23(1):97-110.

[41] Li DR, Cai JH. Methods of isolation, expansion, differentiating induction and preservation of human umbilical cord mesenchymal stem cells. *Chin Med J* (Engl). 2012 Dec; 125(24):4504-10.

[42] Nekanti U, Mohanty L, Venugopal P, Balasubramanian S, Totey S, Ta M. Optimization and scale-up of Wharton's jelly-derived mesenchymal stem cells for clinical applications. *Stem Cell Res*. 2010 Nov; 5(3):244-54.

[43] Balasubramanian S, Venugopal P, Sundarraj S, Zakaria Z, Majumdar AS, Ta M. Comparison of chemokine and receptor gene expression between Wharton's jelly and bone marrow-derived mesenchymal stromal cells. *Cytotherapy*. 2011 Jan; 14(1):26-33.

[44] Nekanti U, Dastidar S, Venugopal P, Totey S, Ta M. Increased proliferation and analysis of differential gene expression in human Wharton's jelly-derived mesenchymal stromal cells under hypoxia. *Int J Biol Sci*. 2010 Sep 09; 6(5):499-512.

[45] Nekanti U, Rao VB, Bahirvani AG, Jan M, Totey S, Ta M. Long-term expansion and pluripotent marker array analysis of Wharton's jelly-derived mesenchymal stem cells. *Stem Cells Dev*. 2009 Jan; 19(1):117-30.

[46] Priya N, Sarcar S, Majumdar AS, SundarRaj S. Explant culture: a simple, reproducible, efficient and economic technique for isolation of mesenchymal stromal cells from human adipose tissue and lipoaspirate. *J Tissue Eng Regen Med*. 2012 Sep; 8(9):706-16.

[47] Hou T, Xu J, Wu X, Xie Z, Luo F, Zhang Z, et al. Umbilical cord Wharton's Jelly: a new potential cell source of mesenchymal stromal cells for bone tissue engineering. *Tissue Eng Part A*. 2009 Sep; 15(9):2325-34.

[48] Kuznetsov SA, Krebsbach PH, Satomura K, Kerr J, Riminucci M, Benayahu D, et al. Single-colony derived strains of human marrow stromal fibroblasts form bone after transplantation *in vivo*. *J Bone Miner Res*. 1997 Sep; 12(9):1335-47.

[49] Waterman RS, Tomchuck SL, Henkle SL, Betancourt AM. A new mesenchymal stem cell (MSC) paradigm: polarization into a pro-inflammatory MSC1 or an Immunosuppressive MSC2 phenotype. *PLoS One*. 2010 Apr 26; 5(4):e10088.

[50] Kim DW, Staples M, Shinozuka K, Pantcheva P, Kang SD, Borlongan CV. Wharton's jelly-derived mesen-chymal stem cells: phenotypic characterization and optimizing their therapeutic potential for clinical applications. *Int J Mol Sci*. 2013 May 31; 14(6):11692-712.

[51] Semenov O, Olah MJ, Stefanovic D. Mechanism of diffusive transport in molecular spider models. *Phys Rev E Stat Nonlin Soft Matter Phys*. 2011 Feb; 83(2 Pt 1):021117.

[52] Lopez Y, Lutjemeier B, Seshareddy K, Trevino EM, Hageman KS, Musch TI, et al. Wharton's jelly or bone marrow mesenchymal stromal cells improve cardiac function following myocardial infarction for more than 32 weeks in a rat model: a preliminary report. *Curr Stem Cell Res Ther*. 2012 Jan; 8(1):46-59.

[53] Raynaud CM, Maleki M, Lis R, Ahmed B, Al-Azwani I, Malek J, et al. Comprehensive characterization of mesenchymal stem cells from human placenta and fetal membrane and their response to osteoactivin stimulation. *Stem Cells Int.* 2012; 2012:658356.

[54] Sabapathy V, Ravi S, Srivastava V, Srivastava A, Kumar S. Long-term cultured human term placenta-derived mesenchymal stem cells of maternal origin displays plasticity. *Stem Cells Int.* 2012; 2012:174328.

[55] Beer AE, Sio JO. Placenta as an immunological barrier. *Biol Reprod.* 1982 Feb; 26(1):15-27.

[56] Hayati AR, Mohamed AE, Tan GC. An immuno-histochemical study of Toll-like receptors 2 and 4 in placenta with and without infection. *Malays J Pathol.* 2010 Jun; 32(1):13-9.

[57] Landers KA, McKinnon BD, Li H, Subramaniam VN, Mortimer RH, Richard K. Carrier-mediated thyroid hormone transport into placenta by placental trans-thyretin. *J Clin Endocrinol Metab*. 2009 Jul; 94(7):2610-6.

[58] Mortimer RH, Landers KA, Balakrishnan B, Li H, Mitchell MD, Patel J, et al. Secretion and transfer of the thyroid hormone binding protein transthyretin by human placenta. *Placenta.* 2012 Apr; 33(4):252-6.

[59] Prusa AR, Marton E, Rosner M, Bernaschek G, Hengstschlager M. Oct-4-expressing cells in human amniotic fluid: a new source for stem cell research? *Hum Reprod*. 2003 Jul; 18(7):1489-93.

[60] Chiavegato A, Bollini S, Pozzobon M, Callegari A, Gasparotto L, Taiani J, et al. Human amniotic fluid-derived stem cells are rejected after transplantation in the myocardium of normal, ischemic, immuno-suppressed or immuno-deficient rat. *J Mol Cell Cardiol*. 2007 Apr; 42(4):746-59.

[61] Kim J, Lee Y, Kim H, Hwang KJ, Kwon HC, Kim SK, et al. Human amniotic fluid-derived stem cells have characteristics of multipotent stem cells. *Cell Prolif.* 2007 Feb; 40(1):75-90.

[62] Roubelakis MG, Pappa KI, Bitsika V, Zagoura D, Vlahou A, Papadaki HA, et al. Molecular and proteomic characterization of human mesenchymal stem cells derived from amniotic fluid: comparison to bone marrow mesenchymal stem cells. *Stem Cells Dev*. 2007 Dec; 16(6):931-52.

[63] Tsai MS, Hwang SM, Tsai YL, Cheng FC, Lee JL, Chang YJ. Clonal amniotic fluid-derived stem cells express characteristics of both mesenchymal and neural stem cells. *Biol Reprod.* 2006 Mar; 74(3):545-51.

[64] Phermthai T, Odglun Y, Julavijitphong S, Titapant V, Chuenwattana P, Vantanasiri C, et al. A novel method to derive amniotic fluid stem cells for therapeutic purposes. *BMC Cell Biol.* 2010 Oct 19; 11:79.

[65] Cai J, Li W, Su H, Qin D, Yang J, Zhu F, et al. Generation of human induced pluripotent stem cells from umbilical cord matrix and amniotic membrane mesenchymal cells. *J Biol Chem*. 2010; 09; 285(15): 11227-34.

[66] In 't Anker PS, Scherjon SA, Kleijburg-van der Keur C, Noort WA, Claas FH, Willemze R, et al. Amniotic fluid as a novel source of mesenchymal stem cells for therapeutic transplantation. *Blood.* 2003; 15; 102(4): 1548-9.

[67] Tsai MS, Lee JL, Chang YJ, Hwang SM. Isolation of human multipotent mesenchymal stem cells from second-trimester amniotic fluid using a novel two-stage culture protocol. *Hum Reprod.* 2004 Jun; 19(6):1450-6.

[68] Miranda-Sayago JM, Fernandez-Arcas N, Benito C, Reyes-Engel A, Carrera J, Alonso A. Lifespan of human amniotic fluid-derived multipotent mesenchymal stromal cells. *Cytotherapy*. 2011 May; 13(5):572-81.

[69] Zagoura DS, Roubelakis MG, Bitsika V, Trohatou O, Pappa KI, Kapelouzou A, et al. Therapeutic potential of a distinct population of human amniotic fluid mesenchymal stem cells and their secreted molecules in mice with acute hepatic failure. *Gut.* 2011; 61(6):894-906.

[70] Liu T, Huang Y, Guo L, Cheng W, Zou G. CD44+/CD105+ human amniotic fluid mesenchymal stem cells survive and proliferate in the ovary long-term in a mouse model of chemotherapy-induced premature ovarian failure. *Int J Med Sci*. 2012; 9(7):592-602.

[71] Beeravolu N, McKee C, Alamri A, Mikhael S, Brown C, Perez-Cruet M, et al. Isolation and Characterization of Mesenchymal Stromal Cells from Human Umbilical Cord and Fetal Placenta. *J Vis Exp*. 2017 Apr 3(122).

[72] Margossian T, Reppel L, Makdissy N, Stoltz JF, Bensoussan D, Huselstein C. Mesenchymal stem cells derived from Wharton's jelly: comparative phenotype analysis between tissue and *in vitro* expansion. *Biomed Mater Eng*. 2012; 22(4):243-54.

[73] Wang M, Yang Y, Yang D, Luo F, Liang W, Guo S, et al. The immunomodulatory activity of human umbilical cord blood-derived mesenchymal stem cells *in vitro. Immunology*. 2009 Feb; 126(2):220-32.

[74] Arutyunyan I, Elchaninov A, Makarov A, Fatkhudinov T. Umbilical Cord as Prospective Source for Mesenchymal Stem Cell-Based Therapy. *Stem Cells Int.* 2016; 2016:6901286.

[75] Li X, Bai J, Ji X, Li R, Xuan Y, Wang Y. Comprehensive characterization of four different populations of human mesenchymal stem cells as regards their immune properties, proliferation and differentiation. *Int J Mol Med.* 2014 Sep; 34(3):695-704.

[76] Richardson SM, Kalamegam G, Pushparaj PN, Matta C, Memic A, Khademhosseini A, et al. Mesenchymal stem cells in regenerative medicine: Focus on articular cartilage and intervertebral disc regeneration. *Methods.* 2015 Apr 15; 99:69-80.

[77] Ostergaard M, Ejbjerg B, Stoltenberg M, Gideon P, Volck B, Skov K, et al. Quantitative magnetic resonance imaging as marker of synovial membrane regeneration and recurrence of synovitis after arthroscopic knee joint synovectomy: a one year follow up study. *Ann Rheum Dis.* 2001 Mar; 60(3):233-6.

[78] Morito T, Muneta T, Hara K, Ju YJ, Mochizuki T, Makino H, et al. Synovial fluid-derived mesenchymal stem cells increase after intra-articular ligament injury in humans. *Rheumatology* (Oxford). 2008 Aug; 47(8): 1137-43.

[79] McGonagle D, Jones E. A potential role for synovial fluid mesenchymal stem cells in ligament regeneration. *Rheumatology (*Oxford). 2008 Aug; 47(8):1114-6.

[80] Hegewald AA, Ringe J, Bartel J, Kruger I, Notter M, Barnewitz D, et al. Hyaluronic acid and autologous synovial fluid induce chondrogenic differentiation of equine mesenchymal stem cells: a preliminary study. *Tissue Cell.* 2004 Dec; 36(6):431-8.

[81] Gronthos S, Mankani M, Brahim J, Robey PG, Shi S. Postnatal human dental pulp stem cells (DPSCs) *in vitro* and *in vivo*. *Proc Natl Acad Sci USA.* 2000 Dec 05; 97(25):13625-30.

[82] Huang GT, Gronthos S, Shi S. Mesenchymal stem cells derived from dental tissues vs. those from other sources: their biology and role in regenerative medicine. *J Dent Res.* 2009 Sep; 88(9):792-806.

[83] Kadar K, Kiraly M, Porcsalmy B, Molnar B, Racz GZ, Blazsek J, et al. Differentiation potential of stem cells from human dental origin - promise for tissue engineering. *J Physiol Pharmacol.* 2009 Dec; 60 Suppl 7:167-75.

[84] Seifrtova M, Havelek R, Cmielova J, Jiroutova A, Soukup T, Bruckova L, et al. The response of human ectomesenchymal dental pulp stem cells to cisplatin treatment. *Int Endod J.* 2011 May; 45(5):401-12.

[85] Sedgley CM, Botero TM. Dental stem cells and their sources. *Dent Clin North Am.* 2012 Jul; 56(3):549-61.

[86] Abu Kasim NH, Govindasamy V, Gnanasegaran N, Musa S, Pradeep PJ, Srijaya TC, et al. Unique molecular signatures influencing the biological function and fate of post-natal stem cells isolated from different sources. *J Tissue Eng Regen Med.* 2012 Dec; 9(12): E252-66.

[87] Martens W, Bronckaers A, Politis C, Jacobs R, Lambrichts I. Dental stem cells and their promising role in neural regeneration: an update. *Clin Oral Investig*. 2013 Dec; 17(9):1969-83.

[88] Martens W, Wolfs E, Struys T, Politis C, Bronckaers A, Lambrichts I. Expression pattern of basal markers in human dental pulp stem cells and tissue. *Cells Tissues Organs*. 2012; 196(6):490-500.

[89] Nosrat IV, Smith CA, Mullally P, Olson L, Nosrat CA. Dental pulp cells provide neurotrophic support for dopaminergic neurons and differentiate into neurons *in vitro*; implications for tissue engineering and repair in the nervous system. *Eur J Neurosci*. 2004 May; 19(9): 2388-98.

[90] Ab Kadir R, Zainal Ariffin SH, Megat Abdul Wahab R, Kermani S, Senafi S. Characterization of mono-nucleated human peripheral blood cells. *Scientific World Journal*. 2012; 2012:843843.

[91] Chong PP, Selvaratnam L, Abbas AA, Kamarul T. Human peripheral blood derived mesenchymal stem cells demonstrate similar characteristics and chondro-genic differentiation potential to bone marrow derived mesenchymal stem cells. *J Orthop Res*. 2011 Apr; 30(4): 634-42.

[92] Trivanovic D, Kocic J, Mojsilovic S, Krstic A, Ilic V, Djordjevic IO, et al. Mesenchymal stem cells isolated from peripheral blood and umbilical cord Wharton's jelly. *Srp Arh Celok Lek*. 2013 Mar-Apr; 141(3-4):178-86.

[93] Hematti P. Human embryonic stem cell-derived mesenchymal stromal cells. *Transfusion*. 2011 Nov; 51 Suppl 4:138S-44S.

[94] Lian Q, Lye E, Suan Yeo K, Khia Way Tan E, Salto-Tellez M, Liu TM, et al. Derivation of clinically compliant MSCs from CD105+, CD24- differentiated human ESCs. *Stem Cells*. 2007 Feb; 25(2):425-36.

[95] Liu YP, Seckin H, Izci Y, Du ZW, Yan YP, Baskaya MK. Neuroprotective effects of mesenchymal stem cells derived from human embryonic stem cells in transient focal cerebral ischemia in rats. *J Cereb Blood Flow Metab*. 2009 Apr; 29(4):780-91.

[96] Sze SK, de Kleijn DP, Lai RC, Khia Way Tan E, Zhao H, Yeo KS, et al. Elucidating the secretion proteome of human embryonic stem cell-derived mesenchymal stem cells. *Mol Cell Proteomics*. 2007 Oct; 6(10):1680-9.

[97] Trivedi P, Hematti P. Derivation and immunological characterization of mesenchymal stromal cells from human embryonic stem cells. *Exp Hematol*. 2008 Mar; 36(3):350-9.

[98] Villa-Diaz LG, Brown SE, Liu Y, Ross AM, Lahann J, Parent JM, et al. Derivation of mesenchymal stem cells from human induced pluripotent stem cells cultured on synthetic substrates. *Stem Cells*. 2012 Jun; 30(6):1174-81.

[99] Griffiths MJ, Bonnet D, Janes SM. Stem cells of the alveolar epithelium. *Lancet*. 2005 Jul 16-22; 366(9481): 249-60.

[100] Beltrami AP, Barlucchi L, Torella D, Baker M, Limana F, Chimenti S, et al. Adult cardiac stem cells are multipotent and support myocardial regeneration. *Cell.* 2003 Sep 19; 114(6):763-76.

[101] Lama VN, Smith L, Badri L, Flint A, Andrei AC, Murray S, et al. Evidence for tissue-resident mesen-chymal stem cells in human adult lung from studies of transplanted allografts. *J Clin Invest*. 2007 Apr; 117(4): 989-96.

[102] Hoogduijn MJ, Crop MJ, Peeters AM, Van Osch GJ, Balk AH, Ijzermans JN, et al. Human heart, spleen, and perirenal fat-derived mesenchymal stem cells have immunomodulatory capacities. *Stem Cells Dev*. 2007 Aug; 16(4):597-604.

[103] Ullah I, Subbarao RB, Rho GJ. Human mesenchymal stem cells - current trends and future prospective. *Biosci Rep.* 2015 Apr 28; 35(2).

[104] Schuring AN, Schulte N, Kelsch R, Ropke A, Kiesel L, Gotte M. Characterization of endometrial mesenchymal stem-like cells obtained by endometrial biopsy during routine diagnostics. *Fertil Steril.* 2010 Jan; 95(1):423-6.

[105] Jiao F, Wang J, Dong ZL, Wu MJ, Zhao TB, Li DD, et al. Human mesenchymal stem cells derived from limb bud can differentiate into all three embryonic germ layers lineages. *Cell Reprogram.* 2012 Aug; 14(4):324-33.

[106] Rotter N, Oder J, Schlenke P, Lindner U, Bohrnsen F, Kramer J, et al. Isolation and characterization of adult stem cells from human salivary glands. *Stem Cells Dev*. 2008 Jun; 17(3):509-18.

[107] Bartsch G, Yoo JJ, De Coppi P, Siddiqui MM, Schuch G, Pohl HG, et al. Propagation, expansion, and multilineage differentiation of human somatic stem cells from dermal progenitors. *Stem Cells Dev*. 2005; 14(3): 337-48.

[108] Riekstina U, Muceniece R, Cakstina I, Muiznieks I, Ancans J. Characterization of human skin-derived mesenchymal stem cell proliferation rate in different growth conditions. *Cytotechnology*. 2008 Nov; 58(3): 153-62.

[109] Kita K, Gauglitz GG, Phan TT, Herndon DN, Jeschke MG. Isolation and characterization of mesenchymal stem cells from the sub-amniotic human umbilical cord lining membrane. *Stem Cells Dev*. 2009 Apr; 19(4):491-502.

[110] Moretti P, Hatlapatka T, Marten D, Lavrentieva A, Majore I, Hass R, et al. Mesenchymal stromal cells derived from human umbilical cord tissues: primitive cells with potential for clinical and tissue engineering applications. *Adv Biochem Eng Biotechnol*. 2009; 123: 29-54.

[111] Bernardo ME, Fibbe WE. Mesenchymal stromal cells: sensors and switchers of inflammation. *Cell Stem Cell*. 2013 Oct 3; 13(4):392-402.

[112] Waterman RS, Henkle SL, Betancourt AM. Mesenchymal stem cell 1 (MSC1)-based therapy attenuates tumor growth whereas MSC2-treatment promotes tumor growth and metastasis. *PLoS One*. 2012; 7(9):e45590.

[113] Mounayar M, Kefaloyianni E, Smith B, Solhjou Z, Maarouf OH, Azzi J, et al. PI3kalpha and STAT1 Interplay Regulates Human Mesenchymal Stem Cell Immune Polarization. *Stem Cells*. 2015 Jun; 33(6):1892-901.

[114] Machado Cde V, Telles PD, Nascimento IL. Immunological characteristics of mesenchymal stem cells. *Rev Bras Hematol Hemoter*. 2013; 35(1):62-7.

[115] Haddad R, Saldanha-Araujo F. Mechanisms of T-cell immunosuppression by mesenchymal stromal cells: what do we know so far? *Biomed Res Int*. 2014; 2014: 216806.

[116] Abdel Aziz MT, Atta HM, Mahfouz S, Fouad HH, Roshdy NK, Ahmed HH, et al. Therapeutic potential of bone marrow-derived mesenchymal stem cells on experimental liver fibrosis. *Clin Biochem*. 2007 Aug; 40 (12):893-9.

[117] Picinich SC, Mishra PJ, Glod J, Banerjee D. The therapeutic potential of mesenchymal stem cells. Cell- & tissue-based therapy. *Expert Opin Biol Ther*. 2007 Jul; 7(7):965-73.

[118] Mets T, Verdonk G. *In vitro* aging of human bone marrow derived stromal cells. *Mech Ageing Dev*. 1981 May; 16(1):81-9.

[119] Colter DC, Class R, DiGirolamo CM, Prockop DJ. Rapid expansion of recycling stem cells in cultures of plastic-adherent cells from human bone marrow. *Proc Natl Acad Sci USA*. 2000 Mar 28; 97(7):3213-8.

[120] Colter DC, Sekiya I, Prockop DJ. Identification of a subpopulation of rapidly self-renewing and multi-potential adult stem cells in colonies of human marrow stromal cells. *Proc Natl Acad Sci USA*. 2001 Jul 03; 98(14):7841-5.

[121] Sekiya I, Larson BL, Smith JR, Pochampally R, Cui JG, Prockop DJ. Expansion of human adult stem cells from bone marrow stroma: conditions that maximize the yields of early progenitors and evaluate their quality. *Stem Cells*. 2002; 20(6):530-41.

[122] Smith JR, Pochampally R, Perry A, Hsu SC, Prockop DJ. Isolation of a highly clonogenic and multipotential subfraction of adult stem cells from bone marrow stroma. *Stem Cells*. 2004; 22(5):823-31.

[123] Settleman J. Tension precedes commitment-even for a stem cell. *Mol Cell*. 2004 Apr 23; 14(2):148-50.

[124] Haasters F, Prall WC, Anz D, Bourquin C, Pautke C, Endres S, et al. Morphological and immune-cytochemical characteristics indicate the yield of early progenitors and represent a quality control for human mesenchymal stem cell culturing. *J Anat*. 2009 May; 214 (5):759-67.

[125] Delorme B, Ringe J, Gallay N, Le Vern Y, Kerboeuf D, Jorgensen C, et al. Specific plasma membrane protein phenotype of culture-amplified and native human bone marrow mesenchymal stem cells. *Blood*. 2008 Mar 1; 111(5):2631-5.

[126] Udaykumar Kolkundkar SGaASM. Cell Therapy Manufacturing and Quality Control: Current Process and Regulatory Challenges. *J Stem Cell Res Ther.* 2014; 4(9).

[127] Panchalingam KM, Jung S, Rosenberg L, Behie LA. Bioprocessing strategies for the large-scale production of human mesenchymal stem cells: a review. *Stem Cell Res Ther.* 2015 Nov 23; 6:225.

[128] Lechanteur C BS, Janssens ME, Giet O, Briquet A, Baudoux E, Beguin Y. Large-Scale Clinical Expansion of Mesenchymal Stem Cells in the GMP-Compliant, Closed Automated Quantum® Cell Expansion System: Comparison with Expansion in Traditional T-Flasks. *J Stem Cell Res Ther.* 2014; 4(6).

[129] Meng X, Leslie P, Zhang Y, Dong J. Stem cells in a three-dimensional scaffold environment. *Springerplus.* 2014; 3:80.

[130] Osiecki MJ, Michl TD, Kul Babur B, Kabiri M, Atkinson K, Lott WB, et al. Packed Bed Bioreactor for the Isolation and Expansion of Placental-Derived Mesenchymal Stromal *Cells. PLoS One.* 2015; 10(12): e0144941.

[131] Wang S, Qu X, Zhao RC. Clinical applications of mesenchymal stem cells. *J Hematol Oncol.* 2012 Apr 30; 5:19.

[132] Doorn J, Moll G, Le Blanc K, van Blitterswijk C, de Boer J. Therapeutic applications of mesenchymal stromal cells: paracrine effects and potential improvements. *Tissue Eng Part B Rev.* 2011 Apr; 18(2): 101-15.

[133] Meirelles Lda S, Fontes AM, Covas DT, Caplan AI. Mechanisms involved in the therapeutic properties of mesenchymal stem cells. *Cytokine Growth Factor Rev.* 2009 Oct-Dec; 20(5-6):419-27.

[134] Salgado AJ, Reis RL, Sousa NJ, Gimble JM. Adipose tissue derived stem cells secretome: soluble factors and their roles in regenerative medicine. *Curr Stem Cell Res Ther.* 2009 Jun; 5(2):103-10.

[135] Fajardo-Orduna GR, Mayani H, Montesinos JJ. Hematopoietic Support Capacity of Mesenchymal Stem Cells: Biology and Clinical Potential. *Arch Med Res.* 2015 Nov; 46(8):589-96.

[136] Tsuchiya A KY, Ikarashi SS, Watanabe Y, Kawata Y, Terai S. Clinical trials using mesenchymal stem cells in liver diseases and inflammatory bowel disease. *Inflammation and Regeneration.* 2017; 37(16).

[137] Amorin B, Alegretti AP, Valim V, Pezzi A, Laureano AM, da Silva MA, et al. Mesenchymal stem cell therapy and acute graft-versus-host disease: a review. *Hum Cell.* 2014 Oct; 27(4):137-50.

[138] Kurtzberg J, Prockop S, Teira P, Bittencourt H, Lewis V, Chan KW, et al. Allogeneic human mesenchymal stem cell therapy (remestemcel-L, Prochymal) as a rescue agent for severe refractory acute graft-versus-host disease in pediatric patients. *Biol Blood Marrow Transplant.* 2013 Feb; 20(2):229-35.

[139] P. J. Martin JPU, R. J. Soiffer, H. Klingemann, E. K. Waller, A. S. Daly, R. P. Herrmann, P. Kebriaei. Prochymal Improves Response Rates in Patients with Steroid-Refractory Acute Graft Versus Host Disease (SR-GVHD) Involving the Liver and Gut: Results of a Randomized, Placebo-Controlled, Multicenter Phase III Trial in GVHD. *Biology of Blood and Marrow Transplantation.* 2010; 16(2).

[140] Prasad VK, Lucas KG, Kleiner GI, Talano JA, Jacobsohn D, Broadwater G, et al. Efficacy and safety of *ex vivo* cultured adult human mesenchymal stem cells (Prochymal) in pediatric patients with severe refractory acute graft-versus-host disease in a compassionate use study. *Biol Blood Marrow Transplant.* 2010 Apr; 17(4):534-41.

[141] Kim N, Cho SG. Clinical applications of mesenchymal stem cells. *Korean J Intern Med.* 2013 Jul; 28(4):387-402.

[142] Le Blanc K, Rasmusson I, Sundberg B, Gotherstrom C, Hassan M, Uzunel M, et al. Treatment of severe acute graft-versus-host disease with third party haploidentical mesenchymal stem cells. *Lancet.* 2004 May 01; 363 (9419):1439-41.

[143] Sanina C, Hare JM. Mesenchymal Stem Cells as a Biological Drug for Heart Disease: Where Are We With Cardiac Cell-Based Therapy? *Circ Res.* 2015 Jul 17; 117(3):229-33.

[144] Karantalis V, Hare JM. Use of mesenchymal stem cells for therapy of cardiac disease. *Circ Res.* 2015 Apr 10; 116(8):1413-30.

[145] Aurich H, Sgodda M, Kaltwasser P, Vetter M, Weise A, Liehr T, et al. Hepatocyte differentiation of mesen-chymal stem cells from human adipose tissue *in vitro* promotes hepatic integration *in vivo*. *Gut.* 2009 Apr; 58(4):570-81.

[146] Liu WH, Song FQ, Ren LN, Guo WQ, Wang T, Feng YX, et al. The multiple functional roles of mesenchymal stem cells in participating in treating liver diseases. *J Cell Mol Med.* 2014 Mar; 19(3):511-20.

[147] Ortiz LA, Dutreil M, Fattman C, Pandey AC, Torres G, Go K, et al. Interleukin 1 receptor antagonist mediates the anti-inflammatory and antifibrotic effect of mesenchymal stem cells during lung injury. *Proc Natl Acad Sci USA.* 2007 Jun 26; 104(26):11002-7.

[148] Kim JK, Park YN, Kim JS, Park MS, Paik YH, Seok JY, et al. Autologous bone marrow infusion activates the progenitor cell compartment in patients with advanced liver cirrhosis. *Cell Transplant.* 2010; 19(10): 1237-46.

[149] Saito T, Okumoto K, Haga H, Nishise Y, Ishii R, Sato C, et al. Potential therapeutic application of intravenous autologous bone marrow infusion in patients with alcoholic liver cirrhosis. *Stem Cells Dev.* 2011 Sep; 20(9):1503-10.

[150] Terai S, Ishikawa T, Omori K, Aoyama K, Marumoto Y, Urata Y, et al. Improved liver function in patients with liver cirrhosis after autologous bone marrow cell infusion therapy. *Stem Cells.* 2006 Oct; 24(10):2292-8.

[151] Wang L, Li J, Liu H, Li Y, Fu J, Sun Y, et al. Pilot study of umbilical cord-derived mesenchymal stem cell transfusion in patients with primary biliary cirrhosis. *J Gastroenterol Hepatol*. 2013 Aug; 28 Suppl 1:85-92.

[152] Zhang Z, Lin H, Shi M, Xu R, Fu J, Lv J, et al. Human umbilical cord mesenchymal stem cells improve liver function and ascites in decompensated liver cirrhosis patients. *J Gastroenterol Hepatol.* 2012 Mar; 27 Suppl 2:112-20.

[153] Joyce N, Annett G, Wirthlin L, Olson S, Bauer G, Nolta JA. Mesenchymal stem cells for the treatment of neurodegenerative disease. *Regen Med*. 2010 Nov; 5(6): 933-46.

[154] Tanna T, Sachan V. Mesenchymal stem cells: potential in treatment of neurodegenerative diseases. *Curr Stem Cell Res Ther.* 2014; 9(6):513-21.

[155] Mazzini L, Ferrero I, Luparello V, Rustichelli D, Gunetti M, Mareschi K, et al. Mesenchymal stem cell transplantation in amyotrophic lateral sclerosis: A Phase I clinical trial. *Exp Neurol.* 2009 May; 223(1):229-37.

[156] Saccardi R, Kozak T, Bocelli-Tyndall C, Fassas A, Kazis A, Havrdova E, et al. Autologous stem cell transplantation for progressive multiple sclerosis: update of the European Group for Blood and Marrow Transplantation autoimmune diseases working party database. *Mult Scler.* 2006 Dec; 12(6):814-23.

[157] Caplan AI, Dennis JE. Mesenchymal stem cells as trophic mediators. *J Cell Biochem*. 2006 Aug 1; 98(5): 1076-84.

[158] Chen L, Tredget EE, Wu PY, Wu Y. Paracrine factors of mesenchymal stem cells recruit macrophages and endothelial lineage cells and enhance wound healing. *PLoS One*. 2008 Apr 2; 3(4):e1886.

[159] Si Y, Zhao Y, Hao H, Liu J, Guo Y, Mu Y, et al. Infusion of mesenchymal stem cells ameliorates hyperglycemia in type 2 diabetic rats: identification of a novel role in improving insulin sensitivity. *Diabetes.* 2012 Jun; 61(6):1616-25.

[160] Xie QP, Huang H, Xu B, Dong X, Gao SL, Zhang B, et al. Human bone marrow mesenchymal stem cells differentiate into insulin-producing cells upon micro-environmental manipulation *in vitro. Differentiation*. 2009 Jun; 77(5):483-91.

[161] Moriscot C, de Fraipont F, Richard MJ, Marchand M, Savatier P, Bosco D, et al. Human bone marrow mesenchymal stem cells can express insulin and key transcription factors of the endocrine pancreas developmental pathway upon genetic and/or microenvironmental manipulation *in vitro. Stem Cells.* 2005 Apr; 23(4):594-603.

[162] Zang L, Hao H, Liu J, Li Y, Han W, Mu Y. Mesenchymal stem cell therapy in type 2 diabetes mellitus. *Diabetol Metab Syndr*. 2017; 9:36.

[163] Compagna R, Amato B, Massa S, Amato M, Grande R, Butrico L, et al. Cell Therapy in Patients with Critical Limb Ischemia. *Stem Cells Int*. 2015; 2015:931420.

[164] Gremmels H, Fledderus JO, Teraa M, Verhaar MC. Mesenchymal stromal cells for the treatment of critical limb ischemia: context and perspective. *Stem Cell Res* Ther. 2013; 4(6):140.

[165] Gupta PK, Chullikana A, Parakh R, Desai S, Das A, Gottipamula S, et al. A double blind randomized placebo controlled phase I/II study assessing the safety and efficacy of allogeneic bone marrow derived mesenchymal stem cell in critical limb ischemia. *J Transl Med.* 2013 Jun 10; 11:143.

[166] Motukuru V, Suresh KR, Vivekanand V, Raj S, Girija KR. Therapeutic angiogenesis in Buerger's disease (*thromboangiitis obliterans*) patients with critical limb ischemia by autologous transplantation of bone marrow mononuclear cells. *J Vasc Surg*. 2008 Dec; 48(6 Suppl):53S-60S; discussion S.

[167] Nizankowski R, Petriczek T, Skotnicki A, Szczeklik A. The treatment of advanced chronic lower limb ischaemia with marrow stem cell autotransplantation. *Kardiol Pol.* 2005 Oct; 63(4):351-60; discussion 61.

[168] Tateishi-Yuyama E, Matsubara H, Murohara T, Ikeda U, Shintani S, Masaki H, et al. Therapeutic angiogenesis for patients with limb ischaemia by autologous transplantation of bone-marrow cells: a pilot study and a randomised controlled trial. *Lancet.* 2002 Aug 10; 360(9331):427-35.

[169] Wyles CC, Houdek MT, Behfar A, Sierra RJ. Mesenchymal stem cell therapy for osteoarthritis: current perspectives. *Stem Cells Cloning.* 2015; 8:117-24.

[170] Gupta PK, Chullikana A, Rengasamy M, Shetty N, Pandey V, Agarwal V, et al. Efficacy and safety of adult human bone marrow-derived, cultured, pooled, allogeneic mesenchymal stromal cells (Stempeucel(R)): preclinical and clinical trial in osteoarthritis of the knee joint. *Arthritis Res Ther*. 2016 Dec 20; 18(1):301.

[171] Cui GH, Wang YY, Li CJ, Shi CH, Wang WS. Efficacy of mesenchymal stem cells in treating patients with osteoarthritis of the knee: A meta-analysis. *Exp Ther Med.* 2016 Nov; 12(5):3390-400.

[172] Keating A. Mesenchymal stromal cells: new directions. *Cell Stem Cell.* 2012 Jun 14; 10(6):709-16.

[173] Maumus M, Jorgensen C, Noel D. Mesenchymal stem cells in regenerative medicine applied to rheumatic diseases: role of secretome and exosomes. *Biochimie.* 2013 Dec; 95(12):2229-34.

In: Manipulation of Stem Cells for Disease Benefits
Editor: Prasad Koka
ISBN: 978-1-53615-468-9

Chapter 3

COMPARISON OF CANCER CELL TROPISM OF VARIOUS MESENCHYMAL STEM CELL TYPES

Sushilkumar Ramdasi**, *Chandra Viswanathan*, *Rohit Kulkarni and Abhijit Bopardikar
Research & Development Team, ReeLabs Private Limited,
Andheri West, Mumbai, India

ABSTRACT

Tumor tropism of Mesenchymal Stem Cells confers them an added characteristic. Possibly, one can explore inherent anticancer potentials to deliver anti-cancer agents to the site of the tumor. It is a well-established fact that Mesenchymal Stem Cells (MSCs) are equipped with traits like multi-lineage differentiation potential, immune privilegedness and probably some affinity for tumors. The scientific community has been debating pro-cancer or anticancer nature of MSCs. It is believed that MSCs, by virtue of their reparative function, acts as a tumor-promoting entity by expressing several growth factors and helps formation of new vessels by a process called angiogenesis. However, MSCs are also reported to play an anti-cancer role by expressing molecules like TRAIL (Tumor Necrosis Factor-related Apoptosis Inducing Ligand) and DKK1 (Wnt pathway inhibitor) and many other tumor suppressor molecules. Extensive literature is available on tumor specific migration and anti-cancer nature of MSCs derived from either bone marrow or adipose tissue. The behavior of mix of MSCs derived from perinatal tissues viz. umbilical cord tissue, placenta and amniotic sac for these investigations is least explored. The advantages of utilizing perinatal tissue as a source of MSCs are obvious, which include the ease of procurement process, their abundant availability and the naive nature of cells as compared to other sources studied so far.

We present here a comparative study of migration capabilities of MSCs derived from umbilical cord tissue alone (UCMSC), a subtype of the UCMSC called MSC1, adipose tissue derived Mesenchymal stem cells (ATMSC) and a mixture of MSCs (Mixed MSCs)

* Corresponding Author's E-mail: sushbiotech@gmail.com.

derived from perinatal tissues namely the umbilical cord tissue, placenta and the amniotic sac.

Keywords: tropism, migration, stem cells, anti-cancer, cancer stem cells

INTRODUCTION

Mesenchymal stem cells are increasingly tested for anti-cancer potential owing to their properties like immune privileged nature [1], multilineage differentiation potential [2], ease of availability and maintenance in culture and most importantly, a tropism for the site of injury [2].

MSCs are immune privileged in nature since they do not express MHC class II molecules but express negligible amount of MHC class I. Further to that, there is no expression of co-stimulatory molecules like CD40 and CD80. Negligible MHC class I expression protects MSCs from NK cell surveillance [2]. However, in a tumor microenvironment, pro-inflammatory MSCs may be more beneficial to act on tumors through an immune system elicitation.

MSCs get attracted to the site of injury through cytokine cues released by injured cells of the tissue and recruit themselves to serve a reparative function [3]. The MSC tropism towards injury is also reported *in vivo* when MSC engineered with human gene infused systemically into irradiated mice and engineered gene was detected in tissues of the mice [4]. According to one convention, tumors are 'Wounds that do not heal' [5] which explains the analogy between tumors and injury. Maestroni et al. in 1999 unraveled evidence of MSC tropism to the site of tumor [6]. For the first time, MSC tropism to glioma was put forth by rat MSC implantation into syngeneic glioma rats [7].

Tumor microenvironment plays a crucial role in coordination with cancer cells in the establishment, growth and dissemination of the tumor. Among cells of the microenvironment, Mesenchymal stem cells (MSCs) and their ability to evolve into cancer associated fibroblasts (CAFs) have recently generated a major interest in the field. Numerous studies have described the potential pro- or anti-tumorigenic action of MSCs. In a tumor microenvironment, tumor cells continuously secret cytokines and chemokines [5] thereby attracting and recruiting respondent cell types including MSCs. This tumor tropic potential of MSC has been shown in a few cancer cell lines [8] like melanoma [9], breast & colon cancer [10], malignant glioma [11], ovarian cancer [12] and pancreatic cancer [13].

CYTOKINES AND FACTORS AFFECTING TROPISM

The underlying mechanism of tumor-tropic migration of MSCs needs extensive investigation, research and understanding, but it appears that it is primarily dependent on the 'tumor niche' [14]. Integration of MSCs into the tumor stroma is mediated by high concentration of inflammatory chemokines and growth factors secreted into the tumor microenvironment. Since a tumor mimics a "wound," its microenvironment becomes the site of chronic inflammation [5] and cytokines are the major factors for eliciting MSC migration to tumors since they are abundantly produced in tumor sites [15] (Refer Diagram no. 1). Many soluble factors are secreted in to the tumor microenvironment which subsequently attracts MSCs. These include but not limited to Stromal-Derived Growth Factor-1α (SDF-lα/CXCL12), Vascular Endothelial Growth Factor-A (VEGF-A), Epidermal Growth Factor (EGF), Inter-leukin-6 (IL-6), Interleukin-8 (IL-8), Granulocyte-Macrophage Colony-Stimulating Factor (GM-CSF), Angiopoietin 1, Monocyte Chemoattractant Protein-1 (CCL2), Platelet-Derived Growth Factor (PDGF), Granulocyte Colony-Stimulating Factor (GCSF), Fibroblast Growth Factor (FGF), Urokinase Dependent Plasminogen Activator, Transforming Growth Factor Beta-1 (TGF-β1) and Hepatocyte Growth Factor[2] (HGF).

Besides cytokines, several other factors are also probably involved in MSC tropism. It has been suggested that HGF (Hepatocyte Growth Factor) and Cyclophilin B are two factors responsible for MSC tropism [16]. An aggressive brain cancer glioma was found to secrete Neurotrophin-3 (NT-3) and Transforming growth factor-ss1 (TGF-ss1) which play major role in tropism of MSCs [17]. In the tumor microenvironment, inflammatory cells and MSCs are recruited by fibrinolytic factors such as uPAR secreted by MSCs. The release of this factor results in creation of a proteolytic environment which in turn activates another cascade of proteolytic enzymes like Matrix Metalloproteinases (MMPs), which enable the release of cytokines and chemokines [18]. It has also been observed that MMP-1 produced by MSCs plays a significant role in tropism through CXCL12/CXCR4 axis [19].

This tumor tropism property of MSC could be exploited to deliver anti-tumor genes into the tumor microenvironment. In fact, one study reported their observations on the behavior of two sub-types of MSCs referred as MSC1 and MSC2 [20]. In this study, researchers claim that MSC1 are pro-inflammatory while MSC2 are immunosuppressive in nature. The same group in another study demonstrated that MSC1 are anti-tumorigenic and MSC2 are pro-tumorigenic in nature [21].

Mesenchymal Stem Cell therapy plays a crucial role in regenerating or repairing tissue or organ damage restoring defective functions [22]. The most common regenerative indications which could potentially be treated with MSC therapy include ischemic diseases, cardiovascular disorders, liver diseases, diabetic ulcers, and orthopedics [23]. Despite the fact that perinatal tissue is a good source of MSCs, free of any ethical concerns, the available literature is mainly concentrated on research conducted on MSCs derived from bone marrow and a few from adipose tissue.

Thus, the present study was focused on evaluation of *in vitro* migration capabilities of MSCs derived from umbilical cord tissue (UCMSC mainly through its subtype MSC1) and a mix of MSCs from perinatal tissue and adipose tissue (ATMSC) towards two cancer cell lines, A549 (Lung carcinoma) and PC-3 (Prostate carcinoma).

Material and Methods

Isolation of MSCs

MSCs from Umbilical Cord Tissue

MSCs were isolated from human umbilical cord tissues and as reported previously [24] [25] after an appropriate informed consenting procedure. The protocol and informed consent was approved by Independent Ethics Committee. Briefly, for umbilical cord tissue MSC isolation, clean and non-contaminated cord tissue of seven to eight centimeters length was washed with Phosphate-buffered saline (Invitrogen, USA) supplemented with antibiotics. Cord was cut open longitudinally and blood vessels removed. Blood clots, if any, were removed and the cord tissue was minced into small explants and placed onto tissue culture grade petri dishes containing expansion media [DMEM/F12 (Invitrogen, USA) with 10% Fetal Bovine Serum (Hyclone, USA), and 2 ng/ml bFGF (Sigma, USA)]. Cells were then allowed to grow from explants incubated at 37°C with 5% CO_2. The media was changed every alternate day; cells were passaged upon 80 - 90% confluence. Cells were characterized appropriately.

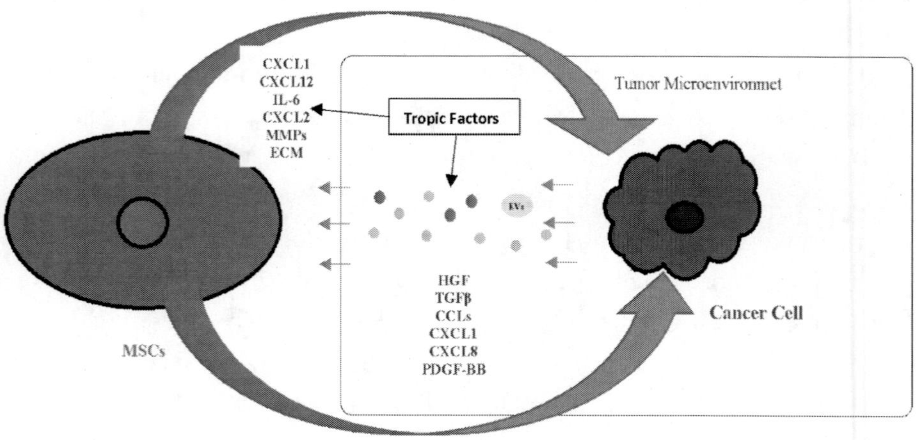

Diagram 1. Cytokines and Factors Responsible for MSC Tropism towards Tumor.

MSCs from Placenta

MSCs from placenta were isolated following an in-house developed enzymatic digestion protocol [24]. Briefly, MSCs from the placental tissue were derived by enzymatic digestion using 0.4% collagenase type IV (Gibco, USA) and 0.01% DNase (Roche, Germany). This mixture was incubated at 37°C for about an hour to achieve complete digestion. The suspension so obtained was washed twice with PBS (Cellclone, Genetix, India) and seeded into a tissue culture treated flask in expansion media containing DMEM/F12 (Gibco, USA) with 10% serum (Gibco, USA) and 2 ng/ml bFGF (Invitrogen, USA). The cells were allowed to grow and further expanded in a monolayer culture at 37°C and 5% CO_2. The media was changed every second day and cells were sub-cultured upon confluence and characterized at every passage.

MSCs from Amniotic Sac

MSCs from amniotic sac were isolated following in-house developed enzymatic digestion protocol [24]. Briefly, the amniotic tissue was extracted from the fetal side to avoid maternal cell contamination. The tissue was mechanically fragmented and the resultant tissue pieces were washed with PBS (Cellclone, Genetix, India) multiple times. The tissue pieces were then subjected to enzymatic digestion in two stages. The first stage was to remove epithelial amniotic cells by incubation with recombinant Trypsin (Trypsol-AOF®, Biogenomics, India) at 37°C for 5 minutes. The second stage was to make a single cell suspension for which collagenase type IV (Gibco, USA) was used at 37°C for 5 minutes. The enzyme was then inactivated by serum. The suspension so obtained was then filtered and washed with PBS (Cellclone, Genetix, India). The cell suspension was seeded into tissue culture treated flask in expansion media containing DMEM/F12 (Gibco, USA) with 10% serum (Gibco, USA) and 2 ng/ml bFGF (Invitrogen, USA). The cells were allowed to grow and further expand into a monolayer culture at 37°C and 5% CO_2. The media was changed every second day and cells were sub-cultured upon confluence and characterized at every passage.

Mixing and Co-Culturing MSCs from Three Perinatal Tissues

The MSCs at passage zero (after primary culture) from all the three sources viz. cord tissue, placental tissue and amniotic sac were co-cultured into a tissue culture-treated flask at a ratio of 1:1:1 in a similar expansion media [24]. The media was changed every second day and cells were sub-cultured upon confluence and characterized at every passage.

MSCs from Adipose Tissue

For MSC isolation from adipose tissue, plastic adherence technique was utilized [25]. Briefly, collagenase type VIII digestion was performed on lipoaspirate obtained from donors after an informed consenting process. The cells were then expanded in expansion media [DMEM/F12 (Invitrogen, USA) with 10% Fetal Bovine Serum (Hyclone, USA), and 2 ng/ml bFGF (Sigma, USA)]. Cells were then allowed to grow by incubating at 37°C with 5% CO_2. The media was changed every alternate day; cells were passaged upon 80 - 90% confluence. Cells were characterized appropriately.

Isolation of MSC1

For studies using MSC1 subtype, [20] [21] we isolated MSC1 for investigating migration capabilities of these sub-types towards tumors. Here, we induced UCMSC with LPS (Lipopolysaccharide) at a concentration of 50 ng/ml for 48 hours and the resultant MSC1 was used to assess migration capabilities. The LPS is utilized to prime TLR-4 (Toll-Like Receptor) in MSCs which in turn conferred pro-inflammatory properties and anti-tumor properties [20] to MSCs.

Characterization of MSCs Using Flow Cytometry

Flow cytometry analysis was performed for MSC cell surface markers. Briefly, MSCs were harvested upon 80 - 90% confluence and approximately 1 million cells were stained with fluorochrome tagged anti-bodies as follows; CD45 PerCp (BD Biosciences, USA), CD90 FITC (BD Pharmingen, USA), CD73 PE (BD Pharmingen, USA), CD105 PE (Caltag laboratories, USA), IDO (Millipore Corporation, Billerica, MA), 7-AAD (BD Biosciences, USA). Isotype controls were used for FITC, PerCp and PE anti-bodies. Rb X Sh IgG FLUOR (Merk) antibody used as secondary antibody to IDO (Indoleamine 2, 3-dioxygenase). Approximately 10,000 events were acquired on FACSCanto II (Beckton Dickinson, USA) and analyzed using BD FACS Diva software provided by Beckton Dickinson, USA. UCMSC, placenta MSCs and amniotic sac MSCs were mixed into Mixed MSC hence separate flow cytometry was not done for the same.

Cancer Cells

Lung carcinoma cell line A549 (ATCC® CCL185TM) and Prostate carcinoma cell line PC-3 (ATCC® CRL1435TM) were chosen as representative for the study. They were obtained from ATCC. Both cancer cell lines were cultured when-ever required using expansion media containing DMEM/F12 (Invitrogen, USA) with 10% Fetal Bovine Serum (Hyclone, USA) supplemented with antibiotics.

Cancer Cell –'Condition Media' Preparation

Both cancer cell lines (A549 and PC-3) were cultured in cancer cell expansion media containing DMEM/F12 (Invitrogen, USA) with 10% Fetal Bovine Serum (Hyclone, USA) supplemented with antibiotics. Cells were grown up to 80 - 90% confluence. The cell supernatant was collected, centrifuged and preserved for Transwell migration assay.

Transwell Migration Assay

Transwell migration assay was performed using 24-well Transwell® chamber (Corning®) with inserts having polycarbonate filters of 8.0 μm porosity. The inserts and their respective bottom wells were pre-incubated with 100μl and 600μl MSC expansion media respectively as per manufacturer's instructions and were incubated at 37°C for not less than one hour for initial equilibrium. MSCs (ATMMSC, UCMSC, Mixed MSC and MSC1) and cancer cell lines (A549 and PC-3) were cultured in their respective expansion media and grown up to 80 - 90% confluence before use in assay. Cells were harvested by enzymatic digestion using TrypLE™ Select (Invitrogen, USA). $1x10^5$ (100000) cancer cells (A549 and PC-3 separately) in 600μl expansion media was added to lower wells and incubated for more than one hour at 37°C with 5% CO_2 without placing inserts; this was for cancer cells to settle to the bottom of the wells. Refer Diagram 2 for schematic representation of the Transwell chamber with insert. In another set of experiments, into the lower well, 600μl cancer cell condition media with MSC expansion media was added at a ratio of 1:1. The Transwell inserts were then placed in all wells and $1x10^5$ (100000) MSCs (ATMSC, UCMSC, Mixed MSC and MSC1 in different sets) added to inserts in 100μl of expansion media. Transwell plates were then incubated at 37°C with 5% CO_2 for 24 hours. Every experiment was carried out in duplicate.

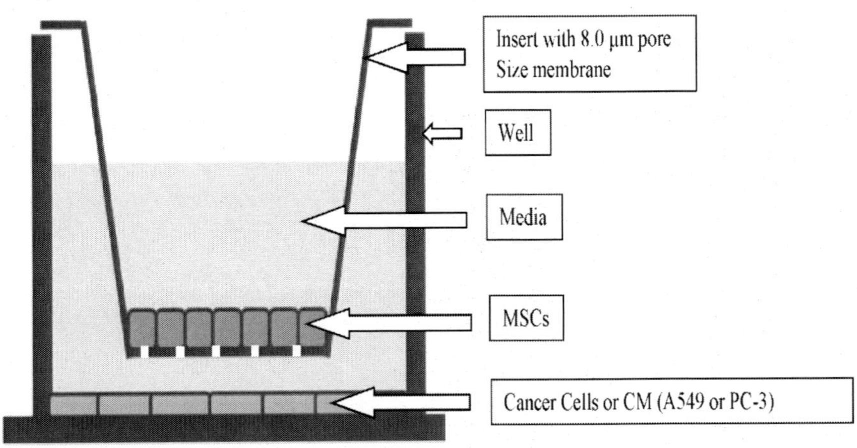

Diagram 2. Schematic Representation of a Transwell Chamber with Insert for Migration Assay.

Evaluation of Migration Activity

Migrated cells were stained, counted and evaluated following the protocol given by the manufacturer with some slight modifications [26, 27]. Briefly, media from the insert and the lower well was aspirated and the insert transferred to a fresh well. The inside of the insert membrane was wiped gently with the help of cotton swab to remove non-migrated cells. After gently washing the insert membrane with Phosphate-buffered saline, the cells on the insert membrane were fixed with 10% Paraformaldehyde (Polysciences, Ink.) for 10 minutes. Post-fixation, the insert membrane was washed with water.

The insert membrane was then stained with Hematoxylin (H&E, Sigma-Aldrich) for 30 minutes. The insert was then washed with water until the water ran clear and inserts were allowed to dry completely. The cells were counted using a light microscope (Olympus CKX41 Inverted), and calculations were performed as per the manufacturer's instructions for evaluating the number of cells migrated [27].

Statistical Analysis

The data was analyzed using student's unpaired 2 tailed t-test using online calculator provided by www.graphpad.com to determine statistical significance. Values are given as mean ± SD (standard deviation).

RESULTS

Morphological Characteristics of MSCs

MSCs were characterized by their property of plastic adherence, morphology and expression of cell surface markers. Morphologically UCMSC, Mixed MSC and MSC1 were spindle shaped, 'fibroblast like cells' growing in monolayers and reaching 80 - 90% confluence in about 6 to 8 days upon initial passage (Refer Figure 1. (a), (b) and (c)). ATMSCs were also 'fibroblast like' elongated cells growing in monolayers and reaching 80 - 90% confluence, in 12 to 16 days upon initial passage (Refer Figure 1. (d)).

Characterization of MSCs Using Flow Cytometry

The flow cytometric analysis revealed that the Mixted MSC, MSC1 and ATMSCs did not express CD45; on the contrary CD90, CD73 and CD105 were expressed by all these MSCs (Figure 2. (a), (b) and (c). IDO initially expressed by Mixed MSCs and ATMSCs at a minimal level was further suppressed by MSC1 as reported earlier [25] (Figure 2. (d)). Suppression of IDO expression is indicative of a pro-inflammatory nature of MSC1.

Morphological Characteristics of Cancer Cells (A549 and PC-3)

Lung carcinoma cell line A549 (ATCC® CCL185TM) grew as adherent cells and revealed epithelial like morphology (Figure 3. (a)). Prostate carcinoma cell line PC-3 (ATCC® CRL1435TM) grew as adherent, epithelial like grade IV adeno-carcinoma cells (Figure 3. (b)).

In Vitro Transwell Migration Assay

Transwell migration assay was performed using a 24-well Transwell® chamber (Corning®) with inserts having polycarbonate filters of 8.0 μm porosity. The migration activity of MSCs was evaluated as is described in the 'Materials and Methods' section of this article. Please refer to Figure 4 (a) for pictures of the stained inserts.

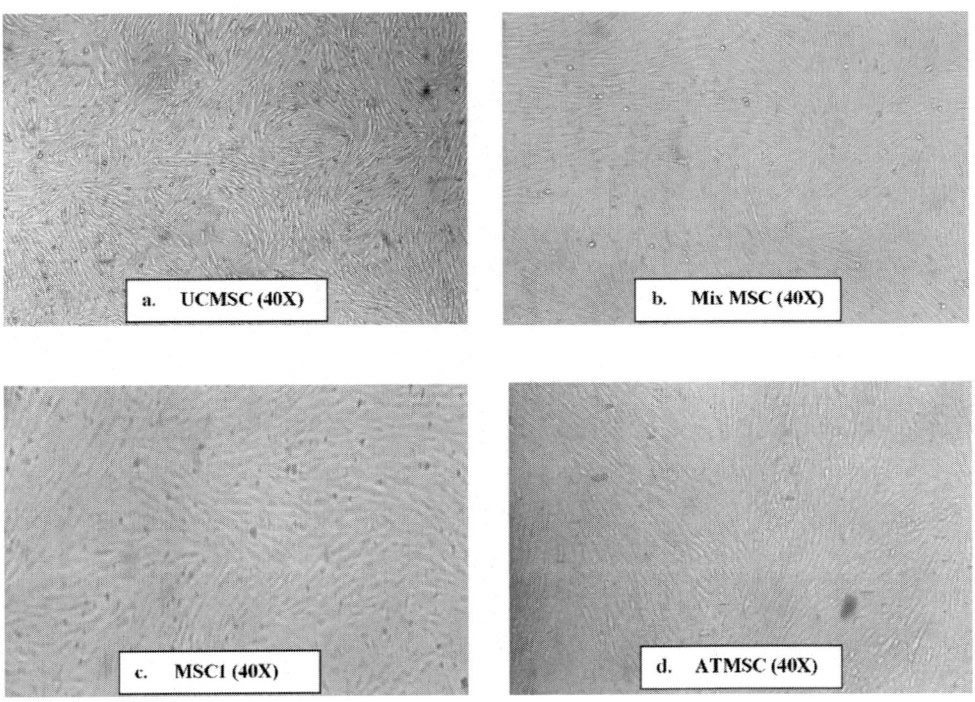

Figure 1. Morphology of MSCs (a) UCMSC (b) Mixed MSC (c) MSC1 (d) ATMSC. MSCs formed monolayers and reflected fibroblast like elongated morphology.

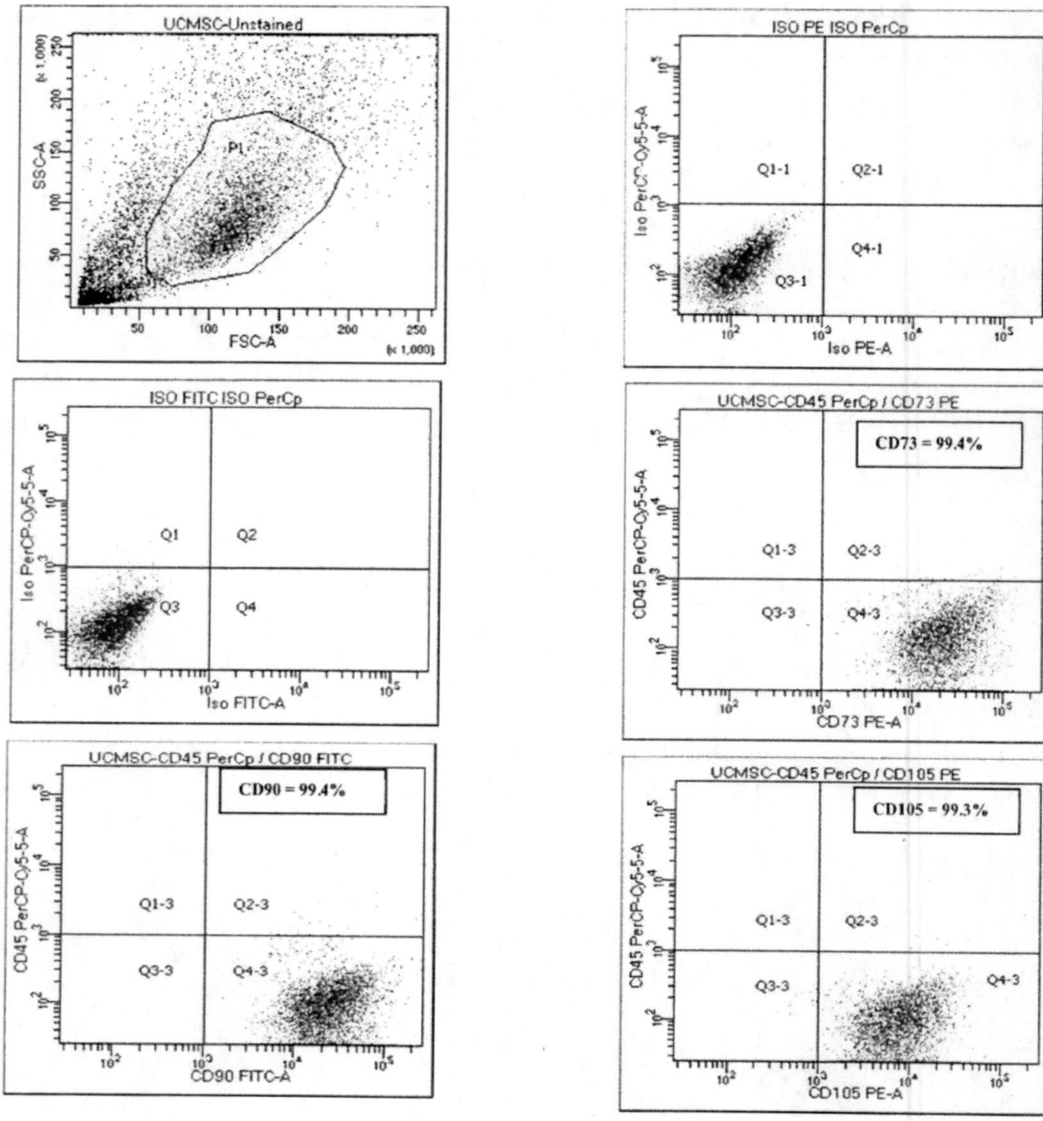

Figure 2a. Immunophenotyping of MSCs by Flow Cytometry. Mixed MSCs: Note the Co-cultivated Mixture of MSCs (Mixed MSCs) were strongly negative for hematopoietic marker CD45 and strongly positive for Mesenchymal markers CD90, CD73 and CD 105.

In this set of assay, Mixed MSCs showed the highest percentage of migration (55.1%) towards A549, and the UCMSC migration was 44.3% ($p = 0.001$). The MSC1 percentage migration was 35.77% ($p < 0.0002$). The percentage migration of Mixed MSC towards CM derived from A549 was 40% ($p = 0.0452$). The percent migration of UCMSC towards conditioned media derived from A549 was 34.0% ($p < 0.0006$). Note that the ATMSC migration towards A549 CM was only 22.37% ($p < 0.0001$) (Figure 4. (b)).

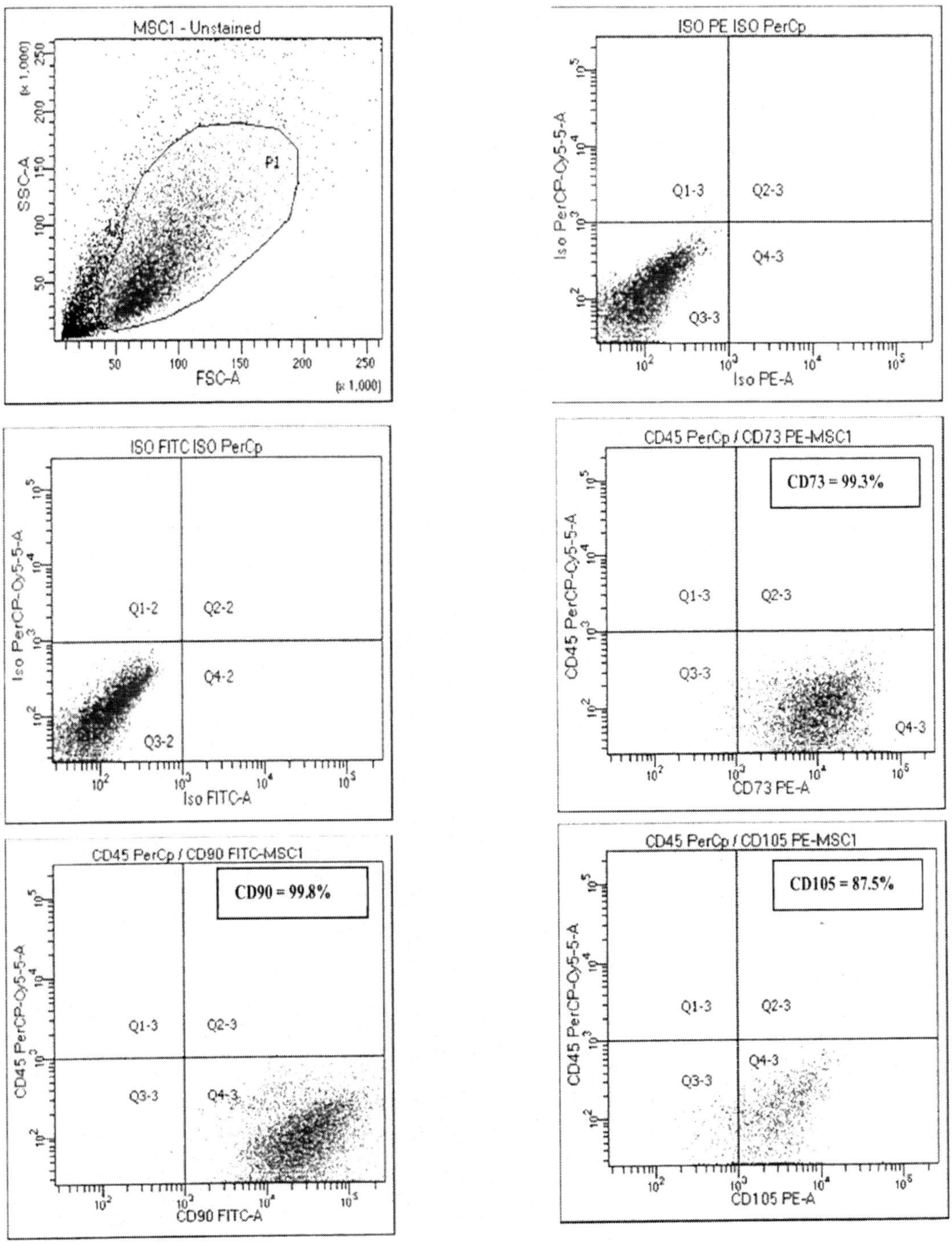

Figure 2b. Immunophenotyping of MSCs by Flow Cytometry. MSC1: MSC1 were strongly negative for hematopoietic marker CD45 and were strongly positive for Mesenchymal markers CD90, CD73 and CD 105.

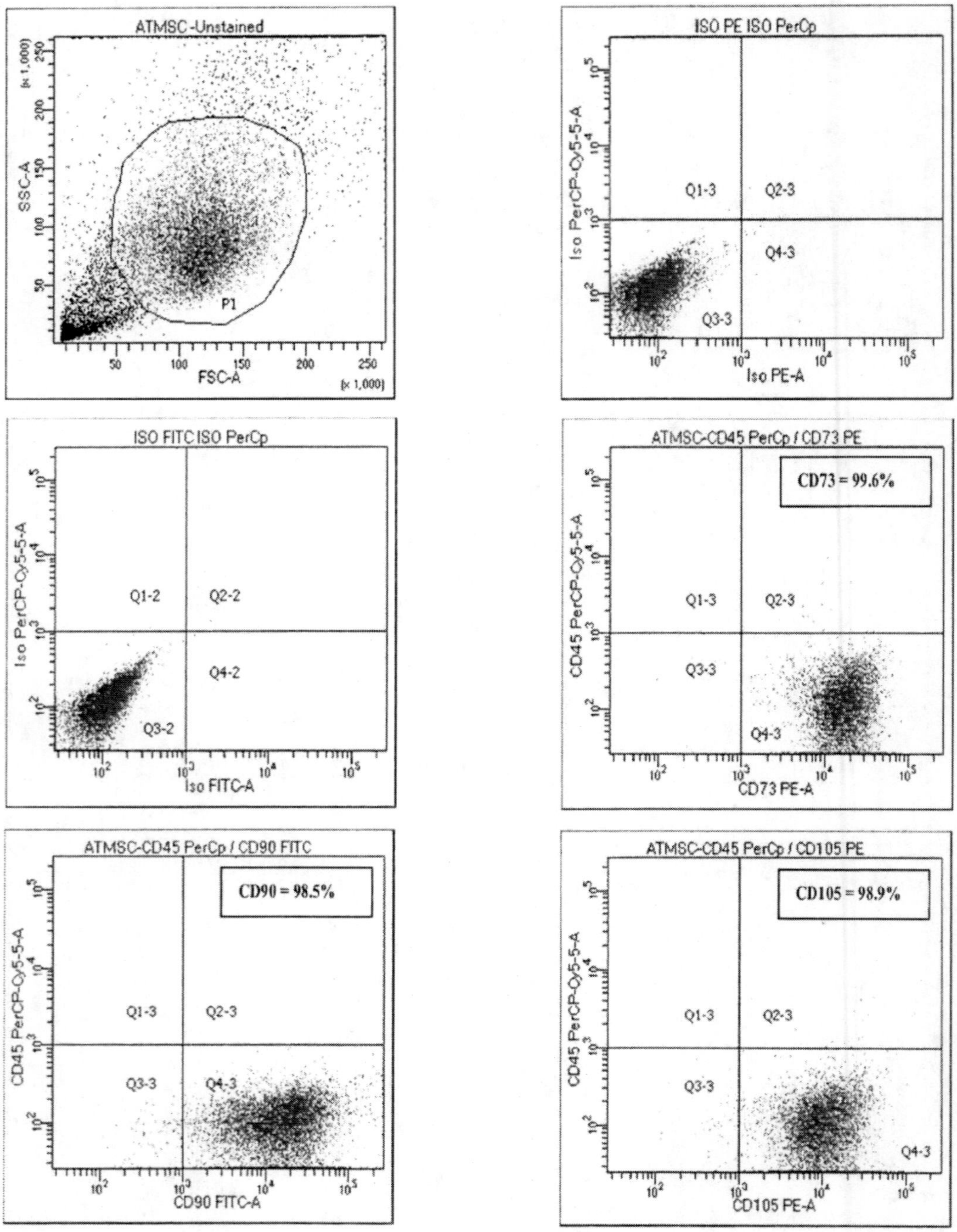

Figure 2c. Immunophenotyping of MSCs by Flow Cytometry. ATMSC: ATMSC were strongly negative for hematopoietic marker CD45 and were strongly positive for Mesenchymal markers CD90, CD73 and CD 105.

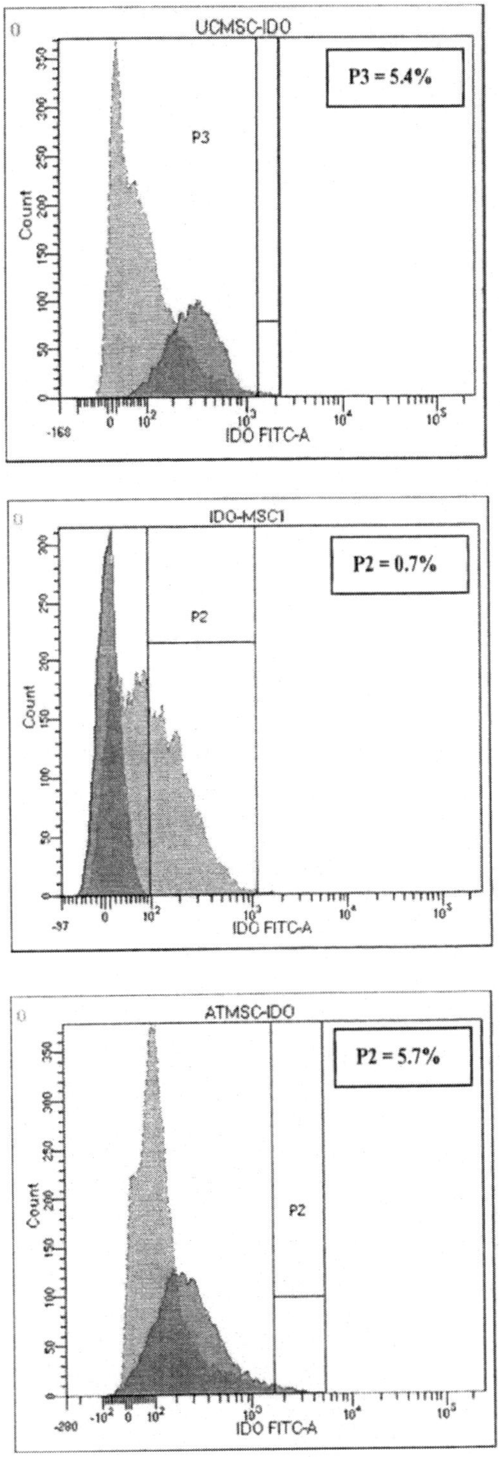

Figure 2d. Immunophenotyping of MSCs by Flow Cytometry. IDO Expression of MSCs: IDO expression by Flow Cytometry by Mixed MSCs, ATMSCs and MSC1-shows 5.4%, 5.7% and 0.7% respectively.

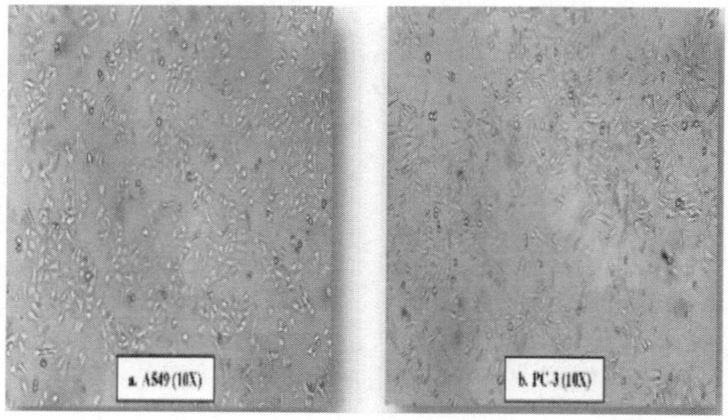

Figure 3. Morphology of cancer cells (a) Lung carcinoma cells A549 were adherent reflecting epithelial like morph-ology (b) Prostate carcinoma PC-3 cells were adherent revealing epithelial like morphology.

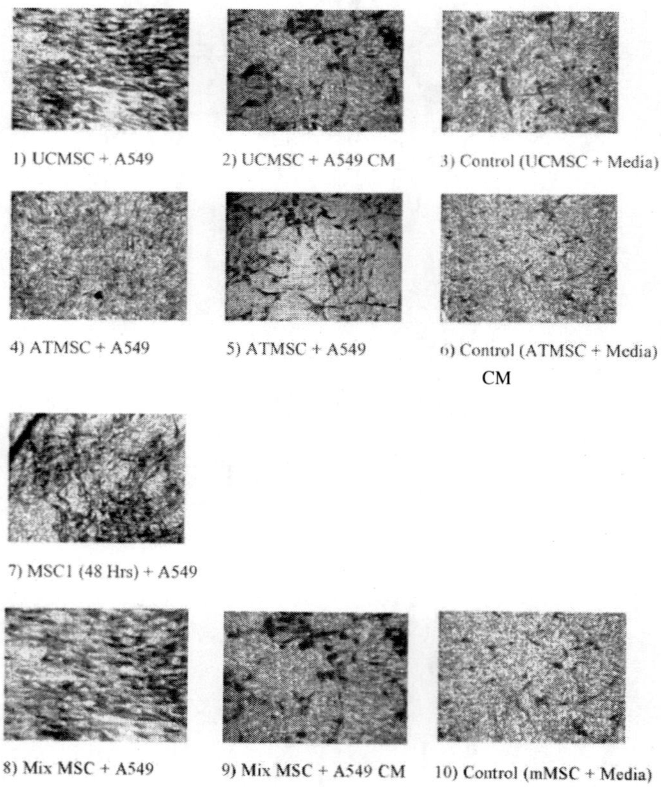

Figure 4 (a). Transwell Migration of MSCs to A549. The number of migrated MSCs were counted under 20X objective. (1) Stained UCMSCs on inserts, the lower well contained A549 cells (2) Stained UCMSCs on inserts, the lower well contained CM derived from A549 cells (3) Stained UCMSCs on inserts, the lower well contained media only (Control) (4) Stained ATMSCs on inserts, the lower well contained A549 cells (5) Stained ATMSCs on inserts, the lower well contained CM derived from A549 cells (6) Stained ATMSCs on inserts, the lower well contained media only (Control) (7) Stained MSC1 cells on inserts, the lower well contained A549 cells. (8) Mixed MSCs on inserts after staining, the lower well contained A549 cells (9) Stained Mixed MSCs on inserts, the lower well contained CM derived from A549 cells (10) Stained Mixed MSCs on inserts, the lower well contained media only (Control). For assay set up refer Diagram 2.

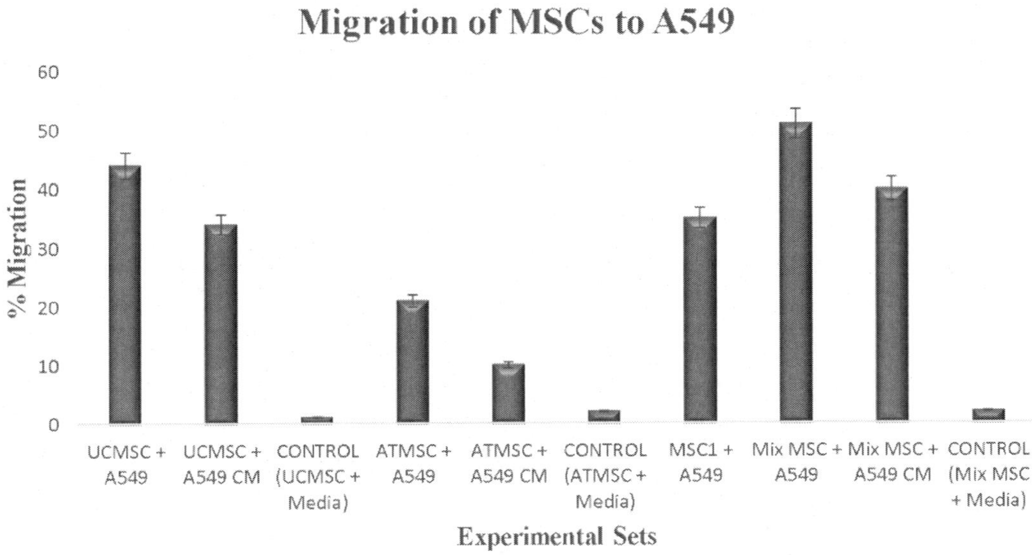

Figure 4 (b). Transwell Migration of MSCs to A549 (b) Percent migration of MSCs towards A549 cells.

In another set of experiments, refer to Figure 5. (a) for pictures of stained inserts. In this set of assay, Mixed MSC & UCMSC shown highest migration percentage (75% and 71% respectively with $p = 0.0161$) towards PC-3, Mixed MSC migration was 51% towards conditioned media derived from PC-3 ($p < 0.0001$). UCMSC migration towards conditioned media derived from PC-3 was 41.51% ($p < 0.001$). MSC1 migrated towards PC-3 with 10.63% only ($p < 0.0001$). In this assay ATMSC migrated towards PC-3 cells and its conditioned media at a 5% and 2% respectively with $p = 0.0705$ (Refer Figure 5. (b)). Refer Diagram 2 for schematic representation of the Transwell chamber with insert.

DISCUSSION

Cancer, is one of the leading causes of mortality worldwide. The hallmark of cancer cells is unregulated and uncontrolled cell multiplication. The stem cells and cancer cells, both possess properties of self-renewal and plasticity, however, the former has strict and regulated control over multiplication and the later loses it [28].

Cancer stem cell can be defined as those cancer cells having capability to regrow tumor from which it is isolated and identified [2]. It needs to be noted that the term 'cancer stem cells' (CSCs) do not mean the stem cell transformed in to cancer [29]. These CSCs are simply cancer cells having the potential to migrate to the distant site in the body, gets adjusted into local milieu and get transformed into local tissue type to form another tumor.

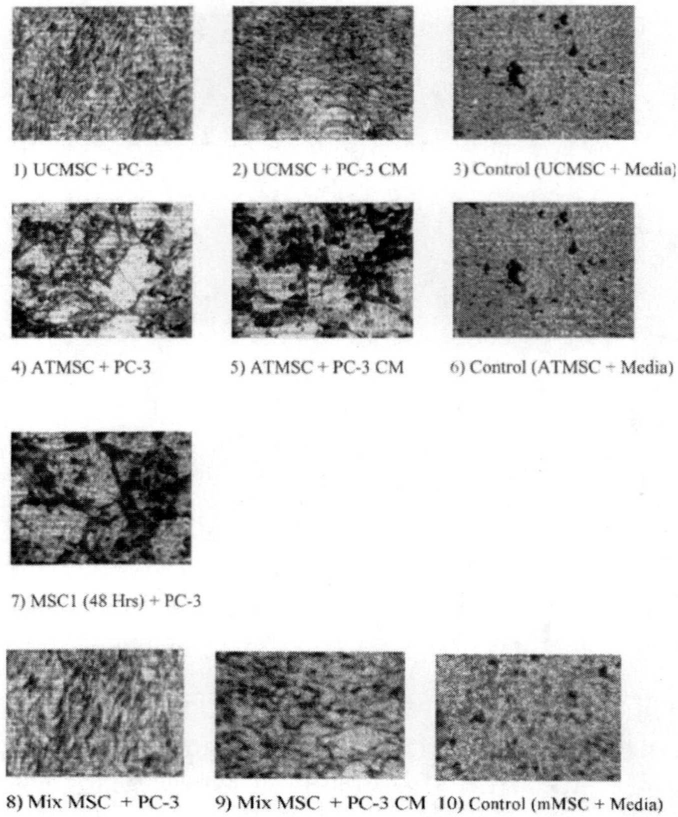

Figure 5 (a). Transwell Migration of MSCs to PC-3. The number of MSCs migrated were counted under 20X objective. (1) Stained UCMSCs on inserts, the lower well contained PC-3 cells (2) Stained UCMSCs on inserts, the lower well contained CM derived from PC-3 cells (3) Stained UCMSCs on inserts, the lower well contained media only (Control) (4) Stained ATMSCs on inserts, the lower well contained PC-3 cells (5) Stained ATMSCs on inserts, the lower well contained CM derived from PC-3 cells (6) Stained ATMSCs on inserts, the lower well contained media only (Control) (7) Stained MSC1 cells on inserts, the lower well contained PC-3 cells. (8) Stained Mixed MSCs on inserts, the lower well contained PC-3 cells (9) Stained Mixed MSCs on inserts, the lower well contained CM derived from PC-3 cells (10) Stained Mixed MSCs on inserts, the lower well contained media only (Control). Refer Diagram 2 for schematic representation of the Transwell chamber with insert.

The current treatment targets only cancer cells and not cancer stem cells and probably results in relapse and metastasis. Though the accurate mechanism of metastasis is poorly understood, it is hypothesized that the cancer stem cells play a crucial role due to their adaptability. This means that the cancer stem cells along with cancer cells need to be targeted while designing cancer therapy approach. Another strategy reported by many scientists is to genetically engineer MSCs to express anti-cancer factors at the site of tumors. Though, it seems like an effective method to deliver anti-cancer agents to the tumor, the stability of such genetically engineered MSC is under exhaustive investigation. The tropism towards cancer stem cells thus seems to be the most challenging problem to researchers and clinicians alike.

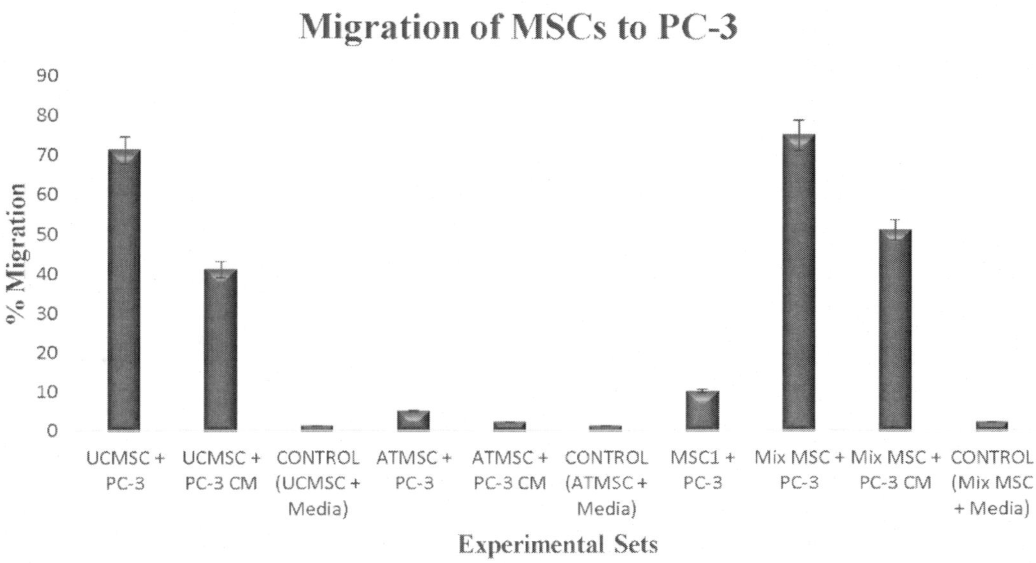

Figure 5(b). Transwell Migration of MSCs to PC-3 (b) Percent migration of MSCs towards PC-3 cells.

The MSC tropism towards tumor depends on various factors like the cancer cell type under investigation, source of MSCs and factors secreted by cancer cells to mediate migration. MSC tropism has been tested *in vivo* in various animal models (Refer Table 1). In most of the migration studies, bone marrow and rarely adipose tissue is utilized as a source of MSCs. The extraction procedures are invasive and MSCs so isolated are partially committed to a certain lineage.

It has been shown by Studeny et al. in melanoma athymic nude mice model that recombinant MSCs expressing IFN-beta gets attracted towards the tumor and exerts an anti-tumor effect only upon getting recruited into the tumor stroma [9]. This probably means that the MSCs could be an ideal vehicle for anti-cancer drug delivery at the tumor site. In the study by Kidd et al. the MSC migration *in vivo* was monitored non-invasively by utilizing *in vivo* bio-luminescent imaging technique with firefly-luciferase expression. The luciferase-expressing MSCs were injected into mice with and without tumor. Interestingly, when injected into mice without any tumor, MSCs accumulated in the lungs and further migrated to the spleen and the liver. However, in the mice with a breast carcinoma, systemic injection of MSCs resulted in migration of these cells to the site of tumor. The same phenomenon was observed in mice with ovarian cancer. This is suggestive of the fact that MSCs possess some potential of migration towards inflammatory signals and towards tumors in animal models [12]. Yet again, in the study by Kidd et al. firefly-luciferase-expressing MSCs were injected into orthotopic pancreatic tumor mice model intraperitoneally and observed that the MSCs migrated to the primary site of tumor and to the metastatic site as well. The MSCs were engineered to express IFN-beta and showed a reduction in tumor size when injected locally. However, when IFN-beta alone was delivered locally, there was no reduction in tumor mass [1]. This is again highlighting the potential of MSCs as a drug delivery vehicle and proves the importance of cell-to-cell contact that is much necessary to exert an anti-tumor effect. The migratory potential of MSCs towards tumors is consistent in highly progressive and invasive cancers – like glioblastoma. In the study conducted by Sasportas et al. in a mouse model of glioblastoma, MSCs were engineered to express TRAIL (Tumor necrosis factor-related Apoptosis Inducing Ligand). These cells not only migrated to the site of the tumor, they also caused regression of tumor mass [11]. The underlying mechanism of migration of MSCs to glioblastoma remained un-elucidated though. Most animal studies showed that MSCs respond to the signaling cues released by tumor stroma and get attracted to the tumor. However, in the absence of tumor or inflammatory-mediated signaling cues, MSCs tend to get accumulated in the lungs.

These encouraging observations lead to the next question as to ‘do MSCs exert anti-tumor effect on their own?’ ‘What prompts them to migrate to the tumor?’ ‘What are the most important factors that govern this?’ These will form the subject matter for the next level of research.

In the present study, we found that the mixed MSCs migrated to the highest maximum towards lung carcinoma (A549) and prostate carcinoma (PC-3) cell lines. This is indicative of a higher degree of affinity of mixed MSCs towards cancer cell lines in comparison to UCMSC alone and its subtype MSC1 and ATMSCs individually. A higher degree of tropic activity by these cells may perhaps be due to the naive nature of this cell type compared to other MSC sources. The variability of degree of migration between various MSCs derived from different sources and towards different cancer cell lines is evident in this study. To check if the mechanism of migration is due to a paracrine effect, our experiments threw up some observations. We found that a pure paracrine mode of tropism is not as effective as a ‘cell-to-cell’ contact. Though migration capability of MSCs is not directly related to any anti-cancer activity, it throws up valuable findings to pin down the right set of cytokines that make this effective. The combination of this with knowledge on the biological influences of the tumor makes this problem even more interesting.

Thus, we need to go a long way to understand the detailed mechanisms and the mechanistic pathways in play that get MSCs attracted towards the tumor, and how sustained that is. A combination of cytokine factors in a certain proportion may work for one tumor and may not for the other; this is dependent on the tumor types and its grade. Our preliminary investigation shows that ‘Mixed’ MSCs migrate better than MSC1 subtype and ATMSCs individually. We, like researchers around the world are intrigued by the probable mechanisms by which MSCs generate CAFs to modulate the growth, response to treatments, angiogenesis, invasion and metastasis of tumors. The evaluation and quantification of various cytokines released by various cells was not a part of this study.

Table 1. *In vivo* Tested Cancer Models for Tumor Tropism of MSCs

Cancer type	MSC cell type	Cancer cell line	Animal model	Mode of MSC infusion	Migrated to the site of tumor	Ref no.
Melanoma	BM-MSC	A375SM	Male athymic nude mice	Subcutaneous into the flank or intra venous into the lateral	Yes	[9]
Lung tumor produced by Breast cancer cell line	MSC	MDAMB231	Non-obese diabetic/severe combined immunodeficient mice with subcutaneous and metastatic tumors	Subcutaneous into the left flank or intra venous into the lateral tail vein	Yes	[10]
Ovarian Cancer	BM-MSC	HEY cells	Balb/C and severe combined (SCID)/CB-17 mice	Immune disorder Intraperitoneal	Yes	[10]
Breast Cancer	BM-MSC	MDAMB231	Balb/C and severe combined immune disorder (SCID)/CB-17	intravenous via tail vein	Yes	[10]
Pancreatic Cancer	MSC	PANC-1	Orthotopic SCID mice	Intraperitoneal	Yes	[11]
Colon Cancer	Rat BM-MSC	colorectal cancer lines HCT-8 and C85	SC nude mice	Subcutaneous in flanks of nude mice	Yes	[12]
Kaposi's sarcoma	BM-MSC	KSIMM	Male athymic nude mice	Intra venous tail vein injection	Yes	[23]
Malignant glioma	BM-MSC	GBM8	Mice	Implanted stereotactically (from bregma, AP: -2 mm, ML: 1.5 m V)	Yes	[13]

ACKNOWLEDGMENTS

We thank the management of ReeLabs Pvt. Ltd. for the support in conducting this laboratory work.

ETHICAL COMPLIANCE

The authors have stated all possible conflicts of interest within this work. The authors have stated all sources of funding for this work. If this work involved human participants, informed consent was received from each individual. If this work involved human participants, it was conducted in accordance with the 1964 Declaration of Helsinki. If this work involved experiments with humans or animals, it was conducted in accordance with the related institutions' research ethics guidelines.

REFERENCES

[1] Dominici M; Le Blanc, K; Mueller, I; et al. Minimal criteria for defining multipotent mesenchymal stromal cells. The International Society for Cellular Therapy position statement. *Cytotherapy*, 2006, 8(4), 315-7.

[2] Ramdasi, S; Sarang, S; Viswanathan, C. Potential of Mesenchymal Stem Cell based application in Cancer. *Int J Hematol-Oncol and Stem Cell Res*, 2015, 9(2), 95-103.

[3] Maxson, S; Lopez, EA; Yoo, D; Danilkovitch-Miagkova, A; LeRoux, MA. Concise Review: Role of Mesenchymal Stem Cells in Wound Repair. *Stem Cells Translational Medicine*, 2012, 1(2), 142-149.

[4] Meyerrose, T; Olson, S; Pontow, S; et al. Mesenchymal stem cells for the sustained *in vivo* delivery of bioactive factors. *Advanced Drug Delivery Reviews*, 2010, 62(12), 10.1016/j.addr.2010.09.013.

[5] Dvorak, HF. Tumors: wounds that do not heal. Similarities between tumor stroma generation and wound healing. *N Engl J Med*, 1986, Dec 25, 315(26), 1650-9.

[6] Maestroni, GJ; Hertens, E; Galli, P. Factors from nonmacrophage bone marrow stromal cells inhibit Lewis lung carcinoma and B16 melanoma growth in mice. *Cell Mol Life Sci*, 1999, 55, 663–667.

[7] Nakamura, K; Ito, Y; Kawano, Y; et al. Antitumor effect of genetically engineered mesenchymal stem cells in a rat glioma model. *Gene Ther*, 2004, 11, 1155–1164.

[8] Sun, XY; Nong, J; Qin, K; et al. Mesenchymal stem cell-mediated cancer therapy: A dual-targeted strategy of personalized medicine. *World J Stem Cells*, 2011, 3(11), 96–103.

[9] Studeny, M; Marini, FC; Champlin, RE; et al. Bone marrow-derived mesenchymal stem cells as vehicles for interferon-beta delivery into tumors. *Cancer Res*, 2002, 62, 3603–3608.

[10] Menon, LG; Picinich, S; Koneru, RM; et al. Differential gene expression associated with migration of mesenchymal stem cells to conditioned medium from tumor cells or bone marrow cells. *Stem Cells*, 2007, 25, 520–528.

[11] Sasportas, LS; Kasmieh, R; Wakimoto, H; et al. Assessment of therapeutic efficacy and fate of engineered human mesenchymal stem cells for cancer therapy. *Proc Natl Acad Sci USA*, 2009, 106, 4822–4827.

[12] Kidd, S; Spaeth, E; Dembinski, JL; et al. Direct evidence of mesenchymal stem cell tropism for tumor and wounding micro-environments using *in vivo* bio-luminescent imaging. *Stem Cells*, 2009, 27, 2614–2623.

[13] Kidd, S; Caldwell, L; Dietrich, M; et al. Mesenchymal stromal cells alone or expressing interferon-beta suppress pancreatic tumors *in vivo*, an effect countered by anti-inflammatory treatment. *Cytotherapy*, 2010, 12, 615–625.

[14] Roisin, MD; Sonja, K; Frank, PB; et al. Advances in mesenchymal stem cell-mediated gene therapy for cancer. *Stem Cell Research & Therapy*, 2010, 1, 25.

[15] Klopp, AH; Spaeth, EL; Dembinski, JL; et al. Tumor irradiation increases the recruitment of circulating mesenchymal stem cells into the tumor micro-environment. *Cancer Res*, 2007, 67, 11687-11695.

[16] Lin, SY; Yang, J; Everett, AD; et al. The isolation of novel mesenchymal stromal cell chemotactic factors from the conditioned medium of tumor cells. *Exp Cell Res*, 2008, 314, 3107-3117.

[17] Birnbaum, T; Roider, J; Schankin, CJ; et al. Malignant gliomas actively recruit bone marrow stromal cells by secreting angiogenic cytokines. *J Neuro Oncol*, 2007, 83, 241-247.

[18] Heissig, B; Dhahri, D; Eiamboonsert, S; et al. Role of mesenchymal stem cell-derived fibrinolytic factor in tissue regeneration and cancer progression. *Cell Mol Life Sci*, 2015, 72, 4759-4770.

[19] Ho, IA; Chan, KY; Ng, WH; et al. Matrix metallo-proteinase 1 is necessary for the migration of human bone marrow-derived mesenchymal stem cells toward human glioma. *Stem Cells*, 2009, 27, 1366-1375.

[20] Waterman, RS; Tomchuck, SL; Henkle, SL; Betancourt, AM. A New Mesenchymal Stem Cell (MSC) Paradigm: Polarization into a Pro-Inflammatory MSC1 or an Immunosuppressive MSC2 Phenotype. *PLoS ONE*, 2010, 5(4), e10088.

[21] Waterman, RS; Henkle, SL; Betancourt, AM. Mesenchymal Stem Cell 1 (MSC1)-Based Therapy Attenuates Tumor Growth Whereas MSC2-Treatment Promotes Tumor Growth and Metastasis. Fiorina P, ed. *PLoS ONE.*, 2012, 7(9), e45590.

[22] Kalinina, NI; Sysoeva, VY; Rubina, KA; Parfenova, YV; Tkachuk, VA. Mesenchymal Stem Cells in Tissue Growth and Repair. *Acta Naturae*, 2011, 3(4), 30-37.

[23] Devang, MP; Jainy, S; Anand, S. Srivastava. Therapeutic Potential of Mesenchymal Stem Cells in Regenerative Medicine. *Stem Cells International.*, 2013, 2013, 15 pages.

[24] Sushilkumar, Ramdasi; Chandra, Viswanathan; Rohit, Kulkarni; Abhijit, Bopardikar; Raghwendra, Kumar; Pradeep, Somalapur; Poonam, Pandey. A Mixture of Mesenchymal Stem Cells from Perinatal Sources Supports Consistent *Ex-vivo* CD34+ Hematopoietic Stem Cell Expansion. *Int J Life Sciences Res.*, Oct – Dec 2018, 6(4), 1-14.

[25] Strioga, M; Viswanathan, S; Darinskas, A; Slaby, O; Michalek, J. Same or not the same? Comparison of adipose tissue-derived versus bone marrow-derived

mesenchymal stem and stromal cells. *Stem Cells Dev*, 2012, Sep 20, 21(14), 2724-52.

[26] Tingting, Ge; Qin, Yu; Wei, Liu; et al. Characterization of bone marrow-derived mesenchymal stem cells from di-methylloxallyl glycine-preconditioned mice: Evaluation of the feasibility of dimethyloxallyl glycine as a mobilization agent. *Mol Med Rep*, 2016, 13(4), 3498-3506.

[27] *Fixation and Staining Procedure for Costar® Trans-well® Inserts by Corning Life Sciences.*

[28] Sushilkumar, Ramdasi. Normal Cell Signaling Pathways Maintains 'Stemness' in Stem Cells But Aberrant Pathways Causes Cells to Transform Into Cancer Cells – A Review. *International Journal of Healthcare Sciences.*, October 2016 - March 2017, 4(2), 77-91.

[29] Clarke, MF; Dick, JE; Dirks, PB; et al. Cancer stem cells — Perspectives on current status and future directions: AACR Workshop on cancer stem cells. *Cancer Res*, 2006b, 66, 9339–9344.

In: Manipulation of Stem Cells for Disease Benefits
Editor: Prasad Koka
ISBN: 978-1-53615-468-9

Chapter 4

THE EFFECT OF 3D-PRINTED POLYCAPROLACTONE (PCL) SCAFFOLD WITH DIFFERENT SURFACE COATINGS ON THE IMMUNOGENICITY OF STEM CELLS FROM HUMAN EXFOLIATED DECIDUOUS TEETH (SHED)

***Nermeen El-Moataz Bellah Ahmed*[1,2,*], *Ahmad Farouk Abd El Azeem*[1,2] *and Faten Sayed Bayoumi*[3,4]**

[1]Department of Oro-Dental Genetics, Medical Research Centre of Excellence, National Research Centre, Cairo, Egypt

[2]Stem Cell Laboratory, Center of Excellence for Advanced Sciences, National Research Centre, Cairo, Egypt

[3]Department of Microbiology and Immunology, Faculty of Pharmacy, October University of Modern Sciences and Arts (MSA), Cairo, Egypt

[4]Department of Immunogenetics, National Research Centre, Cairo, Egypt

ABSTRACT

Biomaterials have allowed many advances in the field of bone tissue engineering (BTE). Polycaprolactone (PCL) is an FDA degradable polymer that has been used for manufacturing scaffolds in bone tissue engineering. Different modifications have been made to PCL scaffold in order to improve its surface properties and osteoinductive abilities. It is essential that any modification of the engineered scaffold should avoid altering the properties of the seeded cells. Stem cells isolated from human exfoliated deciduous teeth (SHED) -similar to all other mesenchymal stem cells (MSCs)- do not express costimulatory molecules on their surface. These molecules are essential for the

* Corresponding Author's E-mail: nermeenkandel@gmail.com.

completion of T cell activation and therefore the lack of their expression accounts for the low immunogenicity of MSCs. In this study, SHED were isolated and seeded on 3D-printed PCL scaffolds which were either non-coated or coated with either nanohydroxyapatite (N-HAp) or multi-walled carbon nanotubes (MWCNTs). Cells cultured without scaffolds were used as a control. After three-day culture, all cells were collected and analyzed by flow cytometry for the expression of surface co-stimulatory molecules; CD40, CD80, and CD86. Results showed that different coating materials evidently affected the immunogenicity of the seeded SHED. The expression of CD40, CD80, and CD86 markers was significantly higher in cells seeded on MWCNTs/PCL scaffolds, followed by cells seeded on N-HAp/PCL scaffolds when compared to cells seeded on non-coated PCL scaffolds. On the other hand, cells seeded on non-coated PCL scaffolds showed no significant difference in their expression to the specified markers when compared to the control group. The data presented in this study are significant when considering allogeneic MSCs treatments in order to avoid immune rejection.

Keywords: stem cells, 3D printing, immunogenicity, polycaprolactone, scaffolds

INTRODUCTION

Bone grafting has been used for repairing large bone defects secondary to severe trauma, tumor resection, cancer, or genetic disorders [1]. Despite being used for decades, allografts, autografts, xenografts, and artificial bone substitutes have many complications [2]. Postoperative pain and swelling, donor site morbidity, wound dehiscence and immune rejection are some of those complications [3].

Over the last decade, the fast-growing field of tissue engineering- which uses stem cells, scaffold, mechanical and biochemical signals- provided better alternatives for the traditional bone grafting methods with the aim to avoid their complications [4-6]. A scaffold is a 3D construct that serves as a temporary support for cells to grow into new tissue and play a key role in housing the cells and directing their growth into specific tissues [7]. In bone tissue engineering, the material, shape, and structure of the scaffold play an important role in successful bone regeneration.

3D-printed biodegradable synthetic polymers, such as poly L-lactic acid (PLLA), poly (lactic-co-glycolic acid) (PLGA), and poly (ε-Caprolactone) (PCL), have been used to construct scaffolds for bone regeneration [8-10]. Synthetic polymers suit several regenerative applications due to their biodegradability and the capability of modifying their mechanical properties. Moreover, they can be fabricated into different shapes with chosen pore size and shape [11].

One of the most used biodegradable synthetic polymers in bone tissue engineering is the FDA approved PCL [12]. Previous studies proved that PCL can promote cell attachment, proliferation, and matrix production [13, 14]. Although PCL degrades by hydrolyses like polylactic-co-glycolic acid (PLGA) and poly L-lactic acid (PLLA), the amount of lactic acid produced by it is minimal when compared to other biodegradable polymers [15]. Many recent studies aimed at improving the properties of PCL scaffolds by using nanoparticles, surface coating, or the combination of both [16, 17].

Stem cells from human exfoliated deciduous teeth (SHED) are multipotent, mesenchymal cells with high proliferative capacity and can differentiate into odontoblasts, adipocytes, neural cells, and osteogenic cells [18]. In previous studies, SHED were used for bone regeneration to repair various bone defects [19, 20]. Moreover, in a recent study, SHED were found to produce the largest osteoid and widely distributed collagen fibers compared to dental pulp and bone marrow stem cells [21].

Immunogenicity of stem cells is an important factor to consider when it comes to using them for clinical applications. It has been reported that mesenchymal stem cells (MSCs) have immuno-modulatory properties [22-24]. Moreover, MSCs were found to express low levels of major histocompatibility class II (MHC II), while they do not express the co-stimulatory molecules CD40, CD80, and CD86 [24, 25]. CD80 and CD86 bind to CD28 on the surface of resting T cells and activate them. Moreover, this leads to activation, proliferation, and differentiation of B cells and induces the secretion of interleukin-6 (IL-6) and interferon-γ (IFN-γ). CD40 molecules increase the proliferation of activated T cells by binding to CD154 on their surface [26]. The low expression of these co-stimulatory molecules in MSCs contribute to their low immunogenicity.

In this study, we investigated the effect of surface coating of 3D-printed PCL scaffold using osteo-inductive materials nanohydroxyapatite (N-HAp) and multi-walled carbon nanotube (MWCNT)- on the immunogenicity of SHED.

MATERIALS AND METHODS

Isolation and Culture of Stem Cells from Human Exfoliated Deciduous Teeth (SHED)

All experimental protocols were performed according to guidelines of the National Research Centre, Cairo, Egypt. Primary teeth were collected randomly from children aged 7-8 years at the Oro-dental Genetics department clinic, National Research Centre. Written informed consents were obtained from the children's guardians. The collected teeth were immediately placed in Dulbecco modified Eagles' medium (DMEM; Sigma-Aldrich, USA) supplemented with 100 units/mL of penicillin/streptomycin (Invitrogen Co., USA). They were then transferred to the laboratory where they were processed within 24 hours of extraction. The teeth were split open using sterile metal weight and the pulp tissue was gently removed using sterile dental tweezers. The collected pulp tissue was then transferred to a 3.5 cm dish and cut into small pieces using sterile scissors. The dissected tissue pieces were then digested in 0.02% collagenase type II (Worthington Biochemical, Lakewood, NJ, USA) for 60 min at 37°C with continuous shaking in a water bath shaker. After complete digestion of the pulp tissue, the enzyme was deactivated by dilution with DMEM supplemented with 15% fetal bovine serum (FBS; Invitrogen, Carlsbad, CA, USA).

The isolated SHED were cultured in DMEM supplemented with 15% FBS, 100 units/mL penicillin, 100 μg/mL of streptomycin, and 0.25 μg/mL of Fungizone. Cells were selected on the basis of their ability to adhere to the tissue culture dish; non-adherent cells were removed during medium replacement after 5-day culture. SHED isolated from the teeth of three different children were used to conduct the subsequent experiment. All isolated cells were regularly monitored using an inverted light microscope (Leica, 6000B-4) using Suite V3 (Leica).

3D Printing of PCL Scaffold

From 100% pure PCL (Sigma, USA, CAS: 24980-41-4), 1.7 mm filaments were made using a Rubik "Prusha I3 Bioprinter" fusion deposition modeling (FDM) desktop printer (Rubik 3D, Egypt). With an accuracy of 200 μm/layer and using a 200 μm sized nozzle at 100°C, three layers of an inter-connected meshwork were printed.

Surface Coating of PCL Scaffolds

All 3D-printed scaffolds were first treated with an alkaline solution (30% NaOH (0.25M):70% absolute ethanol) for 24 hours. For nanohydroxyapatite (N-HAp) coating, the scaffolds were embedded in an absorbable gelatin sponge (EquiSpon, equimedical, Netherlands) filled with 0.25g of nanohydroxyapatite (N-HAp) then were pressed using a sterilization bag sealing machine (DEASIN, China) at around 110°C for 2 mins to form the composite scaffold.

The MWCNT-coated PCL scaffolds were gifts from Dr. Emad Al-ashkar, Spectroscopy Department, National Research Centre. A new technique of surface mechanical alloying (SMA) was used for coating the PCL scaffolds with MWCNT [27].

Seeding of SHED on the Scaffold

Sterile N-HAp/PCL, MWCNT/PCL, and non-coated PCL scaffolds were placed in 3.5 cm plates (Figure 1). The scaffolds were then incubated with 2ml of DMEM overnight. The SHED of the 4th passage of culture were detached by trypsin-ethylenediaminetetraacetic acid (EDTA) treatment. 1 x 10^5 cells were diluted into 500 μl of DMEM supplemented with 15% FBS and homogenously seeded on the top of each scaffold to allow cells to adhere to the scaffold for 2 hours before adding the full volume (2 mL) of the medium. All samples were incubated at 37°C and 5% CO_2 for 3 days and the medium was changed every other day. Cells cultured without scaffold were used as a control.

Detection of Cell Surface Markers of Immunogenicity Using Flow Cytometry

Evaluation of cell surface markers was necessary to detect whether the immunogenicity of SHED cells was affected by the different surface coatings of the 3D printed PCL scaffold. After three days culture, cells were detached from coated and non-coated scaffolds using Accutase (Sigma-Aldrich). The average total number of the harvested cells in the control, non-coated PCL, N-HAp and MWNCT groups was 8 x 10^5, 4.7 x 10^5, 4.4 x 10^5, and 4 x 10^5 respectively.

FcR blocking reagent (human, Miltenyi Biotec, Germany) was used to block and reduce the non-specific FcR binding receptors to increase the specificity of the used antibodies. From each sample, 1x10^5 cells were incubated with FcR blocking reagent (1:500 dilution) for 20 minutes at 4°C. Cells were further incubated with 1µg/ml of; CD40 (APC, mouse, Biolegend, USA), CD80 (FITC, mouse, eBioscience, UK), CD86 (PE-Cy5, mouse, eBio-science, UK), IgG1 isotype control (FITC, mouse, Biolegend, USA) and IgG2b isotype control (PE-Cy5, mouse, Biolegend, USA) for 1 hour, at 4°C. The cells were then washed with PBS supplemented with 20% FBS and then centrifuged at 1300 rpm for 1 min at 4°C. The supernatant was discarded and cells were re-suspended in Hank's solution (Invitrogen) which was supplemented with FBS, and 4-(2-hydroxyethyl)-1-piperazineethanesulfonic acid buffer solution (HEPES) (Invitrogen) to which 2µg/ml propidium iodide (PI) stain (Sigma) was added in order to stain dead cells. Labeled cells were analyzed using FACSAria II flow cytometer (Becton Dickinson, USA). Only viable cells as determined by propidium iodide (PI) (Sigma-Aldrich) exclusion were gated and analyzed.

Three different fluorochromes were used in this experiment (FITC, APC, and PE-CY5), therefore, compensation beads (Thermo fisher Scientific, USA) have been used to confirm that the emission spectra of a given fluorochrome was not within the detector channel of another by mathematically subtracting the fluorescent signal from the fluorochrome that is spilling over into that channel. Control samples immunolabelled with each fluorochrome were used as follows the signal detected from a single fluorochrome in each of the other channels was measured and compensation was performed by beads to remove that signal.

Statistical Analysis

Data were reported as mean ± standard error. Statistical analysis was performed using Microsoft (MS) Office Excel Software. One-way ANOVA was used to assess differences between groups. If a significant difference was detected, Student's t-test was subsequently used, to detect which group is responsible for the significance and to calculate the p-value. Differences were considered statistically significant if the p-value was less than 0.05.

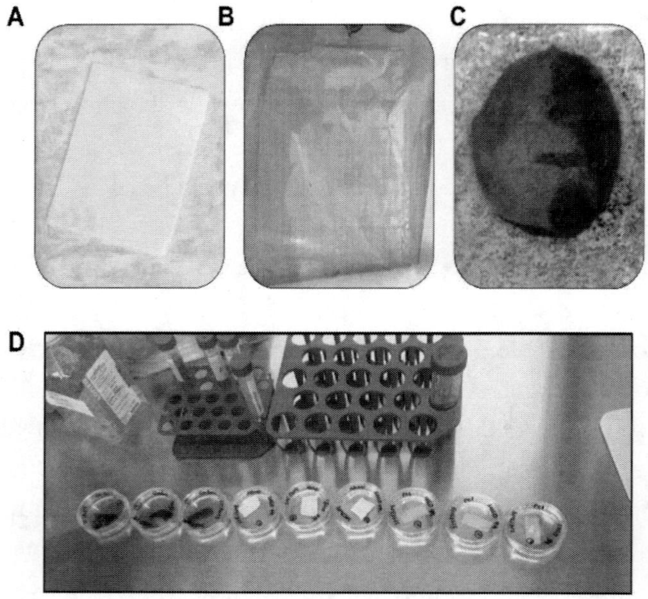

Figure 1. Preparation of different scaffolds. (A) Non-coated-PCL scaffold. (B) N-HAp coated PCL scaffold. (C) MWCNT coated PCL scaffold. (D) Scaffolds in the 3.5cm dishes.

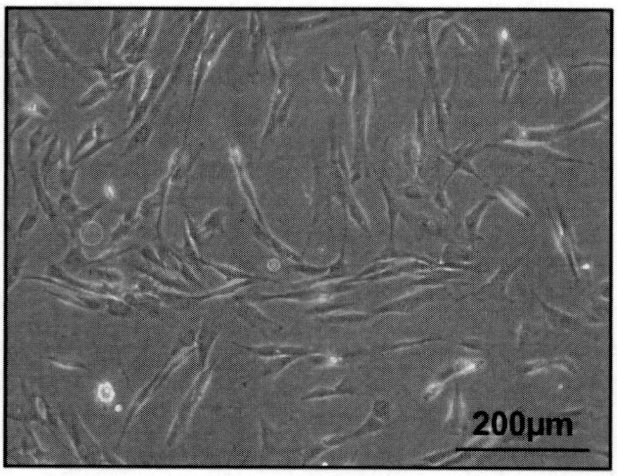

Figure 2. Morphology of the isolated stem cells from human exfoliated deciduous teeth (SHED).

RESULTS

Cells were successfully isolated from the primary teeth, cells adhered to the plastic of the cell culture dish and exhibited small spindle-shaped phenotype (Figure 2). Flow cytometric analysis demonstrated that the type of coating material evidently affects the immunogenicity of the attached cells. The fraction of cells expressing co-stimulatory markers CD40, CD80, and CD86 was markedly affected by different coating materials of the 3D- printed PCL scaffold (Figure 3). The expression of CD40 in cells seeded on non-coated PCL scaffolds was very low similar to that of the control group. Moreover, there was no significant difference between the expression of CD40 in cells seeded on N-HAp/PCL scaffolds and cells in all other groups. On the other hand, the expression of surface antigen marker CD40 was significantly higher in cells seeded on MWCNT/PCL scaffolds (29.2 ± 3.6) than in cells seeded on non-coated PCL scaffolds (8.3 ± 2.5, $p < 0.01$), as well as in cells seeded on N-HAp/PCL scaffolds (14.1 ± 1.1) but without significance.

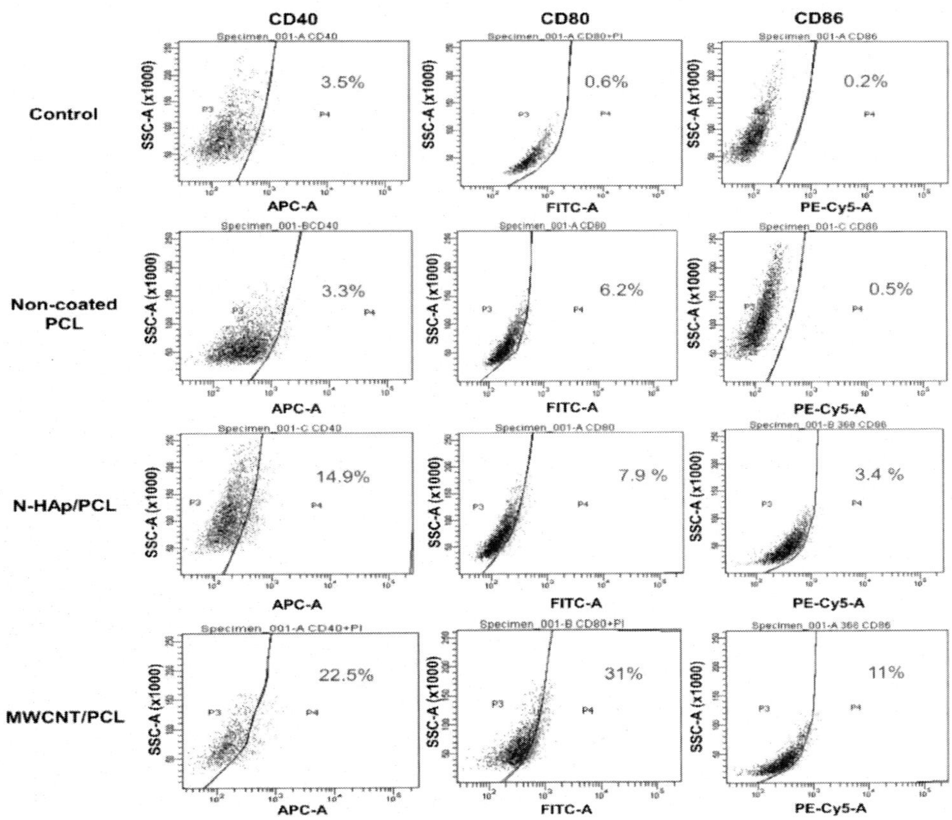

Figure 3. Representative flow cytometry dot plot (marker vs isotype control) showing the percentage of SHED positive to co-stimulatory factors; CD40, CD80, and CD86. Blue dots in P3 area represents the cells negative to the marker and positive to isotype control expression while pink dots in P4 area depict cells with positive marker expression. Numbers represent the percentage of cells positive to the marker.

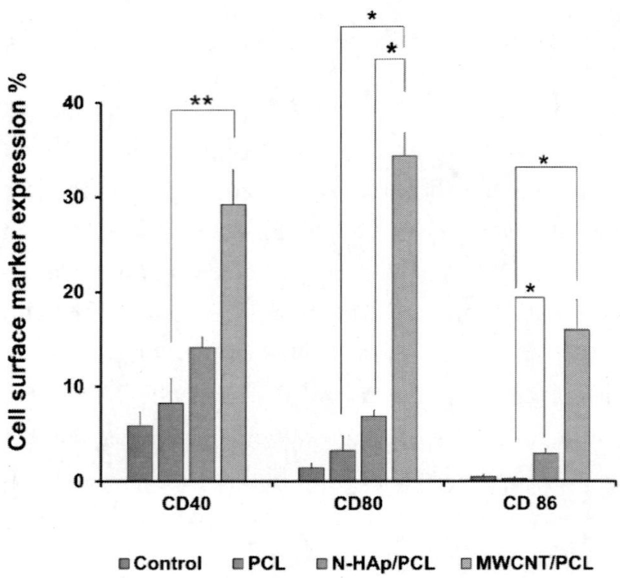

Figure 4. Co-stimulatory markers expression. Significant increase in the co-stimulatory markers expression in cells seeded on MWCNT/PCL scaffold was evident when compared to cells seeded on both N-HAp/PCL and non-coated PCL scaffolds (mean ± S.D., n = 3. *p < 0.05, **p < 0.01).

For CD80 expression, there was no significant difference in the marker expression between cells in non-coated PCL group and control group. The expression of CD80 was higher in cells in N-HAp/ PCL group than those in the non-coated PCL group, however without significance. On the other hand, cells in MWCNT/PCL group (34.4 ± 2.3) expressed CD80 marker significantly higher than N-HAp/PCL group (6.9 ± 0.6, $p < 0.05$), and non-coated PCL group (3.2 ± 1.6, $p < 0.05$).

Similar to CD40 and CD80, CD86 marker expression showed no significant difference between cells seeded on non-coated PCL scaffolds and control groups. However, Cells in the N-HAp/PCL group expressed the CD86 marker higher than those in the non-coated group with a significant difference ($p < 0.05$). CD86 marker was highly expressed in MWCNT/PCL group (15.9 ± 3.1) when compared to N-HAp/PCL (2.9 ± 0.5) without significance while the difference was significant when compared to non-coated-PCL (0.2 ± 0.1, $p < 0.05$).

In general, all examined markers were expressed at the lowest rate in the control group and the highest in MWCNTs group. The non-coated-PCL groups expressed the markers at higher rates than the control groups, however, without significance (Figure 4).

DISCUSSION

In the present study, we evaluated the effect of 3D-printed PCL scaffold coated with either nanohydroxyapatite (N-HAp), multi-walled carbon nanotubes (MWCNTs) or non-coated scaffolds on the immunogenicity of MSCs. One of the most important properties of MSCs is that they lack the expression of major histocompatibility complex I and costimulatory molecules; CD40, CD80, and CD86, which contribute to their low immunogenicity [24, 25]. This property is very important when it comes to their allogeneic transportation for clinical applications, as it can eliminate the need for the prolonged use of immuno-suppressive drugs.

In this study, we used 3D printing technology because it allows the fabrication of custom-designed scaffolds [28]. Moreover, recently, 3D-printed scaffolds have been widely used in bone, cartilage and cardiac tissue engineering [29-31].

In bone tissue engineering (BTE), various degradable polymers have been used as scaffolds [8-10]. PCL has been used by many recent studies due to the material's biodegradability, biocompatibility, plasticity, availability, and relatively low cost [32-34]. Hence, using 3D-printed PCL scaffold for bone tissue engineering (BTE) can be considered a good choice. However, PCL has low osteoinductivity when compared to ceramics [35]. In order to improve the low osteoinductive property of PCL for bone tissue engineering (BTE), PCL based scaffolds were combined with ceramics [32] or coated with other osteoinductive materials [16, 17].

Hydroxyapatite (HAp) is a main inorganic constituent in normal bone. Moreover, nano-hydroxyapatite (N-HAp) has been used in bone tissue engineering (BTE) for its osteoinductivity, biocompatibility and high mechanical strength [36]. Similarly, carbon nanotubes (CNTs) are cylinder nanoparticles that have been recently shown to induce osteogenic differentiation. CNTs have been used in scaffolds for bone tissue engineering (BTE) due to its osteo-inductive ability and outstanding mechanical proper-ties [37]. Moreover, previous studies showed that multiwalled carbon nanotubes (MWCNTs) are biocompatible with bone tissue and can help in bone repair by accelerating its growth, particularly when stimulated by recombinant human bone morphogenetic protein-2 (rhBMP-2) [38, 39]. Furthermore, MWCNT/PLLA composite and MWCNT/PCL composite have been found to improve the mechanical properties of the polymer scaffolds [40, 41]. In the present study, we chose to use N-HAp and MWCNT as coating materials for our 3D printed PCL scaffolds.

While many studies have investigated the effect of different coating materials on the mechanical properties and osteoinductivity of PCL scaffolds, none has investigated their effect on the immunogenicity of the seeded cells [42, 43]. Many studies showed that the immunogenic properties of MSCs can be affected by various factors, for instance; passage number, culture conditions, and oxygen tension [44-46]. Our results demonstrated that with N-HAp and MWCNT coatings, the seeded cells become increasingly immunogenic while in the non-coated-PCL group, the cells' expression of the co-stimulatory factors remained unaffected.

It was obvious that MWCNT had the maximum adverse effect on the seeded MSCs by increasing their expression of co-stimulatory factors; CD80, CD86, and CD40. CD80 was apparently the most affected surface antigen followed by CD40 while CD86 expression was affected to a lesser extent. N-HAp effect on the expression of the costimulatory factors was also evident especially that of the CD86. However, the increase in the CD40 expression was without significance when compared to non-coated PCL groups.

Our results clearly indicate that coating 3D-printed PCL scaffolds with MWCNT strongly increases the immunogenicity of MSCs by increasing their expression of all costimulatory factors, particularly CD80. On the other hand, N-HAp increased the expression of CD86 significantly more than the other costimulatory factors. These results should be put into consideration when designing a scaffold for bone tissue engineering (BTE).

Further *in vitro* and *in vivo* studies should be carried out to investigate the mechanisms by which N-HAp and MWCNT affect the immunogenicity of MSCs. Additionally, it would be interesting to investigate MSCs from other tissue sources.

Conclusion

The data presented in this study are significant when considering allogeneic MSCs treatments for clinical applications. Our results showed that, although the immunogenicity of the cells seeded on a non-coated PCL membrane was not affected, MWCNT coating made them more immunogenic while N-HAp coating had a milder effect on the seeded cells. Hence, the effect of the scaffold coating materials on cell immunogenic properties should not be ignored when clinical applications are considered.

Acknowledgments

The authors would like to thank Al-ashkar E. (Spectroscopy Department) and Ebrahim MR. (Solid State Department), both are members of the National Research Centre, for gifting the MWCNT-coated scaffolds. The authors would also like to acknowledge; Mai Mohsen, Abdul-Rahman Anis, Omar Gamal and Karim Talaat for their technical assistance.

Ethical Compliance

The authors have stated all possible conflicts of interest within this work. The authors have stated all sources of funding for this work. If this work involved human participants, informed consent was received from each individual. If this work involved human participants, it was conducted in accordance with the 1964 Declaration of Helsinki. If this work involved experiments with humans or animals, it was conducted in accordance with the related institutions' research ethics guidelines.

REFERENCES

[1] Yang F, Wang J, Hou J, Guo H, Liu C. Bone regeneration using cell-mediated responsive degradable PEG-based scaffolds incorporating with rhBMP-2. *Biomaterials* 2013; 34: 1514–1528.

[2] Athanasiou VT, Papachristou DJ, Panagopoulos A, Saridis A, Scopa CD, Megas P. Histological comparison of autograft, allograft-DBM, xenograft, and synthetic grafts in a trabecular bone defect: an experimental study in rabbits. *Med Sci Monit.* 2010;16(1):24-31.

[3] Rawashdeh MA. Morbidity of iliac crest donor site following open bone harvesting in cleft lip and palate patients. *Int J Oral Maxillofac Surg.* 2008; 37:223-227.

[4] Al-Ahmady HH, Abd Elazeem AF, Ahmed NEB, Shawkat WM, Elmasry M, Abdelrahman MA, Abderazik MA. Combining autologous bone marrow mononuclear cells seeded on a collagen sponge with nano-hydroxyapatite, and platelet-rich fibrin: Reporting a novel strategy for alveolar cleft bone regeneration. *J Craniomaxillofac Surg.* 2018; 46:1593-600.

[5] Wang X, Li G, Guo J, Yang L, Liu Y, Sun Q, Li R, Yu W. Hybrid composites of mesenchymal stem cell sheets, hydroxyapatite, and platelet-rich fibrin granules for bone regeneration in a rabbit calvarial critical-size defect model. *Exp Ther Med.* 2017;13(5):1891-1899.

[6] Uchiyama H, Yamato M, Sasaki R, Sekine H, Yang J, Ogiuchi H, Ando T and Okano T. *In vivo* 3D analysis with micro-computed tomography of rat calvaria bone regeneration using periosteal cell sheets fabricated on temperature-responsive culture dishes. *J Tissue Eng Regen Med* 2011;5: 483-490.

[7] Seitz H, Rieder W, Irsen S, Leukers B, Tille C. Three-dimensional printing of porous ceramic scaffolds for bone tissue engineering. *J. Biomed. Mater. Res.* 2005;74B: 782-788.

[8] McNeil SE, Griffiths HR, Perrie Y. Polycaprolactone fibers as a potential delivery system for collagen to support bone regeneration. *Curr Drug Deliv.* 2011;8: 448–455.

[9] Hiep NJ, Khon HC, Hai ND, Byong-Taek L, Toi VV, Hung LT. Biocompatibility of PCL/PLGA-BCP porous scaffold for bone tissue engineering applications. *J Biomater Sci Polym* 2017;28(9):864-878.

[10] Salerno A, Fernández-Gutiérrez M, Román del Barrio JS, Domingo C. Bio-safe fabrication of PLA scaffolds for bone tissue engineering by combining phase

separation, porogen leaching and scCO2 drying. *J. Supercrit. Fluid.* 2014;97:238-246.

[11] BaoLin G, MA PX. Synthetic biodegradable functional polymers for tissue engineering: a brief review. *Sci China Chem.* 2014;57(4):490-500.

[12] Petrie AC, Cooper JJ, Sefcik LS, Tholpady SS, Ogle RC, Botchwey EA. Osteogenic differentiation of dura mater stem cells cultured *in vitro* on three-dimensional porous scaffolds of poly (Epsilon-Caprolactone) fabricated via co-extrusion and gas foaming. *Acta Biomater.* 2008;4:1187–1197.

[13] Kim HJ, Lee JH, Im GI. Chondrogenesis using mesenchymal stem cells and PCL scaffolds. *J. Biomed. Mater. Res. A* 2010;92:659–666.

[14] Izquierdo R, Garcia-Giralt N, Rodriguez MT, Caceres E, Garcia SJ, Gomez RJ, Monleon M, Monllau JC, Suay J. Biodegradable PCL scaffolds with an interconnected spherical pore network for tissue engineering. *J. Biomed. Mater. Res. A* 2008;85:25–35.

[15] Luong-Van E, Grondahl L, Chua KN, Leong KW, Nurcombe V, Cool SM. Controlled release of heparin from poly (Epsilon-Caprolactone) electrospun fibers. *Biomaterials* 2006;27:2042–2050.

[16] Zelenková T, Mora MJ, Barresi AA, Granero GE, Fissore D. On the production of chitosan-coated poly-caprolactone nanoparticles in a confined impinging jet reactor. *J Pharm Sci* J 2018;107(4):1157-1166.

[17] Sousa I, Mendes A, Bártolo BJ. PCL scaffolds with collagen bioactivator for applications in tissue engineering. *Procedia Eng* 2013;59:279-284.

[18] Miura M, Gronthos S, Zhao M, Lu B, Fisher LW, Robey PG, Shi S. SHED: stem cells from human exfoliated deciduous teeth. *Proc Natl Acad Sci USA.* 2003;100:5807–5812.

[19] Behnia A, Haghighat A, Talebi A, Nourbakhsh N, Heidari F. Transplantation of stem cells from human exfoliated deciduous teeth for bone regeneration in the dog mandibular defect. *World J Stem Cells.* 2014;6(4): 505-510.

[20] Vakhrushev IV, Antonov EN, Popova AV, Konstantinova EV, Karalkin PA, Kholodenko IV, Lupatov AY, Popov VK, Bagratashvili VN, Yarygin KN. Design of tissue engineering implants for bone tissue regeneration of the basis of new generation poly-lactoglycolide scaffolds and multipotent mesenchymal stem cells from human exfoliated deciduous teeth (SHED cells). *Bull Exp Biol Med.* 2012;153(1):143–147.

[21] Nakajima K, Kunimatsu R, Ando K, Ando T, Hayashi Y, Kihara T, Hiraki T, Tsuka Y, Abe T, Kaku M, Nikawa H, Takata T, Tanne K, Tanimoto K. Comparison of the bone regeneration ability between stem cells from human exfoliated deciduous teeth, human dental pulp stem cells and human bone marrow mesenchymal stem cells. *Biochem Biophys Res Commun.* 2018;497(3):876-882.

[22] Le Blanc, K, Tammik, L, Sundberg, B. Mesenchymal stem cells inhibit and stimulate mixed lymphocyte cultures and mitogenic responses independently of the major histocompatibility complex. *Scand J Immunol* 2003;57(1): 11–20.

[23] Aggarwal, S, Pittenger, MF. Human mesenchymal stem cells modulate allogeneic immune cell responses. *Blood* 2005; 105(4): 1815–1822.

[24] Ryan, JM, Barry, FP, Murphy, JM. Mesenchymal stem cells avoid allogeneic rejection. *J Inflamm* 2005; 2(1): 8.

[25] Di Nicola M, Carlo-Stella C, Magni M, Milanesi M, Longoni PD, Matteucci P, Grisanti S, Gianni AM. Human bone marrow stromal cells suppress T-lymphocyte proliferation induced by cellular or nonspecific mitogenic stimuli. *Blood* 2002;99(10):3838-3843.

[26] Magee CN, Boenisch O, Najafian N. The role of co-stimulatory molecules in directing the functional differentiation of allo-reactive t helper cells. *Am J Transplant* 2012;12(10):2588-2600.

[27] Abouelsayed A, Ebrahim MR, El hotaby W, Hassan SA, Al-Ashkar E. Terhertz acoustic phonon detection from a compact surface layer of spherical nanoparticles powder mixture of aluminum, alumina and multi-walled carbon nanotube, Spectrochim. *Acta A Mol. Biomol. Spectrosc* 2017;185(2017):179-187.

[28] Tarafder S, Koch A, Jun Y, Chou C, Awadallah MR, Lee CH. Micro-precise spatiotemporal delivery system embedded in 3D printing for complex tissue regeneration. *Biofabrication* 2016; 8:025003.

[29] Nyberg E, Rindone A, Dorafshar, A, Grayson WL. Comparison of 3D-printed poly-epsilon-caprolactone scaffolds functionalized with tricalcium Phosphate, hydroxyapatite, bio-oss, or decellularized Bone Matrix. *Tissue Eng. Part A* 2016;23:503–514.

[30] Jeong, CG, Hollister SJ. A comparison of the influence of material on *in vitro* cartilage tissue engineering with PCL, PGS, and POC 3D scaffold architecture seeded with chondrocytes. *Biomaterials* 2010;31:4304–4312.

[31] Ho CM, Mishra A, Lin PT, Ng SH, Yeong WY, Kim YJ, Yoon YJ. 3D printed polycaprolactone carbon nanotube composite scaffolds for cardiac tissue engineering. *Macromol. Biosci.* 2016;17.

[32] Park SA, Lee HJ, Kim KS, Lee SJ, Lee JT, Kim SY, Chang NH. *In vivo* evaluation of 3D-printed poly-caprolactone scaffold implantation combined with -TCP powder for alveolar bone augmentation in a beagle defect model. *Materials* 2018;11(2):238.

[33] Heydari Z, Mohebbi-Kalhori D, Afarani MS. Engineered electrospun polycaprolactone (PCL)/ octa-calcium phosphate (OCP) scaffold for bone tissue engineering. *Mater Sci Eng C Mater Biol Appl* 2017;81: 127-132.

[34] Malikmammadov E, Tanir TE, Kiziltay A, Hasirci V, Hasirci N. PCL and PCL-based materials in biomedical applications. *J Biomater Sci Polym Ed* 2017; 29(7):863-893.

[35] Kinoshita Y, Maeda M. Recent developments of functional scaffolds for craniomaxillofacial bone tissue engineering applications. *Sci. World J* 2013; 863157,21 pages.

[36] Wei G, Ma PX. Structure and properties of nano-hydroxyapatite/polymer composite scaffolds for bone tissue engineering. *Biomaterials* 2004;25(19):4749–4757.

[37] Zancanela DC, de Faria AN, Simao AM, Goncalves RR, Ramos AP, Ciancaglini P. Multi and single walled carbon nanotubes: effects on cell responses and biomineralization of osteoblasts cultures. *J Mater Sci Mater Med* 2016;27(3):62.

[38] Usui Y, Aoki K, Narita N, Murakami N, Nakamura I, Nakamura K, Ishigaki N, Yamazaki H, Horiuchi H, Kato H, Taruta S, Kim YA, Endo M, Saito N. Carbon nanotubes with high bone tissue compatibility and bone formation acceleration effects. *Small* 2008;4(2): 240-246.

[39] Li X, Liu H, Niu X, Yo B, Fan Y, Feng Q, Cui F, Watari F. The use of carbon nanotubes to induce osteogenic differentiation of human adipose-derived MSCs *in vitro* and ectopic bone formation *in vivo*. *Biomaterials* 2012; 33(19): 4818-4827.

[40] Wu D, Zhang Y, Zhang M, Yu W. Selective localization of multiwalled carbon nanotubes in poly (ε-capro-lactone)/polylactide blend. *Biomacromolecules* 2009; 10(2):417-424.

[41] Chen GX, Kim HS, Park BH, et al. Synthesis of poly (L-lactide) functionalized multiwalled carbon nanotubes by ring opening polymerization. *Macromol Chem Phys* 2007;208(4): 389-398.

[42] Mattioli-Belmonte M, Vozzi G, Whulanza Y, Seggiani M, Fantauzzi V, Orsini G, Ahluwalia A. Tuning polycaprolactone–carbon nanotube composites for bone tissue engineering scaffolds. *Mater Sci Eng C 2012*; 32(2):152-159.

[43] Kim JW, Shin KH, Koh YH, Hah MJ, Moon J, Kim HE. Production of poly("-caprolactone)/hydroxyapatite composite scaffolds with a tailored macro/micro-porous structure, high mechanical properties, and excellent bioactivity. *Materials* 2017; 10:1123.

[44] Liu H, Lu K, MacAry PA, Wong KL, Heng A, Cao T, Kemeny DM. Soluble molecules are key in maintaining the immunomodulatory activity of murine mesenchymal stromal cells. *J Cell Sci.* 2012;125(1):200-208.

[45] Patrikoski M, Sivula J, Huhtala H, Helminen M, Salo F, Mannerstrom B, Miettinena S. Different culture conditions modulate the immunological properties of adipose stem cells. *Stem Cells Transl Med* 2014;3(10): 1220-1230.

[46] Ahmed NE-B, Murakami M, Kaneko S, Nakashima M. The effects of hypoxia on the stemness properties of human dental pulp stem cells (DPSCs). *Sci Rep* 2016; 6:35476.

In: Manipulation of Stem Cells for Disease Benefits ISBN: 978-1-53615-468-9
Editor: Prasad Koka

Chapter 5

Role of Glutathione in Balancing Total Antioxidant Status and Generation of Reactive Oxygen Species during Hepatic Differentiation of Bone-Marrow-Derived Mesenchymal Stem Cells

Abdolamir Allameh*[1,*]*, Hamid-Reza Ahmadi-Ashtiani*[1]*,
***Maryam Rezapour*[1] *and Hossein Rastegar*[2]**
[1]Department of Clinical Biochemistry, Faculty of Medical Sciences,
Tarbiat Modares University, Tehran, Iran
[2]School of Pharmacy, Tehran University of Medical Sciences, Tehran, Iran

Abstract

Differentiation of mesenchyal stem cells (MSCs) into biologically active hepatocytes depends on several factors. Glutathione (GSH) and antioxidant enzymes play major role in maintaining the balance between oxidative damage factors and antioxidants during the differentiation. There-fore by adding GSH modifiers to the culture media, we examined the impact of GSH on the process of MSC differentiation into hepatocyte-like cells.

In the present study differentiation of MSCs into hepatocyte-like cells was induced using a 2-step protocol. Then production of reactive oxygen species (ROS), cellular GSH, GSH peroxidase (GPX), GSH reductase (GR) and total antioxidant capacity (TAC) were determined on days 2, 7 and 14 of differentiation onset. Besides, the experiment was carried out in cells treated with glutathione modifiers namely; buthionine sulfoximine (BSO) or N-acetylcysteine (NAC).

Depletion in GSH and GPX due to BSO treatments resulted in elevation of ROS production. In contrast, ROS was substantially decreased in cells having high levels of GSH and GPX following NAC treatments. The results showed that during differentiation,

* Corresponding Author's E-mail: allameha@modares.ac.ir.

the cell proliferation was affected by ROS alterations. Cell proliferation was enhanced when treated with NAC which also increased GSH, GPX and TAC. As a consequence of GSH elevation by NAC, there was a substantial increase in antioxidant activity of the cells undergoing differentiation. This data show that ROS generation and TAC status can be balanced during the process of hepatic differentiation of MSCs by inducing GSH biosynthesis using NAC in the culture media. This action is associated with improved cell proliferation and differentiation.

Keywords: mesenchymal stem cells, oxidative stress, hepatogenic differentiation, glutathione, N-acetylcysteine

Abbreviations

MSCs	Mesenchyal stem cells
GSH	Glutathione
ROS	Reactive oxygen species
GPX	GSH peroxidase
GR	GSH reductase
TAC	Total antioxidant capacity
BSO	Buthionine sulfoximine
NAC	N-acetylcysteine
DMEM-LG	Dulbecco's Modified Eagle's Medium - low glucose
FBS	Fetal Bovine Serum
HGF	Hepatocyte growth factor
DEX	Dexamethasone
OSM	Oncostatin-M
Brdu	Bromodeoxyuridine

Introduction

Mesenchymal stem cells (MSCs) are multipotent cells, which have been isolated from fetal and adult tissues of different sources. They are self-renewable, multipotent cells which can be expanded and differentiated *ex vivo* into specific cell lineages.

MSCs and MSC technology are now considered as important tools for cell therapy in regenerative medicine, tissue repair and immunomodulatory properties (Denu and Hematti, 2016). The *in vitro* and *in vivo* characteristics of MSCs including their immunogenicity, homing ability, banking and cryo-preservation has been reviewed in different articles (Allameh and Kazemnejad, 2012; Ullah et al., 2015).

Due to the low frequency of MSCs in human bone marrow (1 in 100,000 cells) in adult bone marrow), their expansion *in vitro* to obtain sufficient number of cells is essential for cell transplantation. Ageing is considered as an important factor in decreasing the number of MSCs in bone marrow stroma. This has been reported by researchers showing a link between the number of MSC in human bone marrow stroma with the donor age (Landgraf et al., 2011; Seigel et al., 2013).

It has been reported that human bone marrow derived MSCs undergo senescent during long-term culture, manifested by decline in differentiation potential, shortening of the telomere length and morphological alterations (Bonab et al., 2006). Oxidative stress factors such as reactive oxygen species (ROS) exists in every cell, which is part of the cell regulation and signaling. However, in general it has been understood that an increase in the concentration of cellular ROS can inhibit MSC proliferation, increase senescence, enhance adipogenic but reduce osteogenic differentiation, and inhibit MSC immunomodulation (Denu and Hematti, 2016).

ROS signaling has now been recognized as an emerging key regulator of multiple stem cell populations. Under pathological conditions increase in cellular ROS can disrupt the balance of oxidant and antioxidant factors leading to oxidative stress. It has been suggested that oxidative status is a good marker for expansion potential of MSCs and manipulation of this system can affect MSCs life span (Ullah et al., 2015).

Analysis of oxidative status might increase the cost-effectiveness and reduce the rate of unsuccessful advanced cell therapies (Bertolo et al. 2017). The cell proliferation and differentiation into hepatocyte-like cells could be improved by supplementation of culture media with compound having antioxidant activity (Ahmadi-Ashtiani et al., 2012). Furthermore it was demonstrated that manipulation in glutathione in MSCs undergoing hepatic differentiation could alter the efficiency of metabolic function of hepatocytes with emphasize on albumin synthesis (Allameh et al., 2014).

BSO and NAC are well known glutathione modifiers used for manipulation of glutathione and related pathways *in vitro* and *in vivo* studies. N-acetyl cysteine (NAC) is a precursor of glutathione which boosts antioxidant action of glutathione system. In contrast, buthionine sulphoximine (BSO) is an inhibitor of ɣ-glutamylcysteine synthetase leading to suppression of tissue glutathione (GSH) concentrations (Mathan Kumar et al., 2016).

Earlier we reported that hepatogenic differentiation of MSCs is associated with changes in expression of glutathione S-transferase enzymes, particularly the GSH conjugation pathway (Allameh et al., 2009). The present study is focused on the role of glutathione related factors in oxidative stress and antioxidant activities of the MSCs during hepatogenic differentiation. In this study glutathione modifying factors namely BSO and NAC were used as a tool to examine the role of cellular GSH and GSH redox enzymes on ROS production and overall performance of hepatogenic differentiation of MSCs.

MATERIALS AND METHODS

Isolation, Characterization, and Culture of Human Bone-Marrow-Derived MSCs

In this study bone marrow aspiration and biopsy collected from human donors were used as the source of MSCs. The surplus bone marrow samples were collected from the Bone Marrow Transplantation Center, Shariati Hospital (Tehran, Iran) after obtaining an informed consent from the donors. The study has been approved by the Medical Ethics Committee, Ministry of Health, I. R. Iran.

The MSCs were isolated from bone marrow samples as described in our previous publications (Kazemnejad et al., 2008; Ahmadi-Ashtiani et al., 2012). Briefly, the aspirate was diluted with phosphate buffered saline (PBS). The cells were gently overlaid over Ficoll-Hypaque (D = 1.077 g/mL) to separate mononuclear cells which appear on gradient interface. The cells were washed with PBS after centrifugation at 400g for 30 min. The mononuclear cell layer was washed and resuspension in the medium containing DMEM-low glucose (DMEM-LG), supplemented with 15% FBS, 2 mM glutamine, 100 mg/mL streptomycin, and 100 U/mL.

The cells were routinely cultured in 75 Cm^2 polystyrene plastic tissue culture flasks in DMEM-LG medium, at 37°C in a humidified 5% CO2 incubator. The non-adherent cells were removed 3-4 days after the incubation and adherent cell population (MSCs) which was growing as fibroblastic cells in clusters were further cultured and sub-cultured to obtain70–90% confluency. Finally the cells were harvested using trypsin–EDTA solution and transferred to 25 cm^2 plastic flasks at a density of 10^4 cells/cm^2 before inducing hepatic differentiation.

MSCs were characterized by immune phenotyping the cells using flow cytometry and also by assessing their differentiation potential into osteogenic and adipogenic cell linages as described previously (Ahmadi-Ashtiani et al., 2012).

Differentiation of MSCs into Hepatocyte-Like Cells

At passage 3, the MSCs (2 x 10^4 cells/cm^2) were seeded in 24 wells plates as described (Ahmadi-Ashtiani et al., 2012). Then using a 2-stage procedure hepatogenic differentiation was accomplished. Briefly, the cells were differentiated in DMEM-LG supplemented with 15% FBS, 20 ng/mL hepatocyte growth factor (HGF), and 10–7 mol/L dexamethasone (DEX). In the second step (day 7) differentiation was promoted by adding oncostatin-M (OSM;10 ng/mL) and continued for 14 days. During this period the developing hepatocyte- like cells were characterized by their morphological and hepatocyte-specific markers.

Characterization of Hepatocytes Derived from MSCs

Different approaches were used for the characterization of hepatocytes differentiated from human bone marrow MSCs. Morphological observation is a direct approach that confirms formation of polygonal cells from undifferentiated spindal-shaped MSCs. MSC shape changes during differentiation was started from day seven and continued until the end of the culture (fourteen days). Spindle-shaped MSCs were gradually converted into polygonal shaped-hepatocytes. This was further confirmed by estimation of selected hepatic biochemical and molecular markers during differentiation for up to fourteen days in culture. Changes in expression of hepatic markers, particularly albumin, urea, and transferrin together with liver marker enzymes SGOT and SGPT were compared in MSCs before differentiation and hepatocyte-like cells differentiated from the stem cells.

Additionally, expression of albumin and cytochrome P4503A4 (CYP3A4) specific mRNA were detected by using reverse transcription polymerase chain reaction (RTPCR). A detailed description of reverse transcription polymerase chain reaction protocol, as well as the primers used, is as provided in our previous publication (Kazemnejad et al., 2009).

Treatment of the Cells with BSO and NAC

In this experiment which was carried out in 96 well plates the cells were treated with different concentrations of either L-buthionine; BSO (0, 1.0 and 5.0 μM) or NAC (0, 0.1 and 1.0 mM) dissolved in the culture media. For each treatment 3 wells were considered and each assay was performed in duplicate, and at different time intervals the cells counted and used for the assays.

GSH was estimated using a commercially available kit from the Alexis Biochemicals, San Diego, CA, USA. This fluorometric assay is based on reaction of OPA (O-phthalaldehyde) reagent with reduced glutathione (GSH) which generate strong fluorescence for quantification of cellular GSH.

Live cell fluorescent ROS levels was measured using a kit purchased from Marker Gene technologies, Eugene, OR, USA. This kit utilizes the cell permeant reagent 2',7' –dichlorofluorescin diacetate (DCFDA), a fluorogenic dye that measures hydroxyl, peroxyl and other ROS activity within the cell. After diffusion in to the cell, DCFDA is deacetylated by cellular esterases to a non-fluorescent compound, which is later oxidized by ROS into 2', 7' –dichlorofluorescein (DCF) which is a highly fluorescent compound and can be detected by fluorescence spectroscopy at excitation and emission spectra of 495nm and 529nm respectively.

GPX, GR and TAC were measured in cells using commercially available assay kits from the Cayman, Ann Arbor, USA. GPX, Cat. #709001; GR, Cat. #703202 and TAC Cat. #7090001. The basis of these assays are briefly described below:

The GPX assay kit measures glutathione-dependent GPX activity indirectly by a coupled reaction with glutathione reductase (GR). Oxidized glutathione (GSSG), produced upon reduction of an organic hydroperoxide by GPx, is recycled to its reduced state by GR and NADPH. The oxidation of NADPH to NADP+ is accompanied by a decrease in absorbance at 340 nm. The rate of decrease in the absorption at 340 nm is directly proportional to the GPx activity in the samples.

GR activity was estimated by measuring the rate of NADPH oxidation. The oxidation of NADPH to NADP+ is accompanied by a decrease in absorbance at 340 nm. Since GR is present at rate limiting concentrations, the rate of decrease in the absorption is directly proportional to the GR activity in the sample.

Total antioxidant capacity of plasma (TAC) was estimated in the cell lysates based on the ability of antioxidants in the samples to inhibit the oxidation of ABTS® (2,2'-azino-di-[3-ethylbenzthiazoline sulphonate]) to ABTS® • + by metmyoglobin. The capacity of the antioxidants in the sample to prevent ABTS oxidation is compared with that of Trolox, a water-soluble tocopherol analogue, and is quantified as molar Trolox equivalents. The assay was per-formed according to the protocol recommended by the company. The amount of ABTS produced was recorded at 405 nm to produce a standard curve from which the TAC of the cell samples was calculated.

Effects of BSO and NAC on Cell Proliferation (Brdu Assay)

Cell proliferation was estimated in MSC culture at different time intervals (2, 7, and 14 days) using a colorimetric bromodeoxyuridine (Brdu) kit which was purchased from Roche Diagnostics, East Sussex, UK following the procedure described by the manufacturer. In this experiment, to optimize the optical density (OD) in this spectrophotometic assay the number of cells was adjusted for BSO or NAC-treated groups and the rate of cell proliferation was calculated accordingly.

RESULTS

Characterization of undifferentiated MSCs and differentiated hepatocyte-like cells have been performed routinely in our laboratory (Ahmadi-Ashtiani et al., 2012). The data presented in Figure 1 show that the hepatic markers changed during hepatic differentiation. The liver specific markers namely; albumin, SGOT, SGPT, urea and transferrin levels were at minimal levels in MSCs before differentiation, whereas, all these factors elevated significantly in hepatocytes differentiated from them. Typically albumin expression was not detectable in undifferentiated MSCs, but it was elevated by approximately 6 folds ($P < 005$), in hepatocytes 2-3 weeks after differentiation (Figure

1A). Moreover as shown in Figure 1B, albumin expression at mRNA levels was markedly increased in hepatocyte-like cells recovered on day 7 and day 14 of differentiation compared to undifferentiated MSCs (day 0). Likewise, the undifferentiated MSC (0 day) were negative for CYP3A4 (Cytochrome P-4503A4) expression, whereas the expression of this typical liver marker was positive for hepatocyte-like cells 7 and 14 days after differentiation onset (Figure 1C).

A

Hepatic Markers	MSCs before differentiation	Differentiated Hepatocytes
Albumin (μg/ml)	ND	5.9±0.4*
SGPT (IU/L)	0.03±0.01	4.2±1*
SGOT (IU/L)	0.06±0.04	6.9±2*
Urea (mg/dl)	0.06±0.04	14.2±4*
Transferrin (mg/ml)	0.006±0.0002	3.1±0.5*

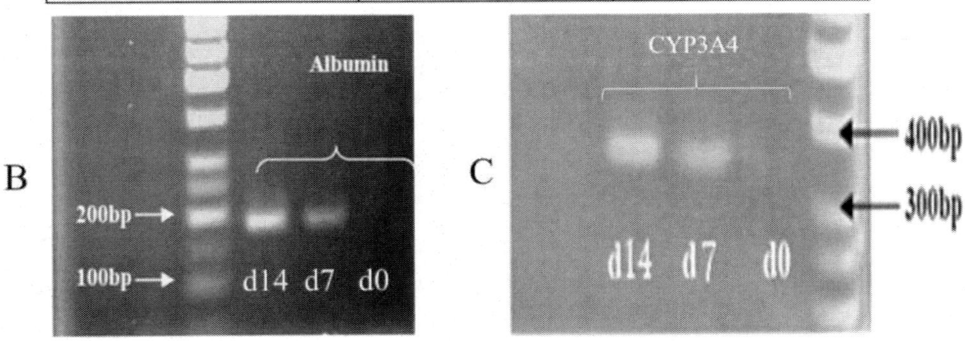

Figure 1. Characterization of hepatocyte-like cells during differentiation from mesenchymal stem cells. Section A, the table summarizes the differences in biochemical markers in differentiated hepatocytes and their progenitor MSCs.* sign shows the statistically difference ($P < 0.05$) between hepatocytes and their progenitor MSCs. Section B, shows the positive expression of albumin (161 bp fragment) at mRNA levels in hepatocytes which was not detectable in undifferentiated MSCs. Section C, shows the expression of CYP3A4 expression (382 bp fragment)in hepatocytes which was not detected in MSCs (day 0). The protocol for hepatic differentiation and assay procedures are as described in methods.

The hepatocytes were proved to be biologically active by showing expression of hepatocyte-specific factors such as albumin, alpha-fetoprotein and cytochrom-P450. The MSCs before undergoing differentiation were also characterized by their morphology and cell surface markers.

Effects of BSO and NAC on Cell Proliferation Following Hepatogenic Differentiation

The data in Figure 2 show the results of Brdu (5-bromo-2'-deoxyuridine) assay obtained from the stem cells undergoing hepatogenic differentiation. This figure compares the relative percentage of cell proliferation after 14 days exposure to either BSO (1.0 and 5 μM) or NAC (0.1 and 1.0 μM). The cell proliferation detected based on BrdU incorporation into newly synthesized DNA. The growth of MSCs using a conventional culture medium without glutathione modifiers are considered as normal and 100% cell proliferation rate. Relative changes (increase/decrease) in the proliferation rate in presence of NAC and BSO were calculated accordingly.

Effects of NAC and BSO on GSH, GPX and GR during Hepatogenic Differentiation of MSCs

As shown in Figure 3, MSCs proliferation and hepatogenic differentiation in presence of NAC (GSH precursor) resulted in a surge in cellular total GSH calculated in terms of nmol/mg protein. Increased GSH was started immediately following hepatogenic differentiation induction. GSH was increased by average about 4, 5 and 6 folds in NAC-treated cells treated for 2, 7 and 14 days respectively compared to respective controls. Increase in GSH was time dependent but less dependent on the concentration of NAC. Under these experimental condition MSCs undergoing hepatogenic differentiation exhibited more resistance to GSH depleting agent (BSO). BSO treatments of cell undergoing hepatic differentiation with two different concentrations of BSO (1 and 5 μM) caused a significant depletion in GSH. GSH depletion in differentiating MSCs was statistically significant ($P < 0.01$) 7 and 14 days after treatment with BSO.

As shown in Figure 4, the changes in cellular glutathione peroxidase (GPX) activity in presence of BSO and NAC were in consistent with the changes in cellular total GSH. BSO (GSH depleting agent) added at two concentration to MSCs on day two of hepatogenic differentiation caused a significant inhibition in GPX activity ($P < 0.01$). This inhibition was further increased with time of differentiation process. The inhibitory effects of BSO on this enzyme was also dependent on the concentration of BSO added to the culture media. The activity of GPX was significantly induced in hepatocyte-like cells recovered 14 days after the differentiation onset ($P < 0.01$). As shown in Figure 4, the activity of GPX started to increase from day 7 of hepatogenic differentiation in cells treated with NAC.

Changes in glutathione reductase (GR) during 14 days of hepatogenic differentiation in presence of BSO or NAC showed a small but not statistically different as compared to that measured in corresponding controls (Figure 5).

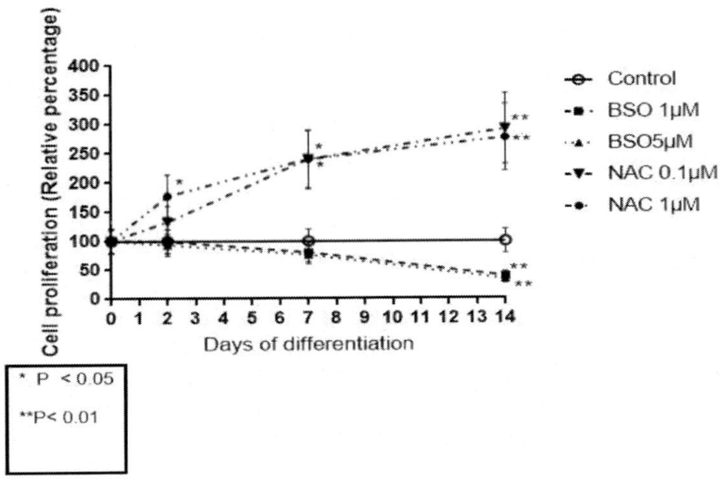

Figure 2. Effects of glutathione modifiers (BSO and NAC) on cell proliferation during hepatic differentiation of MSCs. Details about the MSCs and differentiation protocol is as described under the methods. Cell proliferation was estimated in MSC culture at different time intervals (2, 7, and 14 days) using a colorimetric bromodeoxyuridine (Brdu) kit. Each point is the mean ± SD of 3 samples. The assay was performed in cells at different time points indicated. Cell culture was supplemented with BSO or NAC and cell proliferation was calculated in relation to cell numbers in respective control groups (untreated with BSO/NAC). *sign indicates P < 0.05, statistically different from respective control group.

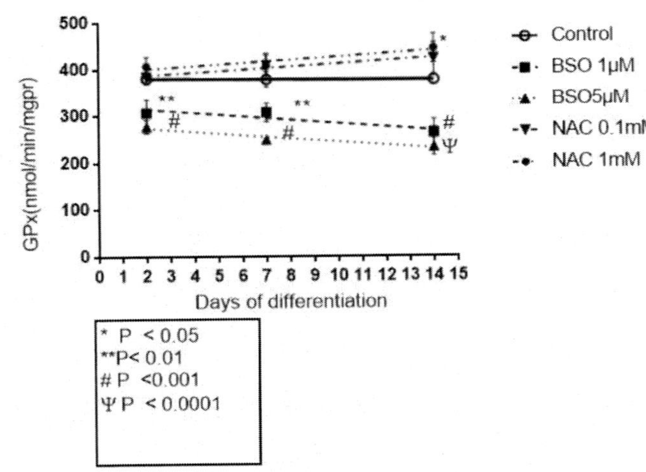

Figure 3. Changes in total glutathione in MSCs during hepatogenic differentiation due to BSO and NAC treatments. Details about the treatments and GSH estimation are described under methods section. Treated cells were exposed to BSO (1.0 and 5.0 μM)(A) or NAC (0.1 and 1.0 mM). Each point in the graph indicates the mean ± SD of 3 samples and results are presented as Mean ± SD. *P < 0.05 shows the difference between treated groups with corresponding controls.

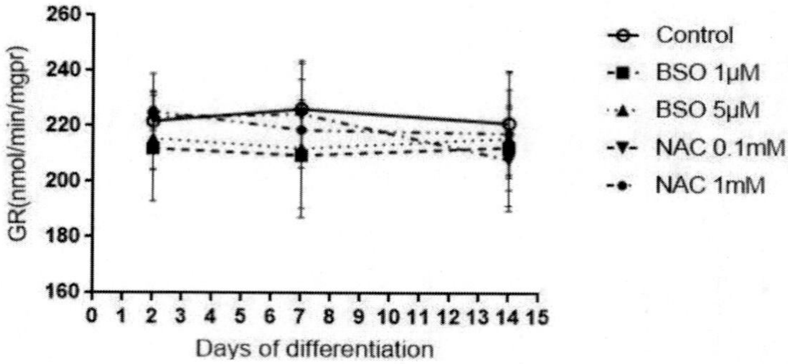

Figure 4. Glutathione peroxidase changes in MSCs undergoing hepatic differentiation in presence of BSO and NAC. Details about the treatments and GPX estimation are described under methods section. Treated cells were treated with BSO (1.0 and 5.0 μM)(A) or NAC (0.1 and 1.0 mM). Each point in the graph indicates the mean ± SD of 3 samples. *P < 0.05 shows the difference between treated groups with corresponding controls.

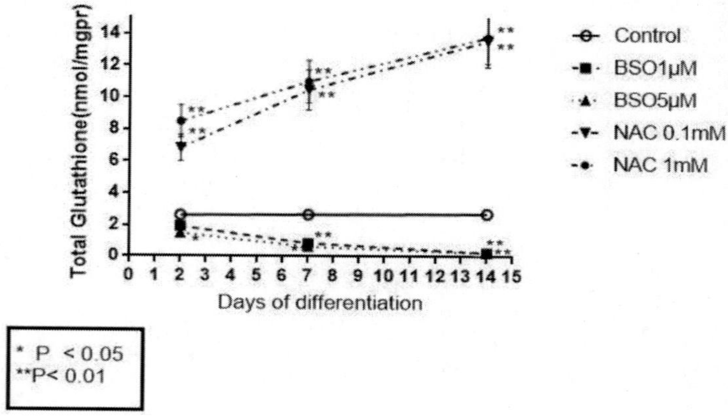

Figure 5. Effects of BSO and NAC treatments on glutathione reductase (GR) during hepatic differentiation of MSCs. Details about the treatments and GR estimation are described under methods section. Cells were treated with BSO (1.0 and 5.0 μM)(A) or NAC (0.1 and 1.0 mM). Each point in the graph indicates the mean ± SD of 3 samples and results are presented as Mean ± SD.

Alterations in Cellular ROS Levels during MSCs Differentiation into Hepatocytes

As shown in Figure 6, the cellular ROS generation in MSCs undergoing hepatogenic differentiation was significantly elevated due to BSO treatments. There was a time-dependent increase in ROS concentration (~2 fold increase; $P < 0.01$) in cells collected 14 days after differentiation onset compared to controls.

In contrast, treatment of MSCs with NAC during hepatogenic differentiation resulted in a significant decrease in ROS levels ($P < 0.05$). Decreased ROS concentration due to NAC was dependent on the concentration of NAC and changes in ROS were significant in cells recovered on days 7 and 14 of differentiation ($P < 0.05$).

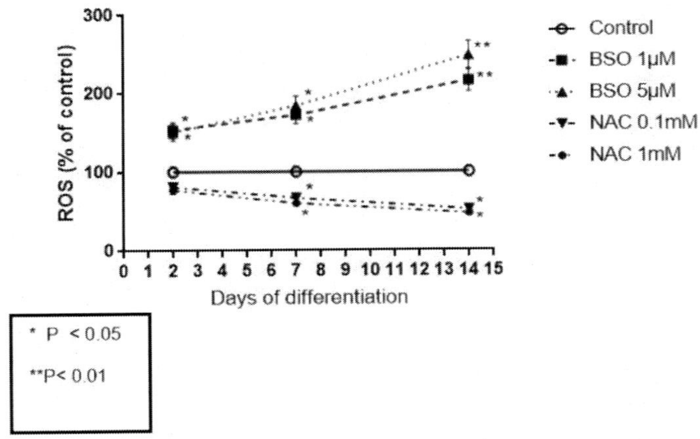

Figure 6. Changes in cellular ROS during hepatogenic differentiation of MSCs in presence of BSO and NAC. Intracellular ROS was measured after washing the cells. Cells were treated with BSO (1.0 and 5.0 μM)(A) or NAC (0.1 and 1.0 mM). Each point in the graph indicates the mean ± SD of 3 samples. *P < 0.05 shows the difference between treated groups with corresponding controls.

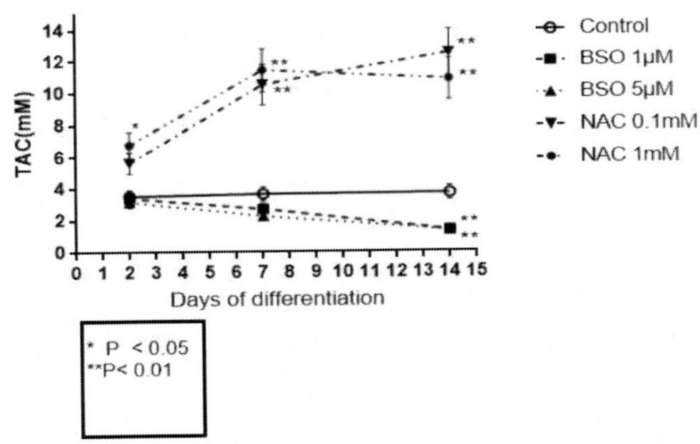

Figure 7. Total antioxidant activity of MSCs during hepatic differentiation in presence of BSO and NAC. Cells were treated with BSO (1.0 and 5.0 μM) or NAC (0.1 and 1.0 mM) before the assay. Data are mean ± SD of 3 cells samples. *P < 0.05 shows the difference between treated groups with corresponding controls.

Influence of BSO and NAC Treatments on Antioxidant Activity of MSCs during Differentiation

The influence of GSH depleting agents (BSO and NAC) on the TAC of MSCs undergoing hepatogenic differentiation is presented in Figure 7. Supplementation of the culture media with BSO resulted in a significant decrease in TAC during differentiation process. TAC suppression was independent of BSO concentration, but the decrease was more significant in cells recovered after 14 days of differentiation (P < 0.01). However there was a surge in TAC in cells treated with NAC during hepatogenic differentiation.

Discussion

Oxidative stress is characterized by deregulated production and/or scavenging of reactive oxygen and nitrogen species (ROS and RNS, respectively). ROS are primarily generated from mitochondrial complexes I and III and NADPH oxidase isoform NOX4 during MSC differentiation (Schroder et al., 2009). ROS generation at physiological levels is necessary and advantageous in order to maintain cellular proliferation, differentiation, and survival, however high levels of ROS and other free radicals can change the fate of the cells by causing damage to biomolecules (Kobayashi and Suda, 2012; D'Autr'eaux and M. B. Toledano, 2007; Atashi et al., 2015).

MSCs which undergo *in vitro* differentiation into hepatocyte-like cells is expected to undergo major morphological and functional changes. Earlier we reported that using a conventional protocol for MSC proliferation, the hepatogenic differentiation of MSCs can result is a time-course increase in lipid peroxidation products and protein carbonyl group formation. This oxidative damage to the cellular components occurs along with down-regulation of antioxidant factors namely; P53 and COX-2 (Khajeniazi et al., 2012).

Evidences show that glutathione (GSH) and GSH related enzymes with antioxidant activity play a major role in protection of cells against oxidative damage. In the present study when hepatogenic differentiation of MSCs was undertaken in presence of GSH modifiers, GSH depletion was associated with a decline in the process of MSC proliferation (Brdu assay; Figure 2). For instance, there was a significant increase in the cell proliferation and differentiation rate in culture supplemented with NAC (GSH precursor and radical scavenging agent). The role of GSH was further elucidated by showing that GSH depletion by BSO resulted in substantial increase in cellular ROS in hepatocytes differentiated from MSCs during 2-week process (Figure 6). This data is in agreement with the reports showing that in MSCs, excess ROS or induced ROS intermediates can impair self-renewal, differentiation capacity, and proliferation (Ko et al., 2012; Meagher et al., 1988; Ito et al., 2004; Alves et al., 2010).

The positive point of this study is that when GSH synthesis is induced in cells treated with NAC, the cell proliferation process was accelerated which apparently affected the hepatic differentiation of MSCs. As a consequence, there was a substantial decrease in ROS generation in hepatocytes at early stage of development. Perhaps suppression of the cellular ROS during differentiation could lead to improvement of the metabolic function of hepatocytes as shown by albumin synthesis (Allameh et al., 2014). Thus it seems that NAC treatment of MSCs that are induced for hepatic differentiation could improve the biological function of hepatocytes and confer protection against ROS-mediated oxidative damage to the cells. This data are also implicated in increasing the safety of procedures involving re-programming of the stem cells. In this connection Ji et al., 2014, reported that supplementation of the antioxidant (NAC) is associated with reduced oxidative stress during reprogramming and early passaging which results in protection of the genome of reprogramming cells from DNA damage and in the iPSCs with fewer overall genomic aberrations.

Investigation of the changes in GSH-related enzymes showed that GPX as an important antioxidant enzyme is induced in presence of NAC during hepatogenic differentiation of MSCs. As shown in Figure 3, changes in GPX were consistent with the pattern of cell proliferation and GSH levels during hepatogenic differentiation. Perhaps GSH and GSH related enzymes are considered important in protection of cells against oxidative stress which is readily inducible in cell culture, on the other hands, suppression of GSH can cause high production of ROS which can makes cells vulnerable to oxidative damages.

The evidences presented in this paper clearly show the direct effects of glutathione modifiers on MSC proliferation which is probably passed on to the hepatocytes derived from them. Evaluation of the antioxidant status of hepatocytes differentiated from MSCs under the influence of NAC is implicated in clinical applications of these cells. Expression of liver specific markers particularly albumin and CYP3A4 in hepatocytes differentiated from their progenitor stem cells in presence of NAC provide additional evidences to explain the influence of NAC or BSO on hepatic differentiation.

The imbalance in cellular GSH system and ROS production was further reflected in the antioxidant status (TAC assay) of the cells during hepatogenic differentiation. TAC was alleviated in cells treated with BSO, whereas, it was promoted when the cells were differentiation in presence of NAC (Figure 7).

Recently we have reported that the hepatogenic differentiation of MSCs derived from umbilical cord tissue using an established protocol, was associated with small changes in ATM expression and DNA damage in hepatocyte-like cells (Esmaeli et al., 2017). However, different studies suggest that depending on the antioxidant status, ROS levels in stem cells can alter the fate of the cells. According to Bigarella et al., (2014), the antioxidant machinery of the cells is maintained by various proteins such as FOXO3 (forkhead box O3), p53 [transformation related protein 53 (TRP53)], HIF1 (hypoxia-inducible factor 1) and ATM (ataxia telangiectasia mutated kinase). Quiescent and/or self-renewing stem cells display low ROS levels due to their strong antioxidant machinery, which is maintained by proteins such as FOXO3, p53 [transformation related protein 53 (TRP53)], HIF1 (hypoxia-inducible factor 1) and ATM (ataxia telangiectasia mutated kinase).

Therefore ROS as a regulatory factor in hepatic differentiation can change the fate of the stem cells. The intermediate ROS levels can prime stem cells for differentiation and some proteins such as p53 and albumin might act as pro-oxidant factors. On the other hands, high ROS levels can cause stem cell senescence and death although all the proteins responsible for senescence and cell death have not been identified.

Conclusion

Although ROS signaling plays a pivotal role in regulation of hepatogenic differentiation of stem cells, but enhancing antioxidant factor, the level of free radicals could be minimized during stem cell development. Overall results may suggest that modulation of ROS generation and TAC status during the process of hepatic differentiation of MSCs is practical by increasing GSH synthesis using NAC in the culture media. This action could be important in reducing cell damage and cell viability in large scale culture and differentiation of MSCs into other cell lineages.

Acknowledgments

This study has also been financially supported by research grant (number 958649) provided by the Elite Research Grant Committee of the NIMAD (National Institute for Medical Research Development), Ministry of Health and Medical Education, I.R. Iran.

Ethical Compliance

The authors have stated all possible conflicts of interest within this work. The authors have stated all sources of funding for this work. If this work involved human participants, informed consent was received from each individual. If this work involved human participants, it was conducted in accordance with the 1964 Declaration of Helsinki. If this work involved experiments with humans or animals, it was conducted in accordance with the related institutions' research ethics guidelines.

References

[1] Ahmadi-Ashtiani, HR, Allameh, A, Rastegar, H, Soleimani, M, Barkhordari, E. Inhibition of cyclo-oxygenase-2 and inducible nitric oxide synthase by silymarin in proliferating mesenchymal stem cell: Comparison with glutathione modifiers. *Journal of Natural Medicines*, 2012, 66, 85–94.

[2] Allameh, A, Ahmadi-Ashtiani, HR, Emami-Aleagha, MS, Rastegar, H. The metabolic function of hepatocytes differentiated from human mesenchymal stem cells is inversely related to cellular glutathione levels. *Cell biochemistry and function*, 2014, 2, 194-200.

[3] Mathan Kumar S, Haridoss M, Swaminathan K, Gopal RK, Clemens D, Dey A. The effects of changes in glutathione levels through exogenous agents on intra-

cellular cysteine content and protein adduct formation in chronic alcohol-treated VL17A cells, *Toxicology Mechanisms and Methods*, 2016; 27:2, 128-135.

[4] Allameh, A, Esmaeli, S, Kazemnejad, S, Soleimani, M. Differential expression of glutathione S-transferases P1-1 and A1-1 at protein and mRNA levels in hepatocytes derived from human bone marrow mesenchymal stem cells. *Toxicology in Vitro*, 2009, 23,674-679.

[5] Allameh, A, Kazemnejad, S. Review article: Safety evaluation of stem cells used for clinical cell therapy in chronic liver diseases; with emphasize on biochemical markers. *Clinical Biochemistry*, 2012, 45, 385-396.

[6] Atashi, F, Modarressi, M, Pepper, SP. The role of reactive oxygen species in mesenchymal stem cell adipogenic and osteogenic differentiation: A review. *Stem Cells and Development,* 2015, 24, 1150–1163.

[7] Bertolo, A, Capossela, S, Fränkl, G, Baur, M, Pötzel, T, Stoyanov, J. Oxidative status predicts quality in human mesenchymal stem cells. *Stem Cell Research & Therapy,* 2017, 8, 3.

[8] Alves, H, Munoz-Najar, U, De Wit, J, Renard, AJS, Hoeijmakers, JHJ, Sedivy, JM, Blitterswijk, CV, De Boer, J. A link between the accumulation of DNA damage and loss of multi-potency of human mesenchymal stromal cells. *Journal of Cellular and Molecular Medicine*, 2010, 14, 2729–2738.

[9] Bigarella, CL, Liang, R, Ghaffari, S. Stem cells and the impact of ROS signaling. *Development*, 2014,141,4206-4218

[10] Bonab, MM, Alimoghaddam, K, Talebian, F, Ghaffari, SH, Ghavamzadeh, A, Nikbin, B. Aging of mesenchymal stem cell *in vitro*. *BMC Cell Biology*, 2006,7,14.

[11] D'Autr'eaux, B, Toledano, MB. ROS as signaling molecules: mechanisms that generate specificity in ROS homeostasis, Nature Reviews. *Molecular Cell Biology*, 2007, 8, 813–824.

[12] Denu, RA, Hematti, P. Review Article: Effects of Oxidative Stress on Mesenchymal Stem Cell. *Biology Oxidative Medicine and Cellular Longevity,* 2016, 2016, 1-9.

[13] Esmaeli, S, Allameh, A, Adelipour, M, Allameh, M, Soleimani, M. The impact of oxidative DNA changes and ATM expression on morphological and functional activities on hepatocytes obtained from mesenchymal stem cells. *Biologicals,* 2017, 47, 52-58.

[14] Ito, K, Hirao, A, Arai, F, Matsuoka, S, Takubo, K, Hamaguchi, I, Nomiyama, K, Hosokawa, K, Sakurada, K, Nakagata, N, Ikeda, Y, Mak, TW, Suda, T. Regulation of oxidative stress by ATM is required for self-renewal of haematopoietic stem cells. *Nature*, 2004, 431,997–1002.

[15] Ji, J, Sharma, V, Qi, S, Guarch, MS, Zhao, P, Luo, Z. Antioxidant supplementation reduces genomic aberrations in human induced pluripotent stem cells. *Stem Cell Reports*, 2014, 2, 44–51.

[16] Kazemnejad, S, Allameh, A, Gharebaghian, A, Soleimani, M, Mohammadi, Y, Amirizadeh, N, Jazayeri, M. Biochemical and molecular characterization of hepatocyte-like cells derived from human bone marrow mesenchymal stem cells on a novel three-dimensional biocompatible nanofibrous scaffold. *Journal of Gastroenterology and Hepatology,* 2009, 24, 278-87.

[17] Khajeniazi, S, Allameh, A., Soleimani, M, Mortaz, E. Changes in COX-2 and oxidative damage factors during differentiation of human mesenchymal stem cells to hepatocyte-like cells is associated with downregulation of P53 gene. *Biological Chemistry*, 2013, 394, 1213-1222.

[18] Ko, E, Lee, KY, Hwang, DS. Human umbilical cord blood-derived mesenchymal stem cells undergo cellular senescence in response to oxidative stress. *Stem Cells and Development,* 2012 21, 1877–1886.

[19] Kobayashi, I, Suda, T. Regulation of reactive oxygen species in stem cells and cancer stem cells. *Journal of Cellular Physiology,* 2012, 227, 421–430.

[20] Landgraf, K, Brunauer, R, Lepperdinger, G, Grubeck-Loebenstein, B. The suppressive effect of mesenchymal stromal cells on T cell proliferation is conserved in old age. *Transplant Immunology*, 2011, 25,167–172.

[21] Meagher, RC, Salvado, AJ, Wright, DG. An analysis of the multilineage production of human hematopoietic progenitors in long-term bone marrow culture: evidence that reactive oxygen intermediates derived from mature phagocytic cells have a role in limiting progenitor cell self-renewal. *Blood,* 1988, 72, 273–281.

[22] Siegel, G, Kluba, T, Hermanutz-Klein, U, Bieback, K, Northoff, H, Schäfer, R. Phenotype, donor age and gender affect function of human bone marrow-derived mesenchymal stromal cells. *BMC Medicine*, 2013, 11,146.

[23] Schröder, K, Wandzioch, K, Helmcke, I, Brandes, RP. Nox4 acts as a switch between differentiation and proliferation in preadipocytes. *Arteriosclerosis, Thrombosis, and Vascular Biology*, 2009, 29, 239–245.

[24] Ullah, I, Subbarao, RB, Rho, GJ. Human mesenchymal stem cells -current trends and future prospective. *Bioscience reports,* 2015, 35, 1-18.

In: Manipulation of Stem Cells for Disease Benefits
Editor: Prasad Koka
ISBN: 978-1-53615-468-9

Chapter 6

The Interplay between Mesenchymal Stem Cells and MicroRNA-133 in Type 1 Diabetic Rats

***Nesma Hussein Abdel-Hay*[1], *Azza Hassan Abou Ghalia*[1], *Dalia Abdel-Wahab Mohammed*[1,*], *Ayman Ragaa Basheer*[1] *and Ansam Aly Seif*[2]**

[1]Medical Biochemistry and Molecular Biology Department, Ain-Shams University, Cairo, Egypt
[2]PhysiologyDepartment, Faculty of Medicine, Ain-Shams University, Cairo, Egypt

Abstract

Background: Stem cells created new hope in regenerative medicine for their ability to repair damaged tissues. This present study examined the effect of bone marrow-derived mesenchymal stem cells (BM-MSCs) on miRNA-133a expression, and their relation to cardiac complications in diabetic rats.

Methods: The current study included three groups of Wistar rats: control rats, type 1 diabetes rat model induced by streptozotocin (STZ), and diabetic rats treated with BM-MSCs. For all rats, fasting blood glucose (FBG), serum insulin as well as cardiovascular functions (heart rate, systolic blood pressure and electrocardiogram) were assessed. All rats were sacrificed after eight weeks. Specimens from cardiac and pancreatic tissues were examined to detect fluorescent labelled BM-MSCs, and their regenerative effect by hematoxylin and eosin stain. Expression of miRNA-133a was assessed in pancreatic and cardiac tissues by quantitative real time polymerase chain reaction (qRT-PCR).

Results: This study revealed that the body weight and serum insulin levels were increased in BM-MSC treated diabetic rats, while FBG didn't reach the euglycemic level.

* Corresponding Author's E-mail: dalia_wahab@ed.asu.edu.eg.

Moreover, improvement of systolic blood pressure and corrected QT (QTc) interval was found. The expression of miR-133a was significantly increased in pancreatic and cardiac tissues of diabetic rats, and correlated with FBG. However, there was no significant difference in its expression after treatment with BM-MSCs.

Conclusion: This study has given evidence for the first time that miR133a was expressed in pancreatic as well as cardiac tissues of diabetic rats in response to hyperglycemia. Also, BM-MSCs had the potential to improve pancreatic and cardiac functions in diabetic rats.

Keywords: type 1 diabetes mellitus, streptozotocin, miRNA-133a, BM-MSCs, cardiovascular complications

INTRODUCTION

Millions of patients, often children, suffer from type 1 diabetes mellitus (T1DM) [1]. Its incidence has increased by 2-5% worldwide, and is characterized by destruction of beta cells of pancreas causing absolute insulin deficiency [2, 3]. Macrovascular complications of diabetes include atherosclerosis in the cerebral, carotid and large arteries of the lower limbs [4]. Moreover, people suffering from diabetes are at a high risk of developing atrial fibrillation [5]. The risk of death from cardiovascular disease (CVD) is more in individuals with long standing diabetes and uncontrolled blood glucose levels [6, 7].

The pathophysiology of CVD with its risk factors, in relation to T1DM is not well understood [8].

MicroRNAs are newly discovered, non-coding regulatory RNAs, 19–23 nucleotides long that modulate gene expression [9]. They form base pairs with their own target messenger RNAs and mediate gene silencing. This ends with translational repression and regulation of multiple proteins within the same biological processes [10]. Bioinformatics analysis indicated that 30% of all mRNAs are likely to be targeted by micro RNAs [11]. Recent studies have started to unveil the powerful role of microRNAs in cardiac physiology and pathophysiology, as well as numerous forms of diseases including the pathogenesis of T1DM and its associated cardiovascular complications [10]. Many studies addressed the role of miR-133a in the pathophysiology of the heart [12]. Rawal et al. [13] reported that miR-133a is one of the most abundant microRNAs in the heart, and they investigated its crucial role in regulation of cardiac ion channels and different cardiovascular diseases. On the other hand, the role of miRNA in relation to pancreatic beta cell function, as well as its expression in the pancreas, in diabetes mellitus is not much addressed in literature. Fred et al. [14] found that miR-133a, induced by hyperglycemia, leads to beta-cell dysfunction and suppression of insulin bio-synthesis. Isaacs et al. [15] highlighted the potential roles of specific miRNAs as therapeutic and prognostic biomarkers of T1DM.

Mesenchymal stem cells (MSCs) are multipotent cells that can migrate selectively to sites of injury and differentiate into multiple cell types [16]. The recent progress in regenerative medicine-especially MSCs therapy- has suggested potential cure for T1DM [17, 18] through preserving beta cell residual mass, improving their viability and regenerating new insulin producing cells. Katuchova et al. [19] added that transplantation of bone marrow derived mesenchymal stem cells (BM-MSCs) reduces hyperglycemia, not only through direct trans-differentiation into insulin producing cells, but also through paracrine influences.

Objectives

The present study aims to investigate the expression of miR133a in pancreatic and cardiac tissues of STZ-induced diabetic rats with cardio-vascular complications, and to evaluate the effect of BM-MSCs on miR133a expression, and their potential improving action on pancreatic islet β cells and cardiac functions.

Materials and Methods

Animals

Twenty four adult male Wistar rats, purchased from an animal farm in Helwan, Cairo, Egypt, and initially weighing 150-200 g were included in the study. Animals were kept at the animal house of the Research Center at the Bilharzial Research unit, Faculty of medicine, Ain Shams University, under standard conditions of boarding: 12 h light/dark cycles, fed on standard chow, and water ad-libitum, throughout the whole period of the study. Rats were left to acclimatize for a week before any intervention. All experimental procedures were performed according to guidelines of the Institutional Animal Care and Use Ethical Committee of the Faculty.

Induction of Diabetes

To establish type 1 diabetic rat model, 35 mg/kg body weight of STZ (Sigma, St Louis, USA) were dissolved in 0.05 M citrate buffer and given as single intra-peritoneal injection [20]. Hyperglycemia was assured by biochemical analysis of blood from rat tails 3 days after induction of diabetes, using glucose strips and a standard automated glucometer (AccuChek Advantage II, Roche, Ireland). Rats were considered diabetic when the random blood glucose was above 200 mg/dL [21]. This step was repeated every week till sacrifice.

Bone Marrow-Derived Stem Cells (BM-MSCs)

These cells were obtained as readily prepared injections from the Unit of biochemistry & molecular biology [UBMB] - Cairo University.

Experiment Protocol

Rats were divided into three groups, eight rats each: Group I (Control group); in which rats received a single intraperitoneal (i.p.) injection of an equivalent amount of 0.05 M citrate buffer, Group II (Diabetic group) in which rats were rendered diabetic by receiving a single intraperitoneal (i.p.) injection of STZ dissolved in 0.05 M citrate buffer in a dose of 35 mg/kg B.W. and Group III (Diabetic group treated with BM-mesenchymal stem cells (BM-MSCs) in which rats were rendered diabetic as in group II, then, four weeks after induction of diabetes, they were treated by a single rat tail intravenous (i.v.) injection of BM- derived mesenchymal stem cells labeled with PKH-26 red fluorescent dye at a dose of 3×10^6 cells per rat [22]. All animals were sacrificed eight weeks after the start of the study. The final body weight was recorded. Samples from retro orbital venous blood were taken for biochemical studies and samples from pancreatic and cardiac tissues were taken for histological studies.

Assessment of Cardiovascular System

Arterial blood pressure was measured every two weeks throughout the experimental period using rat tail electrosphygmomanometer. The average of three arterial blood pressure readings was taken for each pressure recording. ECG was also recorded using the two channel oscillograph (Cardimax FX121, Fukuda Denshi Co., Ltd).

Biochemical Analyses

After sacrifice, fasting blood glucose (FBG) was measured using an automated analyzer (Cobas c 111-Roche, USA). Serum insulin was also detected using insulin ELISA quantitation kit (Rat, INS, Hammerwood Avenue, Sunnyvale, USA) according to the manufacturers' instructions.

Histo-Pathological Examination

The pancreas and heart were carefully dissected and the specimens were immediately immersed in 20% formalin then embedded in paraffin. Thin transverse sections were prepared and stained with hematoxylin and eosin stain [23]. Unstained pancreatic and heart tissue sections from group III were examined with a fluorescence microscope to detect the BM- derived stem cells stained with PKH26 [24].

RNA Isolation from Pancreas and Heart Tissue Samples

Total RNA was extracted from pancreas and heart tissue specimens using the miRN easy Mini kit, according to the manufacturer's instructions (Qiagen, catalog no. 217004, USA). The RNA concentration in each sample was measured by using a NanoDrop™1000 Spectrophotometer (Thermo Fisher Scientific, USA). A ratio of absorbance of 1.8–2.1 (at A260/A280) was accepted as "pure" for RNA.

Reverse transcription was performed by using MiScript RT PCR kits (Qiagen catalog no. 218161, USA) according to manufacturer's instructions by using one step real time PCR (Applied Biosystems, Singapore). Mature miRNAs were polyadenylated by poly (A) polymerase and reverse transcribed into cDNA in the tube itself by reverse transcriptase which uses oligo-dT primers with universal tag. Incubation for 60 min at 3°C was done. To inactivate miScript Reverse Transcriptase, the tubes were incubated for 5 min at 95°C, and then placed on ice. The reverse transcription reactions were stored at −20°C prior to quantitative real-time PCR (qRT-PCR).

Quantitative qRT-PCR for miRNA-133a Expression

Quantitative PCR was carried out using miScript SYBR® Green PCR Kit (Qiagen, catalog no. 218073, USA). The Primer Assays (Qiagen, Germany) were used to amplify miR-133a and SNORD68 as an endogenous reference control. Each primer sequence was derived from NCBI reference sequence data base (https://www.ncbi.nlm.nih.gov/refseq/). Primer sequence for miR-133a was (5'AGCUGGUAAAA UGGAACCAAAU3'). Forty cycles were used, each with denaturation at 94°C for 15 s, annealing 55°C for 30s, and extension at 70°C for 30 s. The expression of miR-133a was defined based on the cycle threshold (Ct). The relative expression levels of miR-133a were calculated as $2^{-\Delta\Delta Ct}$ after normalization to the expression of SNORD68 content in each examined tissue sample [25]. Melting curves were performed to check specificity of PCR products.

Statistical Analysis

The Statistical Package for Social Science version 20 (SPSS Software, SPSS Inc., Chicago, IL, USA) was used to analyze the data. The results were expressed as mean, standard deviation, median and mean rank, and the level of statistical significance was set at $p < 0.05$.

RESULTS

Body Weight, Blood Glucose, and Insulin

Initially, body weight was similar in the three studied groups. Body weight and serum insulin were significantly decreased in diabetic group as compared to the control group. Treatment with BM-MSCs in STZ/ MSC group caused significant increase in the body weight and serum insulin level compared to the diabetic untreated group (Table 1).

Cardiovascular Parameters

Systolic blood pressure was elevated, and QTc interval was prolonged significantly in the diabetic group compared to the control group. These parameters were improved in treated rats, after four weeks of transplantation of BM-MSCs. However, no significant difference was found in the heart rate of the three studied groups (Table 1, Figure 1).

Table 1. Body weight, fasting blood glucose, insulin levels and cardiovascular parameters: Systolic blood pressure (Systolic BP), corrected QT interval (QTc) and heart rate in the studied groups

	Body weight (grams) Mean ± SD	**FBG(mg/dl)**		**Insulin (mIU/L) Mean ± SD**	**Systolic BP (mmHg) Mean ± SD**	**QTc interval (seconds) Mean ± SD**	**Heart rate (beats/min.) Mean ± SD**
		Median (mg/dl)	Mean rank				
Control (n = 8)	339 ± 11.5	88.5	4.5	7.4 ± 2.2	101.7 ± 22.9	0.3 ± 0.01	201.6 ± 18.2
STZ (n = 8)	158 ± 11.5 [a]	404	12.33 [a]	4.4 ± 1.4 [a]	127 ± 12.7 [a]	0.4 ± 0.03 [a]	192.1 ± 29.7
STZ/MSC (n = 8)	232.3 ± 62 [a b]	270.5	11.6 [a]	8.6 ± 1.3 [b]	93 ± 21.9[b]	0.3 5 ± 0.03 [b]	212.6 ± 19.9

[a:] Significance from control group ($P < 0.05$).
[b:] Significance from diabetic (STZ) group ($P < 0.05$).

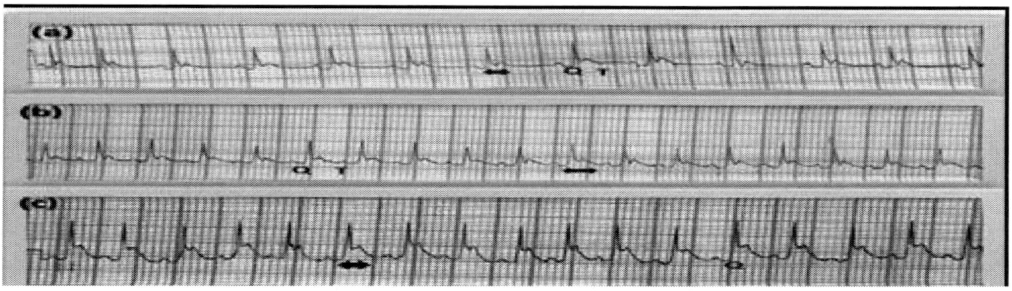

Figure 1. Electrocardiogram showing corrected QT (QTc) interval in the three studied groups; (a) The QTc interval in the control group was 0.24 seconds, (b) whereas in the diabetic (STZ) group, it was significantly prolonged and became 0.45 seconds. (c) Four weeks after injection of MSCs into the STZ induced diabetes; the QTc interval was significantly shortened and became 0.26 seconds.

Analysis of MicroRNA-133a Expression in Pancreatic and Cardiac Tissues

Using quantitative real time PCR (qRT-PCR), the expression of miR-133a was significantly higher in the pancreatic and cardiac tissue specimens obtained from diabetic untreated rats as compared to the control group. Treatment with BM-MSCs didn't significantly affect the expression of miR133a as compared to the diabetic group (Figure 2). Using Spearman's correlation test, there was a significant positive correlation between miR133a expression in pancreatic tissue samples and the FBG level (Figure 3). However, no significant correlation could be found between expression of miR133a and all other studied parameters.

Histological Examination

Homing of the PKH26 labeled BM-MSCs into the injured pancreatic and cardiac tissues appeared as strong red sporadic auto-fluorescence in both Pancreatic (Figure 4A), and cardiac (Figure 4B) tissue specimens obtained from STZ/ MSC group. This confirms homing of these stem cells into the injured cardiac tissues.

The normal architecture of pancreatic tissue specimens from the control group appeared with the hematoxylin and eosin (H&E) staining as exocrine acini (A) and endocrine islets of Langerhans (I) interlacing with a network of ducts (D) and blood vessels.

The endocrine islets of Langerhans were dispersed randomly between the acini as groups of pale stained cells with rounded nuclei. Ducts were interposed between the acini, lined by a single layer of columnar cells, and surrounded by connective tissue (Figure 5A, D).

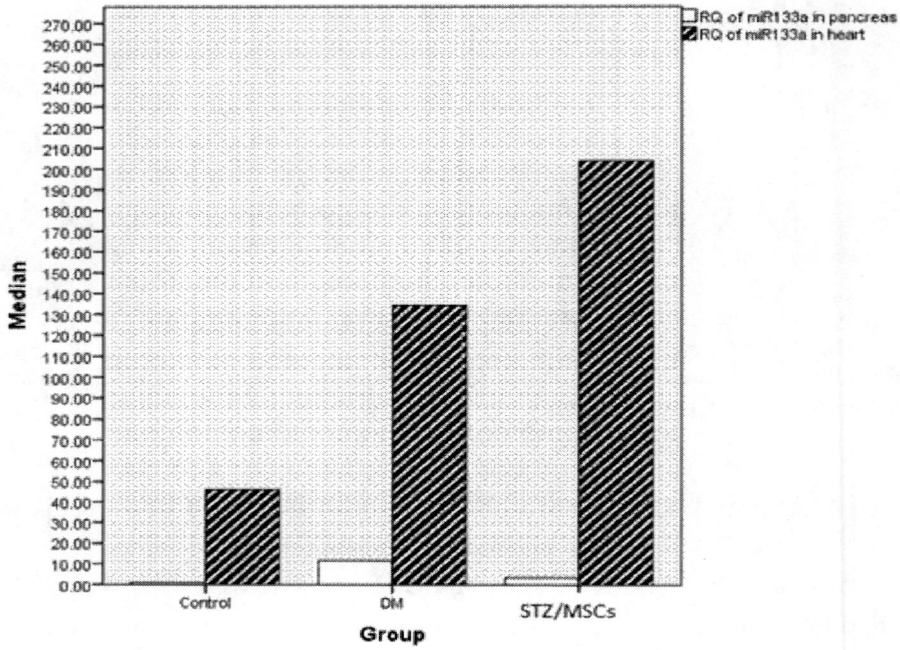

Figure 2. Expression of miR 133a in pancreatic and cardiac tissues obtained from the three studied groups using qRT- PCR.

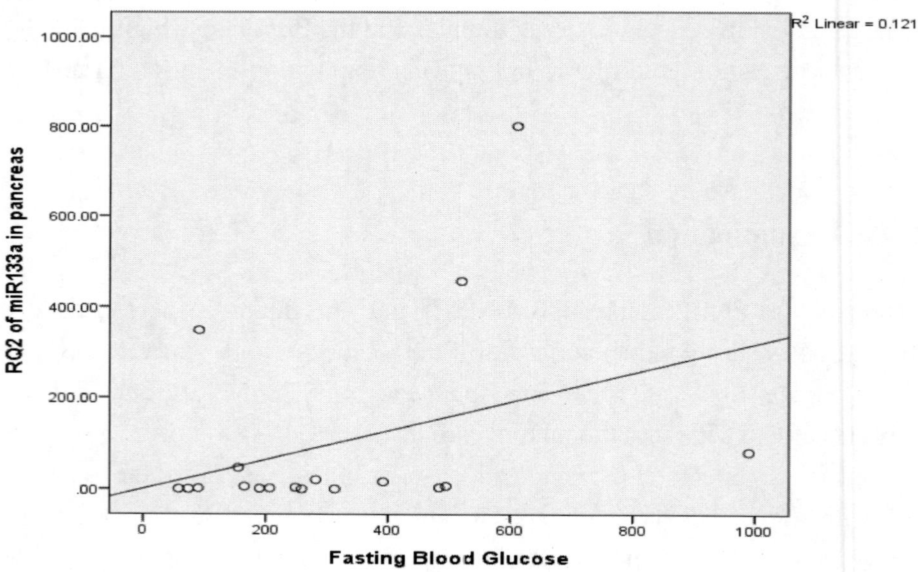

Figure 3. The correlation between the miR133 expression in pancreas and the fasting blood glucose level. A significant positive correlation was found between the two parameters (P < 0.05).

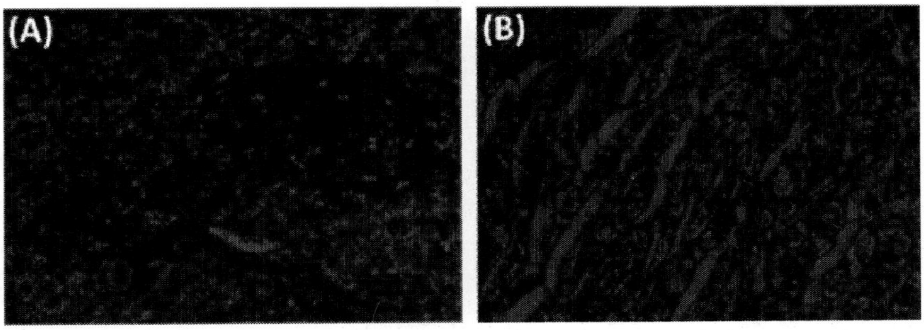

Figure 4. Fluorescent microscope examination of tissue specimens from stem cell treated (STZ/MSC) group showed the PKH26 labeled bone marrow derived mesenchymal stem cells as strong red sporadic auto-fluorescence. This confirms homing of these stem cells into the injured cardiac tissues.
A): Pancreas, (B): Heart.

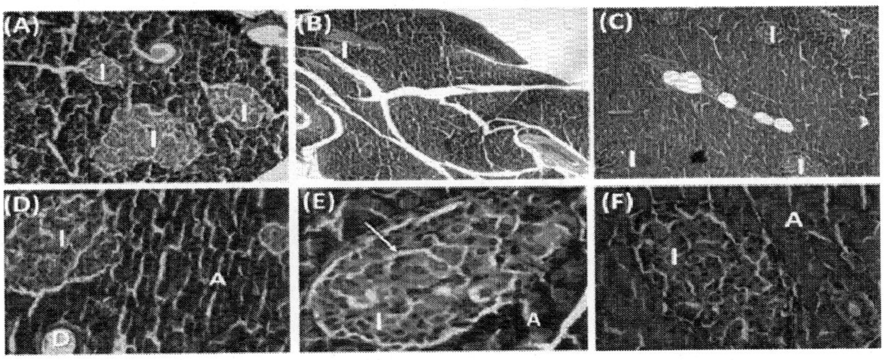

Figure 5. Histopathological examination of photomicrograph of pancreatic tissues stained with Hematoxylin and Eosin [×100]: (A) control, (B) STZ, (C) STZ/MSC groups; [×400]: (D) control, (E) STZ, (F) STZ/MSC groups; Abbreviations: A, acini; I, islets of Langerhans; D, ducts. (A) Normal pancreas showing number of islets of Langerhans (I) by low power field. (B) STZ group: the number of islets of Langerhans per low power field markedly decreased as compared to control group. (C) STZ/MSC group: the number of islets per low power field was increased as compared to STZ group. (D) Normal pancreatic architecture; exocrine acini (A) and endocrine islets of Langerhans (I) (E) Pancreatic tissue from diabetic group showed marked degenerative changes in islets which appear as vacuolations (arrow) and pyknotic nuclei. (F) Pancreatic tissue of treated group showed marked improvement in pancreatic architecture and more vesicular active nuclei.

In STZ group; their number was markedly decreased as detected by low power field as compared to the normal specimens from the control group (hyperactive). Moreover, the degenerative changes were confined mainly to the islet cells (I) in the form of large areas of degeneration and vacuolation. The islet cells showed pyknotic nuclei (dead) alternating with lightly stained vacuolated nuclei (Figure 5B, E).

In STZ/MSC group; 4 weeks after transplantation of BM-MSCs, islets (I) number was markedly increased as detected by low power field as compared to the specimens from the diabetic group Moreover, the pancreas showed partial improvement in its morphology. The islets (I) appeared well defined, highly cellular with prominent vesicular nuclei. (Figure 5C, F).

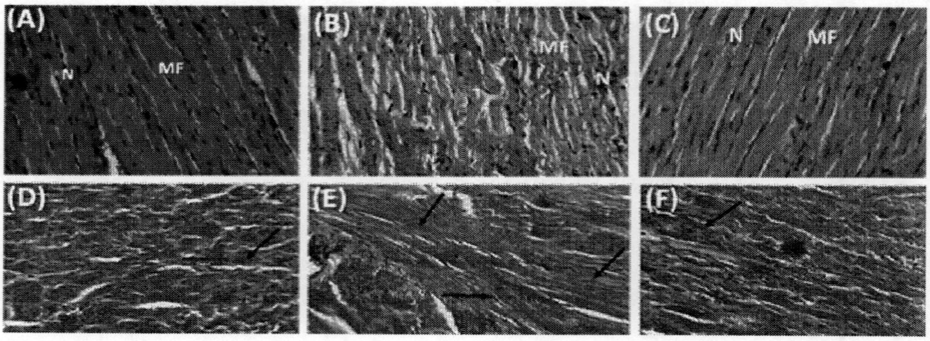

Figure 6. Histopathological examination of photomicrograph of cardiac tissues stained with Hematoxylin and Eosin [×400]: (A) control, (B) STZ, (C) STZ/MSC groups; Photomicrographs of Masson's Trichrome-stained [×400] heart sections of (D) control, (E) STZ, (F) STZ/MSC groups. Abbreviations: MF, Myofibrils; N, Nuceli. (A) Normal cardiac tissue showed regularly arranged cardiac myofibrils (MF) with central nuclei (N). (B) Cardiac tissue from diabetic group showed disarray myofibrils and deformed nuclei. (C) Cardiac tissue from treated group showed more arranged myofibrils (MF) and central nuclei (N) more like the control group. (D) Normal cardiac sections stained with Masson's Trichrome showed normal distribution and normal amount of collagen fibers stained dark blue (arrow). (E) Diabetic rats exhibited excessive fibrous tissue deposition; cardiac muscle fibers almost replaced by fibrous tissues stained dark blue (arrow). (F) MSCs treated rats' cardiac sections revealed mild interstitial fibrosis, which is restricted to small patches (arrow).

Cardiac tissue specimens from the control group stained with H&E appeared as regularly arranged cardiac myofibrils (MF) with single, oval and centrally located nuclei (N) (Figure 6A). In STZ group, the cardiomyocytes showed marked degenerative changes with deformation in sizes, shapes and with the some vesicular active nuclei (Figure 6B). Marked improvement was observed after transplantation of BM-MSCs as the myocytes had regularly arranged MF with centrally located nuclei (Figure 6C). Masson's Trichrome stained cardiac tissues showed normal distribution and normal amount of collagen fibers in control group (Figure 6D), while diabetic rats exhibited excessive fibrous tissue deposition; cardiac muscle fibers almost replaced by fibrous tissues (Figure 6E). However, MSCs treated rats cardiac sections revealed mild interstitial fibrosis, which is restricted to small patches (Figure 6F).

Discussion

As the prevalence of diabetes is increasing worldwide at an alarming rate, it became the 3rd human killer following cancer and cardiovascular disease [1]. In 2017, the International Diabetes Federation estimated that 425 million people were suffering from DM globally [26]. Meanwhile, it has been suggested that certain miRNAs contribute to the pathogenesis of diabetes and may control pancreatic β-cell function [15]. BM-MSCs are capable of homing to specific tissues and differentiation, with stimulation of local repair of damaged tissues, also were used to cure intractable diseases in clinical trials [1, 27]. Thus, their use created hope to regenerate and restore disturbed cell functions [1].

The present study aimed to evaluate the effect of BM-MSCs on cardiac and pancreatic functions, as well as their relation to miRNA 133a expression in rats with diabetic cardiovascular complications. The current study was interested to check the regenerative capacity of BM-MSC on the pancreatic and cardiac functions. Meanwhile, a non - invasive aid for recovery from diabetes was used to inject MSCs. The MSCs were injected into the systemic circulation (rat tail vein) rather than direct injection into these organs, the same as performed by El-Asmar et al. [24], Abdel Aziz et al. [28] and Nakano et al. [29]. The effect of MSCs on the insulin level in STZ diabetic rats is controversial till now [30, 31, 32, 33]. However, the results of the present study revealed that insulin was significantly increased in STZ diabetic rats after treatment with BM-MSCs. This increase in insulin levels might be due to improvement in the pancreatic microenvironment and a shift from pro-inflammatory to anti-inflammatory cytokine expression and secretion [17]. The regenerative ability of BM-MSCs was supported, in this study, by their homing into pancreatic tissues, as shown by fluorescent microscope, as well as by the increased number of islets and improved cellular architecture in H&E stained section. Furthermore, the current results revealed that transplantation of undifferentiated BM-MSCs increased the body weight ($P < 0.05$), and reduced the elevated FBG ($P > 0.05$) in diabetic rats. The lack of return of FBG to the euglycemic level could be attributed to the increased production of free radicals as reported by Mohamed et al. [34] and/or the very high levels of cytokines/ chemokines as Monnerat-Cahli et al. [31] in response to streptozotocin injection. Consequently, we hypothesized that transplantation of BM-MSCs may become more efficient to restore the antioxidant defense, and the function of pancreatic islet cells by one or all the following approaches: a) use of multiple doses of MSCs [22]; b) increasing the dose of MSCs as happened with previous studies [16, 31]; c) use differentiated rather than undifferentiated MSCs [34]; d) direct injection of MSCs into the pancreas [19]. Cardiovascular disease is a major macrovascular complication of diabetes mellitus [35]. In this context, several studies investigated the anti-diabetic benefits of BM-MSCs. Based on the fluorescence microscopic examination and H&E staining, the current study supported the notion that stem cells, after their homing into the heart, were capable of scavenging the myocardium from permanent damage.

As a consequence of energy unbalance seen in diabetes, down regulation of some important cardiac kinases like AMP-activated protein kinase (AMPK) and extracellular signal-regulated kinase 1(ERK1) needed for the normal electrophysiological and mechanical cardiac function have been reported [31, 36, 37]. Also, Pei et al. [37] speculated that transplantation of MSCs may normalize the expression and activity of cardiac AMPK. To further assess the cardiac benefits promoted by MSCs therapy, the blood pressure, heart rate and corrected QT (QTc) interval were measured every 2 weeks throughout the study duration. The results revealed that 4 weeks after MSCs therapy the systolic blood pressure and the QTc interval were improved in STZ/MSC group compared to the STZ group. The decrease in heart rate found in STZ diabetic rats was improved after MSCs therapy, yet with no significant difference ($P > 0.05$). This was supported by the findings of Abdel Aziz et al. [32] and El Said et al. [33], and may indicate partial improvement in systemic metabolic profile with subsequent changes in various cardiac intracellular signaling networks the same as reported by Monnerat-Cahli et al. [31].

A part from the bradycardia, detected in STZ diabetic rats, no other arrhythmias were observed in any of the studied animals. Consequently, further studies with longer duration and higher dose of MSCs may reveal a full benefit from these transplanted cells. MicroRNAs as regulators of protein expression are an evolving research field. By binding to mRNAs, they can induce translational repression leading to lowered protein levels [9]. Target scan software predicted 400- 500 putative miR 133a mRNA targets [38]. In the heart, the most abundant miRNA is miR-133a [12]. It has an essential role in cardiac development, function, and regeneration of cardiomyocytes [39]. Diabetes caused remarkable overexpression of miR133a in cardiac tissues [40]. In accordance with the findings of Xiao et al. [40], the present study revealed significant increase in miR 133a expression in cardiac tissues of diabetic rats, which was correlated with the FBG concentration ($P < 0.05$). Furthermore, it was reported that miR 133a regulates cardiac ion channels. It binds to the 3` UTR of KCNQ1 mRNA that en-codes, Kv7, the pore-forming subunit of the voltage–gated potassium channel, thus slow repolarization, ending in QT prolongation [12, 38, 40, 41]. Consequently, the prolonged QTc interval encountered in untreated diabetic rats, in the present study, can be further explained by the significant increase of miR133a in cardiac tissues of these rats. It was proposed that at least three different miRNAs, including miR 133a, may control translation of insulin mRNA by regulating the expression of polypyrimidine tract binding (PTB) protein in cultured human beta cells [14]. PTB stabilizes insulin mRNA by binding to its 3`untranslated region (UTR), as well as mRNA of proteins involved in insulin secretion [42]. Data about the expression of miR133a in pancreatic tissues of T1DM are scarce. To our knowledge, the present study has given evidence for the first time about the expression of miR 133a in pancreatic tissues of STZ-induced diabetic rats. The results indicated significant positive correlation between miR133a expression in both pancreatic and cardiac tissue samples ($P < 0.05$). Moreover, the positive correlation between FBG and miR 133a found in this study ($P < 0.05$) may be supported by the finding of Fred et al. [14] that prolonged periods of high blood glucose induces miR 133a, in cultured human pancreatic beta cells, with subsequent down regulation of polypyrimidine tract binding (PTB) mRNA and decrease of PTB protein levels. They proposed that this mechanism may explain the dysfunction of pancreatic β cells. The same authors also assumed that uncoupling protein (UCP)-2 is another target of miR 133a, and lowering of its activity results in higher ROS production [14]. Based on the aforesaid findings, the current study suggested that the increase of miR 133a in response to hyperglycemia may be one of the causes of glucotoxicity induced by STZ. Unfortunately, transplantation of BM-MSCs was not able to restore the normal expression level of miR 133a both in pancreatic and cardiac tissues. In contrast, the finding of Chen et al. [43] that miR-133 overexpression enhanced the therapeutic effect of MSCs by suppressing their apoptosis, and mediating their paracrine effects needs further studies to be assessed. In summary, the current study highlights that miR 133a was overexpressed in pancreatic and cardiac tissues of STZ induced diabetic rats, and correlated with the FBG concentration. The increase of miR 133a may explain the abnormalities of insulin, body weight, systolic blood pressure and QTc interval in these rats. Also, the results reinforced the evidence that intravenously injected BM-MSCs were able to home, and have the potential for regeneration of pancreatic β-cells, cardiac tissues, and correction of some of T1DM associated cardiovascular complications. On the other hand, the protocol of BM-MSCs transplantation used in the current study was insufficient to correct the hyperglycemia induced overexpression of miR 133a.

Conclusion

Based on the notion that miRNAs exhibit remarkable stability and protection from endogenous nucleases, this study hypothesized that circulating miR 133a may become an additional biomarker in diagnosis and/or follow up of cardiovascular complications encountered with T1DM. Also, modulation of miR 133a expression and activity using miR 133a inhibitors may facilitate prevention and treatment of T1DM cardiovascular complications. Further studies, combining BM-MSC with miR 133 inhibitors, are clearly needed to confirm that the observed improvement in body weight, serum insulin as well as some of the investigated cardiac functions were due to the effect of the injected MSCs rather than a change in miR 133a expression. Moreover, the effect of BM-MSc on the apoptotic and inflammatory processes induced by STZ needs to be explored in the future studies.

Acknowledgments

This work was supported by Ain Shams Faculty of Medicine Grant's office; *Grants No 2017/16*. All authors shared efforts in the present study. They all read and approved the final manuscript and agreed on publication.

Ethical Compliance

The authors have stated all possible conflicts of interest within this work. The authors have stated all sources of funding for this work. If this work involved human participants, informed consent was received from each individual. If this work involved human participants, it was conducted in accordance with the 1964 Declaration of Helsinki. If this work involved experiments with humans or animals, it was conducted in accordance with the related institutions' research ethics guidelines.

References

[1] Domouky AM, Hegab AS, Al-Shahat A, Raafat N. Mesenchymal stem cells and differentiated insulin producing cells are new horizons for pancreatic regeneration in type I diabetes mellitus. *Int J Biochem Cell Biol.* 2017; 87:77-85.

[2] Shojaeian A, Mehri-Ghahfarrokhi A. An overview of the epidemiology of type 1 Diabetes Mellitus. *Int J Metab Syndr.* 2018; 2: 001-004.

[3] American Diabetes Association. Diagnosis and classification of diabetes mellitus. *Diabetes Care*. 2018; 41:S13–S27.

[4] Adams TD, Arterburn DE, Nathan DM, Eckel RH. Clinical outcomes of metabolic surgery: microvascular and macrovascular complications. *Diabetes Care*. 2016; 39: 912-923.

[5] Sun Y, Hu D. The link between diabetes and atrial fibrillation: cause or correlation? *J Cardiovasc Dis Res*. 2010; 1:10–11.

[6] De Rosa S, Arcidiacono B, Chiefari E, Brunetti A, Indolfi C, Foti DP. Type 2 Diabetes Mellitus and Cardiovascular Disease: Genetic and Epigenetic Links. *Frontiers in Endocrinology*. 2018; 9, 2.

[7] Lee SI, Patel M, Jones CM, Narendran P. Cardio-vascular disease and type 1 diabetes: prevalence, prediction and management in an ageing population. *Ther Adv Chronic Dis*. 2015; 6:347-374.

[8] de Ferranti SD, de Boer IH, Fonseca V, Fox CS, Golden SH, Lavie CJ, Magge SN, Marx N, McGuire DK, Orchard TJ, et al. Type 1 diabetes mellitus and cardio-vascular disease: a scientific statement from the American Heart Association and American Diabetes Association. *Diabetes Care*. 2014; 37:2843-2863.

[9] Galatenko VV, Galatenko AV, Samatov TR., Turchinovich AA, Shkurnikov MY, Makarova JA, Tonevitsky AG. Comprehensive network of miRNA-induced intergenic interactions and a biological role of its core in cancer. *Scientific Reports.* 2 018; 8:2418.

[10] Zampetaki A, Willeit P, Burr S, Yin X, Langley SR, Kiechl S, Klein R, Rossing P, Chaturvedi N, Mayr M. Angiogenic microRNAs Linked to Incidence and

Progression of Diabetic Retinopathy in Type 1 Diabetes. *Diabetes.* 2016; 65:216-227.

[11] Mazzoccoli G, Colangelo T, Panza A, Rubino R., Tiberio C, Palumbo O, Carella M, Trombetta D, Gentile A, Tavano, F, Valvano MR. Analysis of clock gene-miRNA correlation networks reveals candidate drivers in colorectal cancer. *Oncotarget.* 2016; 7:45444- 45461.

[12] Hedley PL, Carlsen AL, Christiansen KM, Kanters JK, Behr ER, Corfield VA, Christiansen M. MicroRNAs in cardiac arrhythmia: DNA sequence variation of MiR-1 and MiR-133A in long QT syndrome. *Sc and J Clin and Lab Invest.* 2014; 74: 485-491.

[13] Rawal S, Manning P, Katare R. Cardiovascular microRNAs: as modulators and diagnostic biomarkers of diabetic heart disease. *Cardiovasc Diabetol.* 2014; 13:44.

[14] Fred RG, Bang-Berthelsen CH, Mandrup-Poulsen T, Grunnet LG and Welsh N. High glucose suppresses human islet insulin biosynthesisby inducing miR133a leading to decreased poly-pyrimidine tract binding protein-expression. *PLoS One.* 2010; 5:e10843.

[15] Isaacs SR, Wang J, Kim KW, Yin C, Zhou L, Mi QS, Craig ME. MicroRNAs in type 1 diabetes: complex interregulation of the immune system, β cell function and viral infections. *Current Diabetes Reports.* 2016; 16: 133.

[16] Bhansali S, Kumar V, Saikia UN, Medhi B, Jha V, Bhansali A, Dutta P. Effect of mesenchymal stem cells transplantation on glycaemic profile and their localization in streptozotocin induced diabetic Wistar rats. *Indian J Med R*es. 2015; 142:63-71.

[17] Ezquer F, Ezquer M, Contador D, Ricca M, Simon V, Conget P. The antidiabetic effect of mesenchymal stem cells is unrelated to their transdifferentiation potential but to their capability to restore Th1/Th2 balance and to modify the pancreatic microenvironment. *Stem Cells.* 2012; 30:1664-1674.

[18] Wu XX, Shao JZ, Xiang C. Generation of pancreatic β cells from mesenchymal stem cells to treat type 1 diabetes. *OA Stem Cells.* 2014; 2:5.

[19] Katuchova J, Harvanova D, Spakova T, Kalanin R, Farkas D, Durny P, Rosocha J, Radonak J, Petrovic D, Siniscalco D et al. Mesenchymal stem cells in the treatment of type 1 diabetes mellitus. *Endocr Pathol.* 2015; 26:95-103.

[20] Sai Varsha MK, Raman T, Manikandan R and Dhanasekaran G. Hypoglycemic action of vitamin K1 protects against early-onset diabetic nephropathy in streptozotocin-induced rats. *Nutrition.* 2015; 31: 1284-1292.

[21] Ventura-Sobrevilla J, Boone-Villa VD, Aguilar CN, Roman-12. Ramos R, Vega-Avila E, Campos-Sepulveda E, Alarcón-Aguilar F. Effect of varying dose and administration of streptozotocin on blood sugar in male CD1 mice. *Proc West Pharmacol Soc.* 2011; 54: 5-9.

[22] Wassef Ma, Fouad H, Sabry D, Afifi N. Use of Differentiated Mesenchymal Stem Cells in Experimental Diabetes Type 1 in Rats. *Med. J. Cairo Univ*. 2015, 83: 1129-1134.

[23] Achliya, GS, Kotagale, NR, Wadodkar SG, Dorle AK. Hepatoprotective activity of Panchagavya Ghrita against carbon tetra chloride induced hepatotoxcity in rats. *Indian Journal of Pharmacology*. 2003; 35: 308-311.

[24] El Asmar MF, Atta HM, Mahfouz S, Fouad HH, Roshdy NK, Rashed LA, Sabry D, Hassouna AA, Taha FM. Efficacy of mesenchymal stem cells in suppression of hepatocarcinorigenesis in rats: possible role of Wnt signaling. *Journal of Experimental & Clinical Cancer Research*. 2011; 30(1):49.

[25] Livak KJ, Schmittgen TD. Analysis of relative gene expression data using real-time quantitative PCR and the 2(-ΔΔCT) method. *Methods.* 2001; 25: 402 - 408.

[26] International Diabetes Federation. 2017; *IDF Diabetes Atlas*, 8th edition. Brussels.

[27] Mathiasen AB, Qayyum AA, Jorgensen E, Helqvist S, Fischer-Nielsen A, Kofoed KF, Haack-Sørensen M, Ekblond A, Kastrup J. Bone marrow-derived mesenchymal stromal cell treatment in patients with severe ischaemic heart failure: A randomized placebo-controlled trial (MSC-HF trial). *Eur Heart J.* 2015; 36: 1744–1753.

[28] Abdel Aziz MT, Wassef MA, Ahmed HH, Rashed L, Mahfouz S, Aly MI, Hussein RE, Abdelaziz M. The role of bone marrow derived-mesenchymal stem cells in attenuation of kidney function in rats with diabetic nephropathy. *Diabetology & Metabolic Syndrome*. 2014; 6(1):34.

[29] Nakano M, Nagaishi K, Konari N, Saito Y, Chikenji T, Mizue Y, Fujimiya M. Bone marrow-derived mesen-chymal stem cells improve diabetes-induced cognitive impairment by exosome transfer into damaged neurons and astrocytes. *Scientific Reports*. 2016;6:24805.

[30] Boumaza I, Srinivasan S, Witt WT, Feghali-Bostwick C, Dai Y, Garcia-Ocana A, Feili-Hariri M. Autologous bone marrow-derived rat mesenchymal stem cells promote PDX-1 and insulin expression in the islets, alter T cell cytokine pattern and preserve regulatory T cells in the periphery and induce sustained normoglycemia. *J Autoimmun*. 20009; 32:33–42.

[31] Monnerat-CahliG, Trentin-Sonoda M, Guerra B, Manso G, Ferreira AC, Silva DL, Coutinho DC, Carneiro-Ramos MS, Rodrigues DC, Cabral-da-Silva MC et al. Bone marrow mesenchymal stromal cells rescue cardiac function in streptozotocin-induced diabetic rats. *Int J Cardiol.* 2014; 171:199-208.

[32] Abdel Aziz MT, El-Asmar MF, Haidara M, Atta HM, Roshdy NK, Rashed LA, Sabry D, Youssef MA, Aziz AT, Moustafa M. Effect of bone marrow-derived mesenchymal stem cells on cardiovascular complications in diabetic rats. *Med Sci Monit*. 2008; 14: BR 249-255.

[33] El Said HE, Gabr HM, Ammar RI. The Effect of human bone marrow mesenchymal stem cells on diabetic heart failure rats. *Life Sci J.* 2013; 10:3413-3425.

[34] Mohamed A, Gabr MM, El-Halawani SM, Ibrahim RY, Khater SM, Refaie AF, Ghoneim MA. Novel evidence of restoring and augmenting antioxidant defense after treatment of diabetic rats using stem cells. *Curr Top Biochem Res.* 2012; 14, 25-37.

[35] Ding Y, Sun X, Shan PF. MicroRNAs and cardiovascular disease in diabetes mellitus. *Biomed Res Int.* 2017:4080364.

[36] Murça TM, Moraes PL, Capuruço CA, Santos SH, Melo MB, Santos RA, Shenoy V, Katovich MJ, Raizada MK, Ferreira AJ. Oral administration of an angiotensin-converting enzyme 2 activator ameliorates diabetes-induced cardiac dysfunction. *Regul Pept.* 2012; 177: 107–115.

[37] Pei H, Qu Y, Lu X, Yu Q, Lian K, Liu P, Yan W, Liu J, Ma Y, Liu Y, Li C. Cardiac-derived adiponectin induced by long-term insulin treatment ameliorates myocardial ischemia/reperfusion injury in type 1 diabetic mice via AMPK signaling. *Basic Res Cardiol.* 2013; 108: 322.

[38] Matkovich SJ, Wang W, T u Y, E schenbacher WH, Dorn LE, Condorelli G, Diwan A, Nerbonne JM, Dorn GW. MicroRNA-133a protects against myocardial fibrosis and modulates electrical repolarization without affecting hypertrophy in pressure-overloaded adult hearts. *Circ Res.* 2010; 106:166-175.

[39] Navickas R, Gal D, Laucevičius A, Taparauskaitė A, Zdanytė M, Holvoet P. Identifying circulating microRNAs as biomarkers of cardiovascular disease: a systematic review. *Cardiovasc Res.* 2016; 111:322–337.

[40] Xiao J, Luo X, Lin H, Zhang Y, Lu Y, Wang N, Zhang Yang B and Wang Z. MicroRNA miR-133 represses HERG K+ channel expression contributing to QT prolongation in diabetic hearts. *J Biol Che.* 2007; 282, 12363– 12367.

[41] Torekov SS, Iepsen E, Christiansen M, Linneberg A, Pedersen O, Holst JJ, Kanters JK and Hansen T. KCNQ1 long QT syndrome patients have hyper-insulinemia and symptomatic hypoglycemia. *Diabetes.* 2014; 63:1315-1325.

[42] Knoch KP, Bergert H, Borgonovo B, Saeger HD, Altkrüger A, Verkade P, Solimena M. Polypyrimidine tract-binding protein promotes insulin secretory granule biogenesis. *Nat Cell Biol.* 2004; 6: 207–214.

[43] Chen Y, Zhao Y, Chen W, Xie L, Zhao ZA, Yang J, Chen Y, Lei W, Shen Z. MicroRNA-133 over-expression promotes the therapeutic efficacy of mesenchymal stem cells on acute myocardial infarction. *Stem cell research and therapy.* 2017; 8:2.

In: Manipulation of Stem Cells for Disease Benefits
Editor: Prasad Koka
ISBN: 978-1-53615-468-9

Chapter 7

EFFECTIVE ENDODERMAL INDUCTION VIA VITRONECTIN-COATED FEEDER-FREE CULTURE

Riham Aly[1,2,*], Takako Yamamoto[3], Chiemi Takenaka[3], Etsu Murakami[3], Mao Arita[3], Miyuki Nakamura[3] and Shin Kawamata[3]

[1]Basic Dental Science Department, Oral and Dental Research Division, National Research Centre, Dokki, Cairo, Egypt

[2]Stem Cell Laboratory, Centre of Excellence for Advanced Sciences, National Research Centre, Dokki, Cairo, Egypt

[3]Foundation Biomedical Research and Innovation (FBRI), Research and Development Center for Cell Therapy, Chuo-ku, Kobe, Japan

ABSTRACT

Current comprehension of endoderm organ development has enabled researchers to successfully direct pluripotent stem cells (PSCs) to differentiate into endodermal lineage which can give rise to cells of the lungs, liver, pancreas, stomach, and intestine. Nevertheless, variations in the differentiation efficiency have been reported mainly due the utilization of poorly defined matrices in the protocols applied. On this basis, the present study investigated the potential role of recombinant human-Vitronectin-N (VN) in inducing differentiation of human induced pluripotent stem cells (hiPSCs) into endodermal lineage. Differentiation was initiated by applying a previously established sequential step wise endodermal differentiation protocol. Expression of endodermal specific genes characteristic of each differentiation stage was investigated and analyzed by qRT-PCR and immunohistochemistry. Our results demonstrated a significant up-regulation of endoderm related markers characteristic of respective stages of differentiation in hiPSCs differentiated on VN coated dishes in comparison to those differentiated on routinely used feeder cells. Analysis of *PDX1* expression in

* Corresponding Author's E-mail: riham.aly@hotmail.com.

differentiated cells illustrated that VN was able to further induce pancreatic progenitors as well. Altogether, our results demonstrated that VN efficiently promoted endodermal differentiation of human induced pluripotent stem cells.

Keywords: vitronectin, endoderm, differentiation, pluripotent stem cells

1. Introduction

Diseases like diabetes and liver cirrhosis result from impairment in cells of endodermal origin. Such diseases pose as social repercussions that dramatically burden the health care systems. The current management of such chronic illnesses ranges from the use of supportive and palliative therapy to organ transplantation. However, the inefficiency of both options justifies the need for an alternative treatment. Current comprehension of endoderm organ development has enabled researchers to successfully direct pluripotent stem cells (PSCs) to differentiate into hepatocyte-like cells and pancreatic β-like cells [1–8]. Induced pluripotent stem cells (iPSCs) specifically forecast an imminent possibility of delivering autologous cells to replace patients own damaged cells and tissues [9]. Several studies have demonstrated induction of endodermal lineage from human embryonic stem cell lines and iPSCs cell lines [10–12]. Nevertheless, variation in the differentiation efficiency was reported either due to the use of chemically undefined components in the differentiation protocols applied or due to the utilization of poorly defined matrices like Matrigel [13, 14]. rh-Vitronectin-N (VN); an extracellular matrix protein that consists of somatomedin B, hemopexin and heparin-binding domain, has been suggested as an alternative to Matrigel and feeder cell layer. It has been reported to enhance cell attachment, growth as well as to maintain the pluripotent state of iPSCs cultures [15–18]. Moreover, Brafman et al., suggested that fibronectin and vitronectin are capable of promoting DE differentiation from human embryonic stem cells [19]. In the present study, we sought to assess the role of recombinant human -Vitronectin-N (VN) on the induction of endodermal lineage differentiation from human iPSCs while comparing its effect to the routinely used feeder layers.

2. Material and Methods

All the experiments conducted in this study used human ESCs and human iPSCs. The work was reviewed and approved by the ethical committee of the Foundation for Biomedical Research and Innovation (FBRI).

2.1. Cell Culture

Human ESC lines KhES-1 (Riken BRC) [20] and human iPSCs lines 201B7 (Riken BRC, Tsukuba, Japan) [21] were cultured with hPSCs culture media on mitomycin C-treated SNL76/7 cells (SIM strain embryonic fibroblast, European Collection of Cell Culture) or with chemical defined medium Essential 8 (Es8, Thermo Fisher Scientific), on recombinant human Vitronectin-N (VN) (Thermo Fisher Scientific)-coated dishes or on Matrigel Growth Factor Reduced (GFR) Basement Membrane Matrix (Corning; Product # 354230) and were incubated at 37°C in a 5% CO2 atmosphere (MCO-19AIC, Panasonic, Osaka, Japan).

The hPSCs culture media comprised DMEM/F-12 (Sigma, Tokyo, Japan) supplemented with 20% knockout serum replacement (KSR; Life Technologies, Carlsbad, CA, USA), 2 mM L-glutamine (Nacalai Tesque, Kyoto, Japan), 1% Non-Essential Amino Acid (NEAA; Life Technologies, Philadelphia, PA, USA), 0.1 mM 2-Mercaptoethanol (Life Technologies Inc, USA), and 5 ng/mL FGF-2 (Reprocell, Kanagawa, Japan). Cells cultured with hPSCs culture media were passaged in clumps using Gentle Cell Dissociation Reagent (GCDR; Stem Cell Technologies) and split at a ratio of 1:3 for iPSCs or 1:3.5 for ESCs. Alternatively, cells were passaged by seeding a single-cell suspension using TrypLE Select (Thermo Fisher Scientific) when cultured with Es8 medium. Cells in single-cell suspensions were seeded at 1×10^5 cells/well in 6-well plates.

2.2. Quantitative RT-PCR (q RT-PCR)

Total RNA was prepared with the RNeasy Micro Kit (74004, QIAGEN, Hilden, Germany) and treated with RNase-free DNase (QIAGEN, Hilden, Germany). A total of 500 ng RNA was used for a reverse transcription (RT) reaction using the QuantiTect Reverse Transcription Kit (205311, QIAGEN, Hilden, Germany). qRT-PCR was carried out in triplicates using SYBR® Select Master Mix (Thermo Fisher Scientific, USA) in StepOnePlus™ (Thermo Fisher Scientific, USA) with the following PCR program: 95°C for 10 min, 40 cycles at 95°C for 15 s, 60°C for 1 min, and 72°C for 15s. The specific primers are listed in (Table 1). RNA from primary human islet used as positive controls in (Figure 5) was kindly provided by Dr. Hirofumi Noguchi of Ryukyu Univ. Japan. Relative quantification was calculated using the 2-ΔΔCt method after normalization to the glycelaldehyde-3-phosphate dehydrogenase (GAPDH).

Table 1. List of primers used in q RT-PCR

Gene		Sequences (5′ to 3′)	
SOX17	F	GGCCGATGAACGCCTTT	Definitive endoderm
	R	TCTTGCTTAGCTCTGCGTTGTG	
CXCR4	F	CACCGCATCTGGAGAACCA	Definitive endoderm
	R	GCCCATTTCCTCGGTGTAGTT	
FOXA2	F	AAAAGCCTCCGGTTTCCACTA	Definitive endoderm
	R	TCAGAATCTGCAGGTGCTTGA	
GATA6	F	GGATTGTCCTGTGCCAACTGT	Definitive endoderm
	R	TCAGAATCTGCAGGTGCTTGA	
HNF1B	F	AACCACCGAAGAGGAAGCAA	primitive gut tube
	R	TCGCATCAGTTTGTTCGATGA	
HNF4A	F	CACCTGATGCAGGAACATATGG	primitive gut tube
	R	CTGTCCGTTGCTGAGGTGAGT	
PDX1	F	GATACTGGATTGGCGTTGTTTG	Posterior foregut
	R	TCCCAAGGTGGAGTGCTGTAG	
GATA4	F	GTTTTTTCCCCTTTGATTTTTGATC	Posterior foregut
	R	AACGACGGCAACAACGATAAT	
HNF6	F	TGCGCAACCCCAAACC	Posterior foregut
	R	TCCACATCCTCCGGAAGGT	
SOX1	F	AAGCCCAGATGGAAATACGTTTAT	Ectoderm
	R	AGGACAAGGAAGGGTGTTGAGA	
MEOX1	F	GGCAGAGTTTGCCCATCATAAC	Mesoderm
	R	GCTCAGAGAGGTCCAGGTTTACC	
GAPDH	F	CCACTCCTCCACCTTTGACG	housekeepin gene
	R	ATGAGGTCCACCACCCTGTT	

2.3. hPSC Scorecard Assay

qRT-PCR for 96 genes were performed with Taqman hPSC Scorecard panel (Thermo Fisher) in accordance with the instruction manual for detection of endoderm lineage-related gene expression in both KhES-1 and 201B7 cell lines in the undifferentiated state. Interpretation of self-renewal, ectoderm, mesoderm, endoderm lineage differentiation was carried out based on the publication (2011, 144, 4390-452, Cell).

2.4. Immunohistochemistry (IHC)

Differentiated cells were fixed on dishes with 4% PFA overnight at 4°C, and then washed 3 times with PBS for 5 min. The cells were permeabilized for 15 min with 2% bovine serum albumin and 0.1% TritonX-100 (Sigma-Aldrich, Tokyo, Japan). The expression of *PDX1* in differentiated cells was detected with the indicated antibody: anti-*PDX1* antibody (1:250; ab84987, Abcam, Japan). Binding was visualized with a secondary antibody labeled with Alexa Fluor 594 (1:500; A11062, Life Technologies, USA), and cells were counterstained with DAPI (D1306, Life Technologies, USA). An Olympus FV1200 laser scanning confocal microscope (Japan) was used for fluorescence detection.

2.5. Statistical Analysis

q RT-PCR experiments were carried out at least three times. Data were presented as the average values ± SEM (standard error of the mean). Statistical significance was analyzed with paired Student t test. Significance levels or P-values are indicated in the figure legends.

3. RESULTS

3.1. Generation of IPSCs-Derived Endoderm

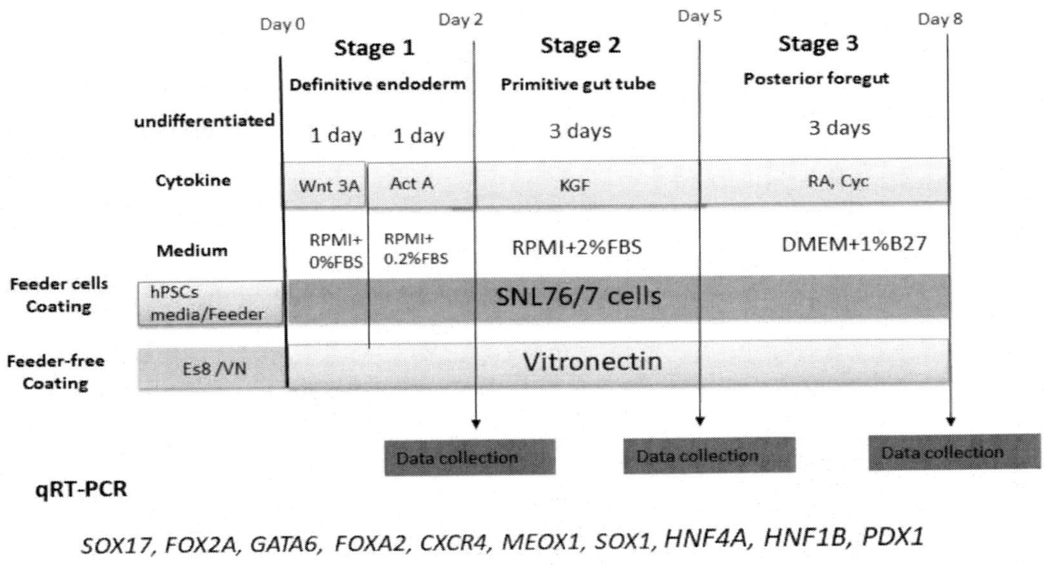

Figure 1. Schematic diagram for endoderm lineage differentiation protocol. Three stages of differentiation are illustrated; growth factors, medium and range of duration for each stage are outlined. In this protocol iPSCs cell line (201B7) were differentiated while cultured either on mitomycin C-treated SNL76/7 feeders (OF) or Vitronectin (VN) coated-dish as feeder-free cultures. Genes related to endoderm differentiation (SOX17, FOX2A, GATA6, FOXA2, CXCR4, MEOX1, SOX1, HNF4A, HNF1B, PDX1) were determine by qRT-PCR. ActA, Activin A; KGF, keratinocyte growth factor CYC, KAAD-cyclopamine; RA, all-trans retinoic acid; VN, Vitronectin; ES8, Essential 8.

Directed differentiation into endoderm followed previously published protocols [22] (Figure 1). In the present study only three stages were applied which involved Definitive Endoderm (DE) induction, primitive gut tube generation and finally posterior foregut specification. Differentiation was initiated as follows; iPSCs were seeded onto 6-well plates covered with mitomycin C-treated SNL76/7 cells or VN. Cells were maintained in iPSCs medium or Essential 8 medium for 3 to 4 days (with daily medium exchange) until they reached 70–80% confluence. Then, the culture medium was changed to RPMI (Mediatech, USA) supplemented with Glutamax, penicillin/streptomycin, and varying concentrations of FBS (Gibco, USA) or 1% (vol/vol) B27 (Life Technologies, USA) supplement where indicated. After a brief wash in PBS (with Mg/Ca) (Nacalai Tesque, Kyoto, Japan), cells were cultured in RPMI (without FBS), 100 ng/ml activin A (Peprotech, NJ, USA) and 50 ng/ml Wnt3a (Peprotech, NJ, USA) for the first day. The next day the medium was changed to RPMI with 0.2% vol/vol FBS and 100 ng/ml activin A, and the cells were cultured for 2 additional days. Next, the cells were briefly washed with PBS (with Mg/Ca) and then cultured in RPMI with 2% vol/vol FBS and 25 ng/ml KGF (Peprotech, NJ, USA) for 3 days.

3.2. Differentiated Cells Demonstrate Endoderm Lineage Characteristics

The first stage of differentiation was set to mimic the events of definitive endoderm (DE) development. hiPSCs were cultured either on feeder, Matrigel or on VN coated dishes in the presence of activin A (Act, a member of the TGF-b superfamily) and Wnt3a for two days. To assess the efficiency of differentiation, mRNA expression levels of stage specific genes was analyzed by qRT–PCR and compared with those of undifferentiated cells. Average of gene expression values for undifferentiated state, ectoderm, mesoderm- or endoderm-related genes of hiPSCs cell line and kHES-1 cell line are shown in comparison with reference standards of TaqMan hPSC Score-card Panel (Supplementary Table 1). In both culture conditions, cells from stage one expressed DE markers *SOX17, FOXA2, CXCR4* and *GATA6*, in comparison to undifferentiated hiPSCs, whereas the expression level of the marker gene of ectoderm marker; *SOX1* and mesoderm marker; *MEOX1* were decreased (Figure 2). The similar initial differentiation process observed in stage 1 was also verified in hESC KhES-1 as show in (Supplementary Figure 1). At stage 2, KAAD-cyclopamine (cyc); a sonic hedgehog signaling inhibitor, was added to allow the transition into primitive gut tube cells. Up-regulation of gut-tube marker genes *FOXA2*, *HNF1b*, and *HNF4a* (hepatocyte nuclear factor 4a) were detected by the end of stage 2 denoting developing gut tube (Figure 3). Transition of expression of genes related to endoderm differentiation of 201B7 cultured on feeder, or on vitronectin-N coated dish at all stages is illustrated in (Supplementary Figure 2).

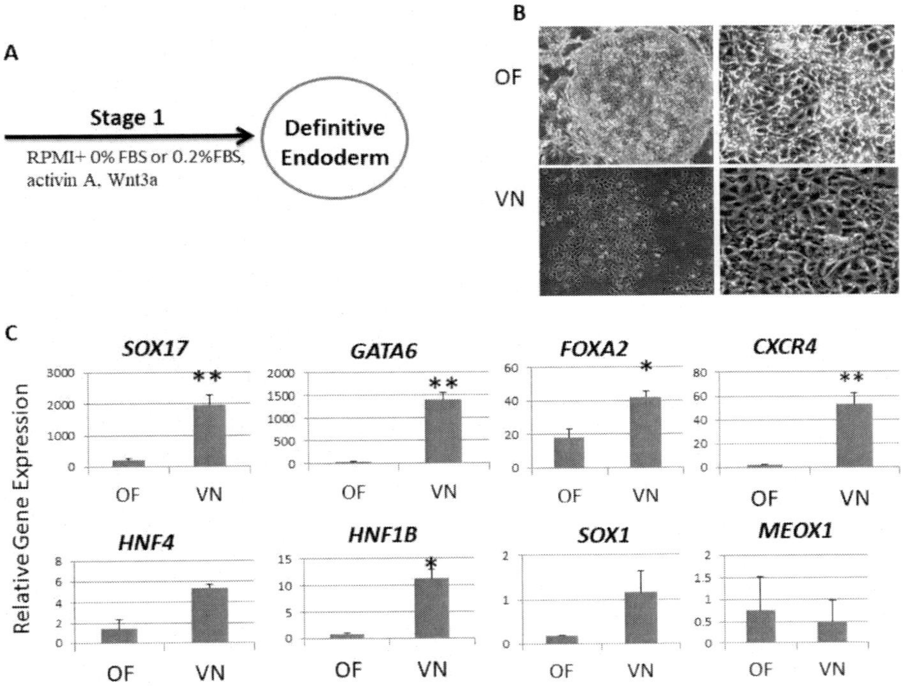

Figure 2. Differentiation of iPSCs into definitive endoderm. (A) Protocol applied for stage 1 of differentiation. (B) Phase contrast microscopic observation of iPSCs cell line 201B7 at the end of stage 1 cultured on mitomycin C-treated SNL76/7 (OF, upper photos) or on Vitronectin-N coated-dish (VN, lower photo). (C)Expression of genes characteristic for definitive endoderm DE (SOX17, FOX2A, GATA6, FOXA2, CXCR4) in addition to mesoderm marker: MEOX1 and ectoderm marker: SOX1 for cells cultured on mitomycin C-treated SNL76/7 (on feeder: OF) or on Vitronectin-N coated-dish (VN) at the end of stage 1 in each graph. The data were analyzed by qRT–PCR and compared with undifferentiated iPSCs. Results are presented as mean ± SEM of three independent experiments (n = 3). *P < 0.05, **P < 0.01. (Scale bars = 200 μM).

3.3. VN-Coated Culture Promotes Endodermal Differentiation

We hypothesized that the differentiation efficiency of pluripotent cells can be affected by the culture system implemented; in terms of the culture medium used, the coating material and the cell seeding density. Therefore, we compared gene expression of cells differentiated while cultured on VN coated dishes to those cultured on different conditions (Figure 2 & 3). q RT-PCR analysis of definitive endoderm-related transcription factor genes (*SOX17, FOXA2, GATA6,* and *CXCR4*) revealed that VN significantly promoted the efficiency of differentiation relative to cultures differentiated on a feeder layer. Similarly, differentiation to more mature endodermal lineages (primitive gut tube and posterior foregut) was assessed and revealed significantly higher expression of *HNF1B* in cells differentiated on VN than those cultured on feeder layer. It was also notable that VN culture condition effectively up regulated DE characteristic genes in the first stage and were effectively down regulated in later stages. Interestingly,

SOX17 was steadily expressed at decreased levels throughout the differentiation. These results demonstrated that culture on VN promoted differentiation efficiency toward endodermal lineages. Morphological changes of the induced cells were also examined daily under phase contrast microscope. Gradually the cells started to assume typical DE cobblestone/petal like appearance, however cells cultured on VN demonstrated a rather uniform appearance than those cultured on feeder cells.

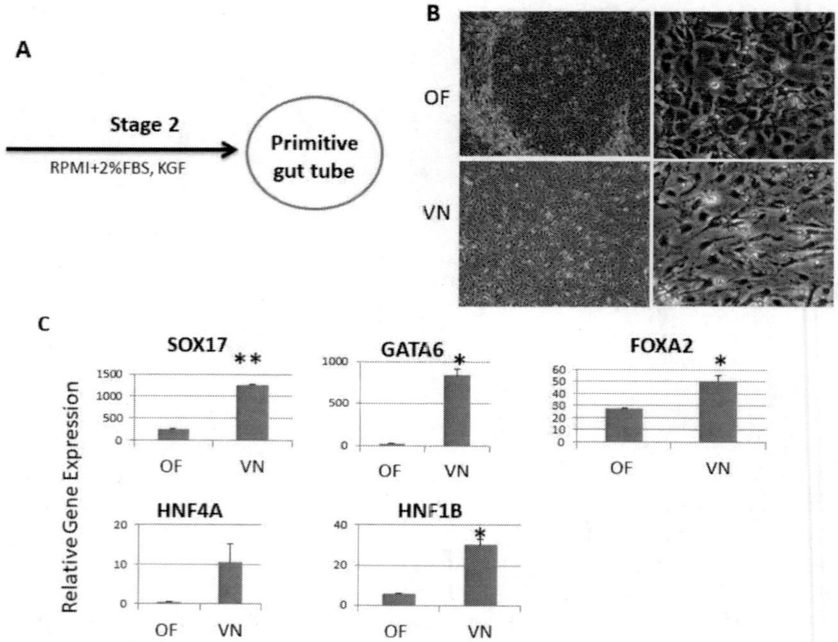

Figure 3. Differentiation of iPSCs into primitive gut tube. (A) Protocol applied for stage 2 of differentiation. (B) Phase contrast microscopic observation of iPSCs cell line 201B7 at the end of stage 2 cultured on mitomycin C-treated SNL76/7 (OF, upper photos) or on Vitronectin-N coated-dish (VN, lower photo). (C) Expression of genes characteristic of primitive gut tube SOX17, GATA6, FOXA2, HNF4A and HNF1B for cells cultured on mitomycin C-treated SNL76/7 (on feeder: OF) or on Vitronectin-N coated-dish (VN) at the end of stage 2 in each graph. The data were analyzed by qRT–PCR and compared with undifferentiated iPSCs. Results are presented as mean ± SEM of three independent experiments (n = 3). *P < 0.05, **P < 0.01. (Scale bars = 200 μM).

3.4. Induction of Pancreatic Progenitors

To determine whether the differentiated iPSCs would further differentiate to endoderm derivatives, we next analyzed pancreatic differentiation through implementing stage three of the previously described protocol [22]. After seven days of culture in endoderm differentiation condition, the medium was changed to DMEM with 1% vol/vol B27 (Invitrogen, USA) supplement, 0.25μM KAAD-cyclopamine (Toronto Research Chemicals, Canada), 1μM all-Trans retinoic acid (RA) (Sigma, Tokyo, Japan) and 30 ng/ml Noggin (R&D, MN, USA) for 3 days to pattern a foregut fate and induce the development of pancreatic progenitors. Gene expression analysis at this stage, revealed a highly significant increase in *PDX1* expression in VN cultures while maintaining significant up-regulation of HNF1B and HNF4A (Figure 4). This combination of gene expression indicated posterior foregut formation.

3.5. Effective Induction of PDX1 via VN Culture

At the end of stage 3, we analyzed *PDX1* expression as a key pancreatic development factor. Gene expression analysis of *PDX1* revealed a consistent increase in VN coated cultures through all stages of differentiation compared to those differentiated via Matrigel or feeder coated dishes (Figure 5). Expression of PDX1 in 201B7 was not detected on either Matrigel condition or on feeder condition by ICH. However, an obvious increase in PDX1 positive cells was demonstrated in cells cultured on VN (Figure 5) which confirmed that iPSCs were efficiently differentiated to pancreatic progenitor cells when cultured on VN-coated dishes. The overall result supported that VN-based culture is more efficient in inducing endodermal derivatives.

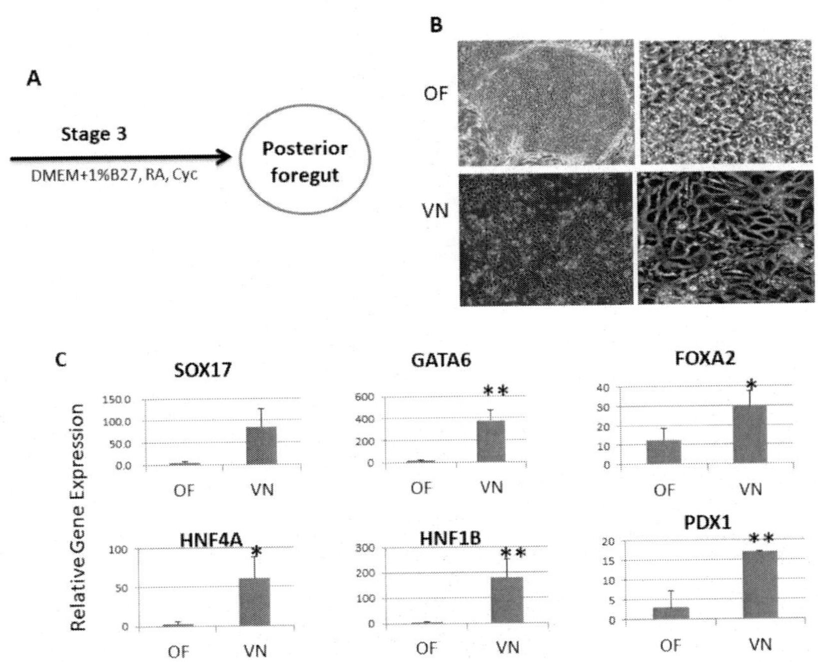

Figure 4. Differentiation of iPSCs into posterior foregut. (A) Protocol applied for stage 3 of differentiation. (B) Phase contrast microscopic observation of iPSCs cell line 201B7 at the end of stage 3 cultured on mitomycin C-treated SNL76/7 (OF, upper photos) or on Vitronectin-N coated-dish (VN, lower photo). (C) Expression of genes characteristic of posterior foregut. (SOX17, GATA6, FOXA2, HNF4A, HNF1B and PDX1) for cells cultured on mitomycin C-treated SNL76/7 (on feeder: OF) or on Vitronectin-N coated-dish (VN) at the end of stage 3 in each graph. The data were analyzed by qRT–PCR and compared with undifferentiated iPSCs. Results are presented as mean ± SEM of three independent experiments (n = 3). *P < 0.05, **P < 0.01. (Scale bars = 200 μM).

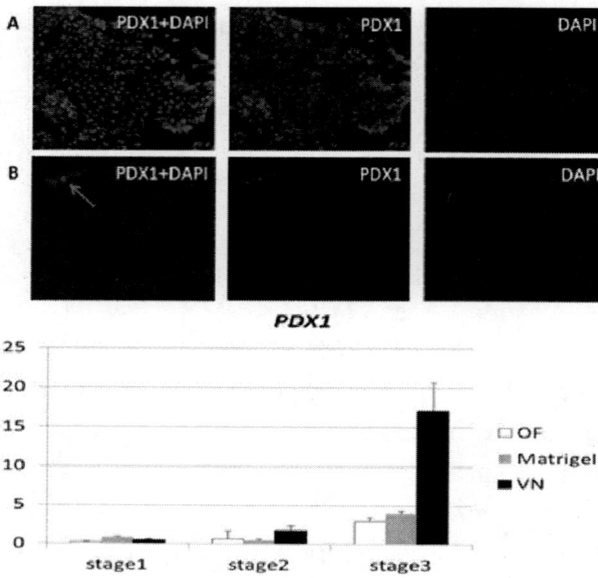

Figure 5. VN coated dishes efficiently induces PDX-1 expression Immunocytochemistry showing increased expression patterns of PDX1-1 (red, pancreatic), positive cells generated at stage 3 on VN coated dish (A) than on mitomycin C-treated SNL76/7 feeder (B) layered dishes. Cells were counterstained with DAPI (blue) (Scale bars = 200 μM). Transition of gene expression of PDX1 in 201B7 cultured on feeder (OF), Matrigel or Vitronectin-N (VN) in stage 1-3 is shown as a fold change of gene expression of cells cultured on VN at stage 2 (n = 3, analytical replicates) (lower photo).

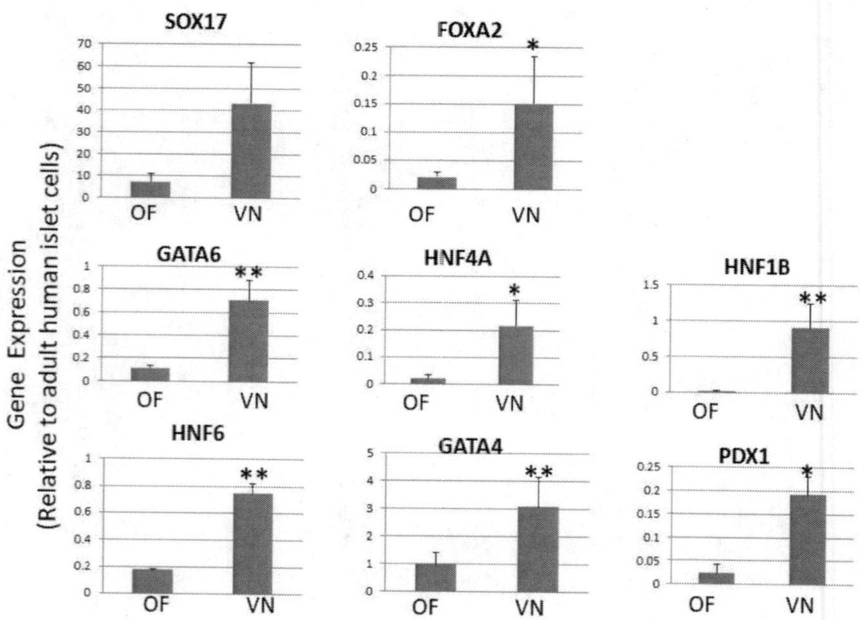

Figure 6. Expression of genes characteristic of stage three relative to adult human islet expression levels by qRT-PCR. Relative mRNA expression levels of (SOX17, GATA6, FOXA2, HNF4A, HNF1B and PDX1) in cells generated at stage three cells and cultured on either mitomycin C-treated SNL76/7 (on feeder: OF) or on Vitronectin-N coated-dish (VN) were compared to pancreatic islet cells. The data were expressed as genes to GAPDH ratio with that of islet arbitrarily set as 1. Results are presented as mean ± SEM of three independent experiments (n = 3). * $P < 0.05$, ** $P < 0.01$.

3.6. Pancreatic Markers Demonstrate Expression Levels Relative to Adult Human Islet Expression

To further elaborate these transcript levels, gene expression of stage three differentiated cells was compared to adult human islets (Figure 6). Remarkably, the majority of the pancreatic markers *(SOX17, GATA6, FOXA2, HNF4A, HNF1B and PDX1)* were significantly up-regulated in cultures differentiated on VN and at comparable levels to human adult islet cells. On the other hand, the same genes were down regulated in cultures differentiated on feeder layer.

4. Discussion

Vitronectin is an efficient coating material essential for the maintenance of pluripotent stem cells and acts as an alternative to feeder layers and Matrigel [23]. However, the role of VN in the induction of endodermal lineage differentiation has not been fully investigated. In this report, we demonstrated that VN effectively promoted endodermal differentiation of iPSCs. Endoderm development is considered a sophisticated and complex process that is controlled by numerous signaling pathways and transcription factor cascades [24]. It is believed that the selection of a successful protocol to differentiate cells is critical to the success of the differentiation. We implemented an established endodermal lineage differentiation protocol that is considered as one of the most efficient protocols [22, 25]. Differentiation was initiated in singly seeded cells cultured on VN in order to allow cells to fully attach to the extra cellular matrix [16]. Konagaya et al. described aggregate culture for generating islet-like aggregates from human iPSCs, however creating these aggregates is complicated in manufacturing and did not increase the efficiency of differentiation [26]. Extracellular matrix plays an important role in endodermal lineage differentiation by allowing cell migration and by guiding primitive streak formation and gastrulation [27, 28]. Recent studies reported that DE cells differentiated from human embryonic stem cells expressed vitronectin integrin alpha-v/ beta-5 receptor, which acts to mediate cell-to-cell and cell-to-ECM interactions [18, 19]. Nagaoka, et al., 2015 reported that a fragment of VN is ample to maintain the pluripotency of hPSCs and aids in the differentiation of the cells towards hepatocyte lineage [29]. We did not consider the use of recombinant human vitronectin-XF (V-XF, Stem Cell Technologies) for this study. V-XF contains various binding motifs compared with recombinant human VN or physiological VN, which may facilitate the binding to various molecules, but at the same time, V-XF might not be optimized to anchor the undifferentiated PSCs and cannot afford to maintain them more than 3 passages with Es8 medium. Thus, we compared feeder-free vitronectin-N-coated condition with that of Matrigel-coated condition and feeder coted condition. Gene expression analysis of markers characteristic of endoderm lineage confirmed the role of VN in promoting endodermal differentiation. The significant up regulation of endoderm markers *CXCR4, FOXA2* and *SOX17* at the end of the first stage was in consistence with previous reports and indicated successful derivation of DE [2, 25, 30]. *CXCR4* is a reliable marker for DE generated from murine and human embryonic stem cells. It indirectly induces pancreatic development through controlling angioblasts migration [31, 32]. *FOXA2* is initially expressed at the anterior region of the primitive streak, where definitive endoderm induction takes place. Co expression of *FOXA2* and *SOX17* is generally used to exclude other lineage differentiation and is considered a defining factor that confirms DE differentiation [33]. The expression of *GATA6* was also maintained throughout the three stages, but with decreasing level which illustrates its critical role in DE formation and in posterior foregut specification [34]. *GATA6* pattern of expression was consistent with recent reports that suggested its critical role in endoderm and pancreas specification [34]. Analysis of the mesoderm marker *MEOX1* and the ectoderm maker *SOX1* expression, revealed decreased expression in differentiated cells relative to cells in the undifferentiated state. This was in consistence with Wong et al., 2010 and indicated that only a relatively small proportion of the differentiated cells differentiated along these alternative lineages [30]. In accordance with previous reports, a considerable up regulation of stage two gut-tube markers; *HNF1B* and *HNF4A* was observed in both culture conditions with advancement of cells cultured on VN over those cultured on a feeder layer. Increased expression of *HNF1B* and *HNF4A* is indicative of posterior foregut specification [25]. At the third stage, retinoic acid (RA) cyclopamine and noggin were administered to induce iPSCs to differentiate into pancreatic progenitor cells and to inhibit hepatic differentiation [31] It has recently been suggested that pancreatic differentiation is achieved through simultaneous suppression of the liver transcriptional factors by *PDX1* [35]. *PDX1* is described as a key pancreatic beta-cell marker and the hallmark for posterior foregut/pancreatic-committed gut endoderm in differentiated cells and human islets [25]. Its expression was significantly high at the end of stage three along with strong positive *PDX1* staining in almost all cells differentiated on VN. Furthermore, gene expression profile at the end of stage 3 in cells differentiated on VN was similar to that of adult islet cells. Overall, these results confirmed the successful differentiation of iPSCs into pancreatic-committed gut endoderm. In conclusion, VN efficiently promoted differentiation of iPSCs into endodermal lineage. Although previous studies suggest that the differentiation of hPSCs into endodermal lineage resembles the developmental process, it was challenging for us to generate mature β cells when subsequent stages of the implemented protocol were attempted. Further improvements are needed in order to produce terminally differentiated tissues. In the future; we plan to completely adapt this protocol to xeno-free conditions and to test the stability of these differentiated cells on *in vivo* models.

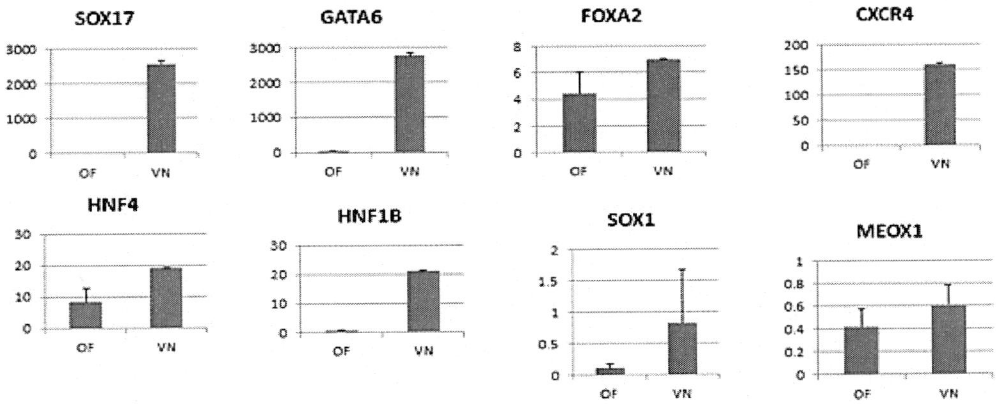

Supplementary Figure 1. Differentiation of iPSCs into definitive endoderm. Expression of genes characteristic for definitive endoderm DE (SOX17, FOX2A, GATA6, FOXA2, CXCR4) in addition to mesoderm marker: MEOX1 and ectoderm marker: SOX1 for cells cultured on mitomycin C-treated SNL76/7 (on feeder: OF) or on Vitronectin-N coated-dish (VN) at the end of stage 1 KhES-1 cell line. The data were analyzed by qRT–PCR and compared with undifferentiated cells.

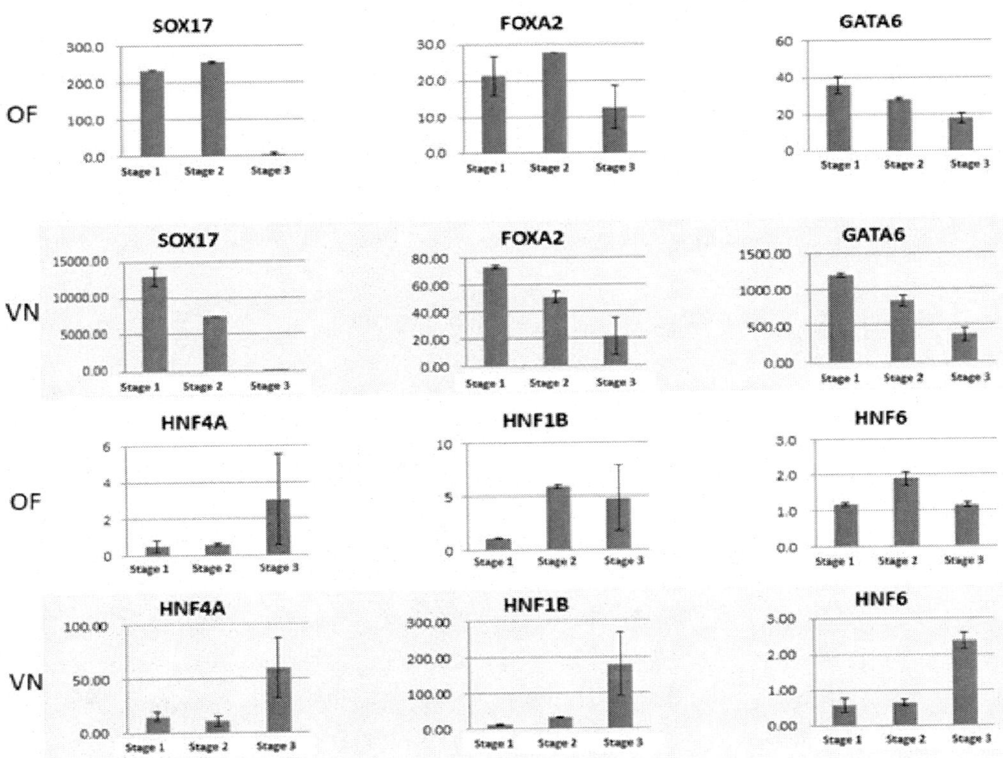

Supplementary Figure 2. Transition of expression of genes related to endoderm differentiation of 201B7 cultured on feeder (OF), or on vitronectin-N coated dish (VN) at stage 1-3.

Supplementary Material to Table 1. Gene expression of endoderm lineage-related molecules in ESC/iPSC in undifferentiated state

Target Name	Category	KhES-1 OF	201B7 OF	KhES-1 Es8	201B7 Es8
AFP	Endoderm	0.00	0.01	0.00	0.00
CABP7	Endoderm	0.82	0.69	0.15	0.08
CDH20	Endoderm	1.75	0.67	0.23	0.35
CLDN1	Endoderm	1.03	1.21	1.09	0.60
CPLX2	Endoderm	5.23	1.60	0.42	0.99
ELAVL3	Endoderm	0.85	1.48	0.62	0.31
EOMES	Endoderm	0.02	0.02	0.03	0.02
FOXA1	Endoderm	0.06	0.32	0.08	0.07
FOXA2	Endoderm	0.01	0.01	1.93	1.87
FOXP2	Endoderm	0.39	0.25	0.22	0.14
GATA4	Endoderm	0.01	0.01	0.01	0.01
GATA6	Endoderm	0.01	0.02	0.00	0.01
HHEX	Endoderm	0.37	0.47	0.11	0.03
HMP19	Endoderm	0.47	0.87	0.41	0.34
HNF1B	Endoderm	0.03	0.05	0.07	0.03
HNF4A	Endoderm	0.00	0.02	0.00	0.00
KLF5	Endoderm	0.76	1.34	0.32	1.50
LEFTY1	Endoderm	0.23	0.11	0.01	0.28
LEFTY2	Endoderm	0.55	0.21	0.02	0.10
NODAL	Endoderm	0.29	0.44	0.04	0.62
PHOX2B	Endoderm	0.03	0.03	0.02	0.02
POU3F3	Endoderm	0.06	0.05	0.03	0.03
PRDM1	Endoderm	0.15	0.20	0.06	0.11
RXRG	Endoderm	0.00	0.08	0.10	0.04
SOX17	Endoderm	0.00	0.00	0.00	0.01
SST	Endoderm	0.42	0.60	0.16	0.87

Target Name	Category	KhES-1 OF	201B7 OF	KhES-1 Es8	201B7 Es8
ABCA4	Mesoderm	0.90	0.48	0.80	0.46
ALOX15	Mesoderm	1.73	1.59	0.86	0.99
BMP10	Mesoderm	0.05	0.42	1.28	0.31
CDH5	Mesoderm	0.15	1.46	1.87	3.69
CDX2	Mesoderm	0.05	0.10	0.26	0.06
COLEC10	Mesoderm	1.08	0.88	0.63	0.57
ESM1	Mesoderm	0.02	0.30	0.01	0.24
FCN3	Mesoderm	0.52	0.90	1.05	0.31
FOXF1	Mesoderm	1.32	0.32	0.31	0.62
HAND1	Mesoderm	0.10	0.04	0.03	0.00
HAND2	Mesoderm	0.78	0.14	0.01	0.29
HEY1	Mesoderm	0.79	0.50	0.91	1.37
HOPX	Mesoderm	0.15	0.30	0.06	0.11
IL6ST	Mesoderm	0.99	1.12	0.80	0.74
NKX2-5	Mesoderm	0.35	0.98	0.24	0.37
ODAM	Mesoderm	0.48	0.71	0.32	2.34
PDGFRA	Mesoderm	0.65	0.48	0.18	0.24
PLVAP	Mesoderm	0.16	0.57	0.36	0.50
RGS4	Mesoderm	0.36	0.14	0.13	0.12
SNAI2	Mesoderm	0.20	0.38	0.21	0.35
TBX3	Mesoderm	0.07	0.08	0.01	0.03
TM4SF1	Mesoderm	1.35	0.44	0.72	2.39
FGF4	Mesendoderm	2.75	1.51	0.12	0.06
GDF3	Mesendoderm	4.62	4.44	2.64	2.60
NPPB	Mesendoderm	0.02	0.38	0.02	0.82
NR5A2	Mesendoderm	174.74	157.80	106.48	165.82
PTHLH	Mesendoderm	0.15	0.87	0.48	4.03
T	Mesendoderm	0.00	0.00	0.00	0.00

Target Name	Category	KhES-1 OF	201B7 OF	KhES-1 Es8	201B7 Es8
CDH9	Ectoderm	0.47	0.32	0.23	0.09
COL2A1	Ectoderm	0.16	0.16	0.62	0.40
DMBX1	Ectoderm	0.21	0.06	0.15	0.08
DRD4	Ectoderm	0.24	0.42	0.04	0.01
EN1	Ectoderm	0.37	0.95	0.01	0.05
LMX1A	Ectoderm	0.10	0.07	0.07	0.11
MAP2	Ectoderm	0.60	1.86	5.07	2.30
MYO3B	Ectoderm	0.93	0.18	0.21	0.18
NOS2	Ectoderm	0.38	0.67	0.60	1.03
NR2F1/NR	Ectoderm	1.64	2.99	0.00	0.02
NR2F2	Ectoderm	0.01	0.26	0.01	0.01
OLFM3	Ectoderm	0.99	0.38	0.59	0.34
PAPLN	Ectoderm	0.27	0.24	0.50	0.20
PAX3	Ectoderm	0.06	0.04	0.04	0.05
PAX6	Ectoderm	0.61	0.30	0.06	0.31
POU4F1	Ectoderm	1.90	0.37	0.22	0.08
PRKCA	Ectoderm	0.69	0.89	0.52	0.67
SDC2	Ectoderm	8.89	10.25	4.21	5.76
SOX1	Ectoderm	0.12	0.06	0.11	0.00
TRPM8	Ectoderm	0.38	2.09	0.53	0.14
WNT1	Ectoderm	0.04	1.14	0.48	0.04
ZBTB16	Ectoderm	0.24	0.19	0.08	0.14

Target Name	Category	KhES-1 OF	201B7 OF	KhES-1 Es8	201B7 Es8
CXCL5	Self-renewal	4.97	3.74	6.45	2.78
DNMT3B	Self-renewal	1.51	1.13	0.55	0.65
HESX1	Self-renewal	0.56	0.53	0.46	0.43
IDO1	Self-renewal	3.06	1.82	0.77	0.24
LCK	Self-renewal	0.69	0.61	1.27	0.99
NANOG	Self-renewal	1.29	1.33	0.91	0.99
POU5F1	Self-renewal	0.76	0.88	1.01	0.76
SOX2	Self-renewal	1.05	1.33	0.81	0.66
TRIM22	Self-renewal	7.51	7.04	2.22	1.30

Fold change legend	
fc>100	Upregulated
10<fc<=100	
2<fc<=10	
0.5<=fc<=2	Comparable
0.1<=fc<0.5	
0.01<=fc<0.1	
fc<0.01	Downregulated
omitted	

Average gene expression of self-renewal (undifferentiated state), ectoderm- mesoderm- or endoderm-related genes is compared with reference standards of TaqMan hPSC Scorecard Panel (Life Technology)

ACKNOWLEDGMENTS

The authors wish to thank Dr. Hirofumi Noguchi of Ryukyu University in Japan for kindly providing RNA from primary human islet cells.

This work is partly supported by the research grant from AMED, Japan to the research titled "Points to Consider to Conduct Tumorigenicity Tests of Pluripotent Stem Cell Derivatives" under the research ID#18bk0104059h0003.

Ethical Compliance

The authors have stated all possible conflicts of interest within this work. The authors have stated all sources of funding for this work. If this work involved human participants, informed consent was received from each individual. If this work involved human participants, it was conducted in accordance with the 1964 Declaration of Helsinki. If this work involved experiments with humans or animals, it was conducted in accordance with the related institutions' research ethics guidelines.

References

[1] D'Amour K a, Agulnick AD, Eliazer S, Kelly OG, Kroon E, Baetge EE. Efficient differentiation of human embryonic stem cells to definitive endoderm. *Nat Biotech.* 2005;23(12):1534–41.

[2] Jiang J, Au M, Lu K, Eshpeter A, Korbutt G, Fisk G, et al. Generation of insulin-producing islet-like clusters from human embryonic stem cells. *Stem Cells.* 2007 Aug;25(8):1940–53.

[3] Wang D, Haviland DL, Burns AR, Zsigmond E, Wetsel R a. A pure population of lung alveolar epithelial type II cells derived from human embryonic stem cells. *Proc Natl Acad Sci USA*. 2007;104(11):4449–54.

[4] Van Vranken BE, Rippon HJ, Samadikuchaksaraei A, Trounson AO, Bishop AE. The Differentiation of Distal Lung Epithelium from Embryonic Stem Cells. In: *Current Protocols in Stem Cell Biology*. 2007.

[5] Spence JR, Mayhew CN, Rankin SA, Kuhar MF, Vallance JE, Tolle K, et al. Directed differentiation of human pluripotent stem cells into intestinal tissue *in vitro*. *Nature*. 2010;470(7332):105–9.

[6] Roelandt P, Pauwelyn KA, Sancho-Bru P, Subramanian K, Bose B, Ordovas L, et al. Human embryonic and rat adult stem cells with primitive endoderm-like phenotype can be fated to definitive endoderm, and finally hepatocyte-like cells. *PLoS One*. 2010;5(8).

[7] Si-Tayeb K, Noto FK, Nagaoka M, Li J, Battle MA, Duris C, et al. Highly efficient generation of human hepatocyte-like cells from induced pluripotent stem cells. *Hepatology*. 2010;51(1):297–305.

[8] Shim JH, Kim SE, Woo DH, Kim SK, Oh CH, McKay R, et al. Directed differentiation of human embryonic stem cells towards a pancreatic cell fate. *Diabetologia*. 2007;50(6):1228–38.

[9] Perez Lopez S, Otero Hernandez *J. Advances in Stem Cell Therapy. Adv Exp Med Biol.* 2017;741:290–313.

[10] Pagliuca FW, Millman JR, Gürtler M, Segel M, Van Dervort A, Ryu JH, et al. Generation of functional human pancreatic β cells *in vitro*. *Cell.* 2014;159(2): 428–39.

[11] Pagliuca FW, Melton DA. How to make a functional β-cell. *Development.* 2013;140(12):2472–83.

[12] Nostro MC, Sarangi F, Yang C, Holland A, Elefanty AG, Stanley EG, et al. Efficient generation of NKX6-1+ pancreatic progenitors from multiple human pluripotent stem cell lines. *Stem Cell Reports.* 2015;4(4).

[13] Chetty S, Pagliuca FW, Honore C, Kweudjeu A, Rezania A, Melton DA. A simple tool to improve pluripotent stem cell differentiation. *Nat Methods.* 2013;10(6): 553–6.

[14] Rodin S, Antonsson L, Hovatta O, Tryggvason K. Monolayer culturing and cloning of human pluripotent stem cells on laminin-521–based matrices under xeno-free and chemically defined conditions. *Nat Protoc.* 2014;9(10):2354–68.

[15] Trubiani O, Piattelli A, Gatta V, Marchisio M, Diomede F, D'Aurora M, et al. Assessment of an Efficient Xeno-Free Culture System of Human Periodontal Ligament Stem Cells. *Tissue Eng Part C-Methods.* 2015;21(1): 52–64.

[16] Takenaka C, Miyajima H, Yoda Y, Imazato H, Yamamoto T, Gomi S, et al. Controlled Growth and the Maintenance of Human Pluripotent Stem Cells by Cultivation with Defined Medium on Extracellular Matrix-Coated Micropatterned Dishes. *PLoS One.* 2015; 10(6):e0129855.

[17] Braam SR, Zeinstra L, Litjens S, Ward-van Oostwaard D, van den Brink S, van Laake L, et al. Recombinant Vitronectin Is a Functionally Defined Substrate That Supports Human Embryonic Stem Cell Self-Renewal via αVβ5 Integrin. *Stem Cells.* 2008 Sep;26(9):2257–65.

[18] Chen G, Gulbranson DR, Hou Z, Bolin JM, Ruotti V, Probasco MD, et al. Chemically defined conditions for human iPSC derivation and culture. *Nat Methods.* 2011 May 10;8(5):424–9.

[19] Brafman DA, Phung C, Kumar N, Willert K. Regulation of endodermal differentiation of human embryonic stem cells through integrin-ECM interactions. *Cell Death Differ.* 2013 Mar 16;20(3):369–81.

[20] Suemori H, Yasuchika K, Hasegawa K, Fujioka T, Tsuneyoshi N, Nakatsuji N. Efficient establishment of human embryonic stem cell lines and long-term maintenance with stable karyotype by enzymatic bulk passage. *Biochem Biophys Res Commun.* 2006;345(3): 926–32.

[21] Takahashi K, Tanabe K, Ohnuki M, Narita M, Ichisaka T, Tomoda K, et al. Induction of Pluripotent Stem Cells from Adult Human Fibroblasts by Defined Factors. *Cell.* 2007 Nov 30;131(5):861–72.

[22] Kelly OG, Chan MY, Martinson LA, Kadoya K, Ostertag TM, Ross KG, et al. Cell-surface markers for the isolation of pancreatic cell types derived from human embryonic stem cells. *Nat Biotechnol*. 2011; 29(8):750–6.

[23] Kaini RR, Shen-Gunther J, Cleland JM, Greene WA, Wang H-C. Recombinant Xeno-Free Vitronectin Supports Self-Renewal and Pluripotency in Protein-Induced Pluripotent Stem Cells. *Tissue Eng Part C Methods*. 2016;22(2):85–90.

[24] Rekittke NE, Ang M, Rawat D, Khatri R, Linn T. Regenerative Therapy of Type 1 Diabetes Mellitus: From Pancreatic Islet Transplantation to Mesenchymal Stem Cells. *Stem Cells Int*. 2016;2016:3764681.

[25] D'Amour K a, Bang AG, Eliazer S, Kelly OG, Agulnick AD, Smart NG, et al. Production of pancreatic hormone-expressing endocrine cells from human embryonic stem cells. *Nat Biotechnol*. 2006 Nov 19;24 (11):1392–401.

[26] Konagaya S, Iwata H. Reproducible preparation of spheroids of pancreatic hormone positive cells from human iPS cells: An *in vitro* study. *Biochim Biophys Acta - Gen Subj*. 2016;1860(9):2008–16.

[27] Brafman DA, Phung C, Kumar N, Willert K. Regulation of endodermal differentiation of human embryonic stem cells through integrin-ECM interactions. *Cell Death Differ*. 2013 Mar 16;20(3):369–81.

[28] Engler AJ, Sweeney HL, Discher DE, Schwarzbauer JE. Extracellular matrix elasticity directs stem cell differentiation. *J Musculoskelet Neuronal Interact*. 2007;7(4):335.

[29] Nagaoka M, Kobayashi M, Kawai C, Mallanna SK, Duncan SA. Design of a Vitronectin-Based Recomb-inant Protein as a Defined Substrate for Differentiation of Human Pluripotent Stem Cells into Hepatocyte-Like Cells. *PLoS One*. 2015;10(8):e0136350.

[30] Wong JCY, Gao SY, Lees JG, Best MB, Wang R, Tuch BE. Definitive endoderm derived from human embry-onic stem cells highly express the integrin receptors alphaV and beta5. *Cell Adh Migr*. 2010;4(1):39–45.

[31] Cai J, Yu C, Liu Y, Chen S, Guo Y, Yong J, et al. Generation of Homogeneous PDX1+ Pancreatic Progenitors from Human ES Cell-derived Endoderm Cells. *J Mol Cell Biol*. 2010 Feb 1;2(1):50–60.

[32] Katsumoto K, Kume S. The role of CXCL12-CXCR4 signaling pathway in pancreatic development. *Theranostics*. 2013;3(1):11–7.

[33] Baetge EE. Production of β-cells from human embryonic stem cells. *Diabetes, Obes Metab*. 2008 Nov; 10:186–94.

[34] Tiyaboonchai A, Cardenas-Diaz FL, Ying L, Maguire JA, Sim X, Jobaliya C, et al. GATA6 Plays an Important Role in the Induction of Human Definitive Endoderm, Development of the Pancreas, and Functionality of Pancreatic β Cells. *Stem Cell Reports*. 2017 Mar 14;8(3):589–604.

[35] Teo AKK, Tsuneyoshi N, Hoon S, Tan EK, Stanton LW, Wright CVE, et al. PDX1 binds and represses hepatic genes to ensure robust pancreatic commitment in differentiating human embryonic stem cells. *Stem Cell Reports.* 2015 Apr 14;4 (4):578–90.

In: Manipulation of Stem Cells for Disease Benefits
Editor: Prasad Koka
ISBN: 978-1-53615-468-9

Chapter 8

GENE-TRACKING OF *IN VITRO* DIFFERENTIATION CAPABILITIES OF ADULT MOUSE NEURAL STEM/PROGENITOR CELLS

K. Ludlow, P. Kumar, G. Simpson and J. Buttigieg*
Department of Biology, University of Regina,
Regina, Saskatchewan, Canada

ABSTRACT

Previous studies have suggested that neurotransmitters may play an important role in influencing neural stem/progenitor cells (NSPCs) differentiation into oligodendrocytes (OL). Differentiated OL are known to aid in remyelination and axonal protection. In order to derive pure lineages of OL, especially for use in regenerative medicine, improved differentiation protocols are required. One potential differentiation cue is the excitatory neurotransmitter glutamate, but, its effect on NSPCs is currently unknown. Using real-time PCR, we examined the *in vitro* ability of glutamate, in combination of growth factors to influence the NSPCs differentiation. Glutamate (200μM) for 14-days did not induce significant changes in the gene expression profile of differentiated cultures. Moreover, the combination of growth factors (FGF2, PDGF, NT3) demonstrated no significant effect on the proportions of differentiated cell types. Although the differentiation media, containing fetal bovine serum, had an effect on appearance of neuronal lineage, the overall expression of mature cell markers continued to decrease by day-14. In contrast, Matrigel-attached cultures, demonstrated significant increase in glial markers, with possible inhibition of neuronal differentiation as observed with spontaneous attachment. Overall, these data suggest that glutamate (200μM) and combination of growth factors had no modulating effect on the gene expression profile of differentiated NSPCs culture.

* Corresponding Author's E-mail: Josef.buttigieg@uregina.ca.

INTRODUCTION

The central nervous system (CNS) consists of neurons that form communicative neural networks with other neurons, and supportive glial cells such as oligodendrocytes (OL) and astrocytes. The long-held dogma has been that the adult CNS had no regenerative capabilities and thus no ability to replace lost or damaged cells [1]. This understanding has now changed, with many studies demonstrating the presence of progenitor cell populations in various niches of the brain, capable of replacing lost or damaged cells (e.g., neurons, or glial cells) [2-8]. One such niche, are those cells derived from the adult subventricular zone (SVZ). These neural stem/progenitor cells (NSPCs) from the SVZ hold great potential *for regenerative medicine* and are being explored for treatment of various neurological disorders such as: Huntington's [9, 10], Parkinson's [11, 12], Multiple Sclerosis [13, 14] and Alzheimer's disease [15, 16]. Although the transplantation of exogenous NSPCs has shown promising results, overall the survival rate of transplanted cells remains poor [17-19]. Thus, a clear understanding of the factors that control and regulate *NSPCs proliferation, survival or differentiation not only has the potential of improving exogenous NSPCs transplantation success, but also may allow for endogenous stem cell therapy.*

Cells surrounding and within the SVZ release various cytokines and growth factors (GF), such as: fibroblast growth factor 2 (FGF), ependymal growth factor (EGF) and platelet derived growth factor AA (PDGFα) [20, 21]. These growth factors play an important role in regulating neural stem cell proliferation and differentiation. During various *in vitro* studies, both FGF and EGF are shown to play an important role in NSPCs differentiation to neuronal [20, 21] or oligodendrocyte lineages, however, FGF and EGF have been found to have no effect on proliferation of NG2+ precursor cells found outside the SVZ [22]. It has also been shown that while PDGFα is a prerequisite for oligodendrogenesis from NSPCs, [23-25] the neutrophic factor 3 (NT3) may play a synergistic role in OL differentiation with PDGFα *in vivo* [23, 26]. Taken together, these studies have demonstrated the proliferative and differentiation potential of various growth factors, however, direct action of these factors on NSPCs *individually and/or in combination,* is of great interest to *promote cell survival and faster remyelination.*

In addition to growth factors involvement in NSPCs development is the major excitatory neuro-transmitter glutamate. Glutamate, which plays an important role in the early development of the CNS [27], has recently been implicated as a regulator, controlling neural stem cell proliferation, migration and differentiation [27, 28]. Adult NSPCs express the metabolic receptors mGluR3, mGluR5, mGluR1 and glutamate transporters, but do not express functional ionotropic receptors (iGluRs), thus suggesting an ability to respond to released glutamate. However, the detailed composition and roles of various glutamate receptors expressed by NPSCs are not fully under-stood and are often reported with conflicting findings [29-31]. Moreover, the effect of the glutamate on NSPCs differentiation and migration remains largely unknown [27-31]. Therefore, further investigation is required to better understand the potential age-related/ region-specific variations and steps governing NSPCs differentiation in response to glutamate.

In this study, we utilized adult NSPCs derived from the SVZ of the mouse brain. We stimulated these cells using a panel of candidate molecules previously implicated in stem cell proliferation and differentiation. We included glutamate, FGF2, PDGF, NT3, and 2% fetal bovine serum (FBS) as a control.

MATERIALS AND METHODS

Isolation and Culture of Primary Cells

Adult NSPCs were isolated from C57/Bl6 mice. Mice were housed at the UofR animal facility accord-ing to the Canadian Council on Animal Care (CCAC) regulations. All animal care and experimental protocols were approved by the University of Regina's President's Council on Animal Care following CCAC guidelines. To culture NSPCs *in vitro,* brains and spinal columns were excised and placed in ice cold phosphate buffered saline (PBS) containing 1% penicillin/streptomycin, under sterile conditions. The SVZ were dissected, enzymatically digested with 25 mg/mL type IV collagenase and 12.5% trypsin (Gibco; Burlington, ON, Canada) and then mechanically broken up into single cells with a glass Pasteur pipette.

For stock neurosphere suspension cultures, isolated NSPCs were thawed quickly and placed in uncoated culture dishes with serum free NSPCs growth media consisting of 20 ng/mL FGF2, 20 ng/mL EGF, 0.5 mg/mL heparin and 2% B27 supplement added to NSPC stock media: equal proportions of DMEM/F-12 HAMS (Gibco), 4 mL 30% Glucose, 1% penicillin/streptomycin, 2 mM glutamine, and 5 mM HEPES. Cultures were passaged every 7-10 days based on neurosphere size and media additions or 70% media changes were conducted every 3-4 days. A minimum of 100,000 cells/mL was plated during cell passage. To improve the propensity of the NSPCs to differentiate towards the OL lineage, a driving media based on Neri et al., (2010) [23] was used for 48 h before differentiation. Driving media consisted of NSPCs stock media with 2% B27, 10 ng/mL FGF2, 20 ng/mL PDGF-AA, 20 ng/mL NT3 (FPN media). Differentiation media (FBS+/GF-) consisted of NSPC stock media, 2% B27, and 2% fetal bovine serum (FBS). Coverslips were treated with a thin coating of a complex extracellular matrix substrate, specifically, 0.5 mg/mL Matrigel (BD Biosciences; Mississauga, ON, Canada) in DMEM at room temperature for 30 min.

Glutamate Dose Response Curve

To test the effect of glutamate on NSPCs survival, dose response curves were performed on floating neurosphere cultures as well as during attachment to a Matrigel coated dish. Neurospheres were briefly plated at 100,000 cells/mL in triplicate wells at each time point with a gradient (0-1000 μM) of glutamate (Sigma-Aldrich) added to the regular NSPCs growth media 24 h after plating. After addition of glutamate, cultures grew for 24 h, 72 h, and 120 h, dissociated with TrypLE (Gibco) and mechanical triterating. Cell viability was determined using trypan blue exclusion method for each well separately. A similar protocol for attached neuro-spheres was used except dissociated cultures were plated onto Matrigel coated wells at 39,500 cells/cm^2 and 10μM glutamate was also used.

Attachment, Treatment and Differentiation Experiments

For treatment groups, one week prior to plating an experimental trial, stock NSPCs cultures were split into four dishes. Five days later, 48 h before plating, sets of two dishes were combined, centrifuged at 250 × g for 2.5 min to perform a 70% media change with either FPN media or NSPC growth media. To plate the experiment, termed day 0 (0 d), FPN+ or FPN- dishes were created accordingly, centrifuged at 300 × g for 3 min, resuspended in 2 mL NSPCs stock media. Cells were plated into 6-well dishes (Corning, NY, USA) in triplicate per treatment in 0.5 mg Matrigel coated wells at 50,000 cells/well (~26,315 cells/cm^2). Treatments consisted of NSPCs growth media with and without 200 μM glutamate on FPN- cells, differentiation media (FBS+/GF-) with and without 200 μM glutamate on both FPN+ and FPN- cells. Partial media was changed on days 3, 7, and 10.

RNA Isolation, cDNA Synthesis, and Reverse Transcription Quantitative PCR (QPCR)

Total RNA was extracted using RNeasy Plus Mini Kit (Qiagen) according to the manufacturer's protocol from spontaneously attached, FPN+/- cultures at day 0, and from each treatment at day 7 and 14. Briefly, each well was lysed with 350 μL lysis buffer containing β-mercaptoethanol, triplicates were combined and the sample homogenized using a motorized pestle (VWR). Pure RNA was eluted with 50 μL or 30 μL of RNase-free water for day 0 and day 7/14 samples, respectively. RNA purity and approximate concentration was determined using a Nanodrop 1000 (ThermoFisher Scientific); however, samples only underwent RNA precipitation, if 260/230 < 1.4. RNA integrity was determined using the RNA 6000 Nano Kit on the Bioanalyzer 2100 (Agilent; Santa Clara, CA, USA) according to manufacturer's instructions. If a sample's RNA concentration was above the quantitative range (5-500 ng/μL), a 10-fold dilution with RNase-free water was used to determine quality and for cDNA synthesis. RNA integrity numbers (RINs) ranged from 6.2 to 10. Most samples had an RIN around 8. Concentrations obtained from the Bioanalyzer were used for reverse transcription. Reverse transcription of 200 ng RNA was performed using the ProtoScript II Reverse Transciptase kit (NEB), to produce cDNA and NRT samples. To reach the volume of cDNA required for QPCR, Sso Advanced PreAmp Supermix (BioRad) was used, according to the manufacturer's instructions.

Quantitative polymerase chain reaction (QPCR) was performed with 1.5 μL cDNA template using PerfeCTa SYBR Green Supermix with ROX (Quanta Biosciences; Gaithersburg, MD, USA), and 300 nM optimized primer pairs (Table 1) in 20 μL reactions on CFX Connect and CFX96 Touch real-time PCR detection systems (BioRad; Mississauga, Canada). The threshold line to determine the quantitative cycle (Cq) was set using baseline subtracted curve fit. The reference genes used for normalization for spontaneous attachment experiments were eukaryotic elongation factor 2 (eEF2) and 26S proteasome non-ATPase regulatory subunit 4 (PSMD4). As necessary, wells for inter-run sample calibration (IRC) for a given target on different plates were included on each run with cDNA from juvenile mouse brain used as template for IRCs. Stable reference genes, non-POU domain containing, octamer-binding protein (Nono) and transferrin receptor protein 1 (Tfrc) were selected from 14 genes on M96 PrimePCR reference gene plates (BioRad). Synthetic DNA and RNA templates were provided to test for inhibitors in the QPCR re-action and RT reaction efficiency, respectively. Selected reference genes were ordered as preoptimized PrimePCR assays, but acceptable amplification efficiency and R2 was verified.

Data Analysis

Raw quantification cycle (Cq) qPCR data was exported from CFX 3.1 software (Biorad) and analyzed using MCMC.qpcr package [32] in R (version 3.4.3) and R studio (version 1.1.423). The package uses a Poisson-lognormal generalized linear mixed model to compare differences in fold changes in target genes in response to fixed factors and variation due to random differences in technical replicates. A Bayesian Markov Chain Monte Carlo sampling scheme is used, including reference genes as priors. Using this method negates the variability discovered in the reference genes utilized in this study. We present several reference gene expression in the results to demonstrate this variability.

Calibrated normalized relative quantities (CNRQs) of attached and control samples were log transformed and compared using an unpaired test with two-sided significance ($p < 0.05$) and false discovery rate (FDR) correction was used for testing multiple hypotheses.

Table 1. Primers used for RT QPCR analysis

Target	Primer Sequence (5' to 3') Forward/Reverse	Amplicon (bp)	% E	% E preamp	Design
SOX2	ACAGCATGTCCTACTCGCAG	60	101.1	97.7	Exonic
	CCTCGGACTTGACCACAGAG				
Nestin	GCTACATACAGGACTCTGCTGG	133	101.2	98.3	Exon-exon
	GGTGCTGGTCCTCTGGTATC				
NG2	AACGGACGGATCGCCTTGAG	106	97	92.5	Exon-exon
	CCAGGGCTCCTCTGTGTGAGA				
PDGF	AGTGGCTACATCATCCCCCT	91	103.2	N/A	Exon-exon
	CCGAAGTCTGTGAGCTGTGT				
CNP	GCAGGAGGTGGTGAAGAGAT	148	99.6	100.4	Exon-exon
	GGCAGATGGCTTGTCCAGAT				
MBP	GTACAAGGACTCACACACGAGA	217	93	95.0	Exon-exon
	GCCTCCGTAGCCAAATCCTG				
GFAP	CACGAACGAGTCCCTAGAGC	84	105.5	100.0	Exon-exon
	GCAAGTGCCTCCTGGTAACT				
NeuroD1	GAAGGCAAGGTGTCCCGAGG	83	96.4	98.7	Exon-exon
	GGTCATGTTTCCACTTCCTGTTGTT				
Dcx2	AACGACCAAGACGCAAATGGAA	138	104.3	N/A	Exon-exon
	ATCCAATGACAGCGGCAGGT				
Dcx4	AAGCTGGACAAGGCACTAGGAC	127	105.7	N/A	Exon-exon
	CTGGTTGGGTGGAGATGCTGA				
β3 tubulin	CACGCAGCAGATGTTCGATG	198	107.1	93.7	Exonic
	TCACACACGGCTACCTTGAC				
eEF2	CTTCAAGGTGTTCGACGCCA	198	107.9	N/A	Exon-exon
	GTGACGGGGGATGGTAAGTG				
PSMD4	CTG AAG ACT CGG ATG ACG CCC	107	101.2	N/A	Exon-exon
	GGCGATCTGCTCTTCCTCAGT				
RpL37	CGTTCCCTTCGTCATCTTGCTT	82	105.4	N/A	Exon-exon
	CTTATCCACAGGAAGTGGCGG				
Nono	Assay ID: qMmuCED0040697	96	N/A	87.3	Exonic
Tfrc	Assay ID: qMmuCID0039655	104	N/A	90.2	Intron spanning

Amplification efficiencies were determined from standard curves for cDNA template (%E) and pre-amplified cDNA template (%E preamp) with N/A indicating %E was not calculated with that template type. QPCR was performed with 300nM and 250nM for cDNA and pre-amplified cDNA reactions, respectively. Most primer sets have one primer spanning an exon-exon junction, except Tfrc, which is intron spanning, and Nono, SOX2, and β3 tubulin which have both primers in the same exon. Reference genes, Nono and Tfrc, were Prime PCR assays (BioRad; Ontario), but the rest of the primers were ordered from Invitrogen (Ontario)

Due to the multiple factors involved in the treatment groups, the best fitting general linear model (GLM) was used for each gene to determine factors or interactions that had significant effects ($p < 0.05$) overall on mRNA levels. The model with the best fit included a gamma distribution with a log-link function, all factors' full effects and interactions with time, and standard error (SE) weighted to the inverse proportion of the propagated SE:

CNRQ ~ Timepoint + FBS + FPN + Glutamate +
Timepoint: FBS + Timepoint: FPN +
Timepoint: Glutamate.

For each treatment and gene, main effects are reported with their log estimates and critical t value and were plotted as CNRQ mean point estimates ± 95% confidence intervals over the time points included in the study. Experimental trials were repeated four times, but data were combined across all treatments to measure the full effects for each factor. Outliers were determined by graphical analysis of the following residual plots: residuals vs. fitted values, scale location, normal Q-Q, and residuals vs. leverage. Since factors with a priori hypotheses (FPN and Glutamate) returned no significant results at the full effects level, further directed hypothesis tests were not conducted. Statistical analysis was performed in R Studio (R Core Team) using the visual packages "ggplot2" and "effects."

RESULTS

NSPCs Development in the Presence of Glutamate, FPN, and FBS

To test the effect of glutamate on NSPCs, a dose response curve was performed on floating neurospheres and attached cultures to a Matrigel coated dish. Glutamate (200 µM - 1 mM) was found to have no effect on cell viability of NSPCs cultures, when floating or attached to Matrigel. Similar trends were observed without the addition of glutamate. However, increasing the dosage of glutamate had an overall negative effect on cell viability. After 120 h, a concentration of 10 mM glutamate caused a 63% decrease in cell survival compared to 0 µM glutamate (Figure 1). For this study, we have selected 200 µM of glutamate as the concentration to use in our tests, based on both the dose response curve (Figure 1), in addition to electrophysiological findings from our previously published studies [33, 34]. Addition of 200 µM glutamate increased cell proliferation, requiring more frequent passages of cell cultures. During cell counts, this resulted in a 27.4 ± 0.29% (n = 10) fold increase in counted cells. The presence of glutamate had an effect on several genes responsible for both stem cell proliferation as well as differentiation (Figure 2). In general, cells not exposed to glutamate (Glu-) demonstrated an overall tendency to have no significant change in any gene expression over time. The only exception being SOX, whose expression increased after 14 days compared to day 1. This could be attributed to increases in cell number as cells divided over the time course of the study. When cells were exposed to glutamate (Glu+), we found an overall tendency to increase the expression of genes involved in stem cell proliferation. For example, cells treated with glutamate saw nestin expression levels start to decrease by day 14, compared to controls (Glu+ = -0.43, t = -1.68, p = 0.01). Whereas, without glutamate present, nestin mRNA levels continued to increase by day 14 (Figure 2). Further effects demonstrated a tendency for an increased expression of cells that have started the expression of genes involved in oligodendroglial expression. For example there was a significant increase in both Olig2 and CNPase expression in Glu+ treated cells compared to controls. Not surprisingly there was no significant difference in MBP expression between the two groups. It takes several weeks for oligodendroglial differentiation to occur and, in the two weeks of this study, we would not expect to observe MBP expression at this early stage (Figure 2).

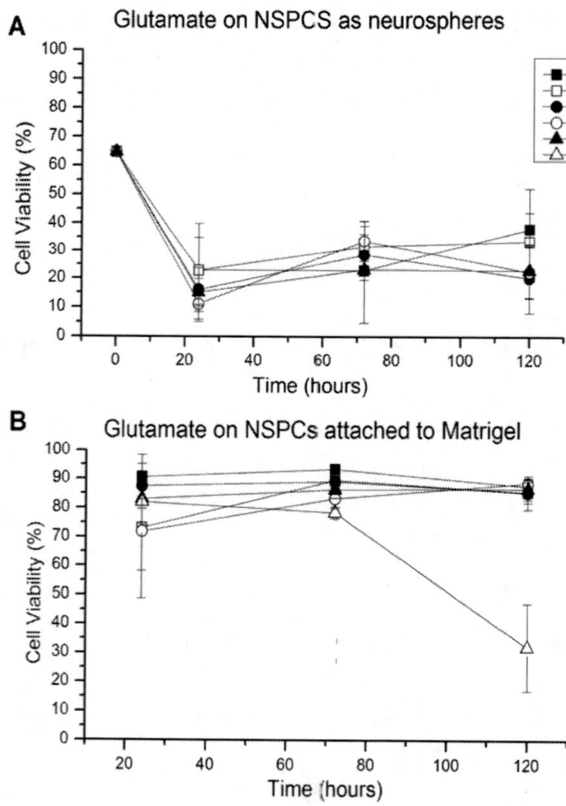

Figure 1. Glutamate does not affect NSPCs survival. A gradient of glutamic acid concentrations (0-1000 μM, 10 mM in B) was added to NSPCs working media for 5 days while cultures were either A) floating neurospheres or B) attached to Matrigel coated dishes. Survival was determined by counts using the trypan blue exclusion method and calculating percent cell viability at 24h, 72h, and 120h after addition of glutamic acid. Measurements were averaged from three separate wells serving as technical replicates; therefore, graphs A and B contain means ± SD.

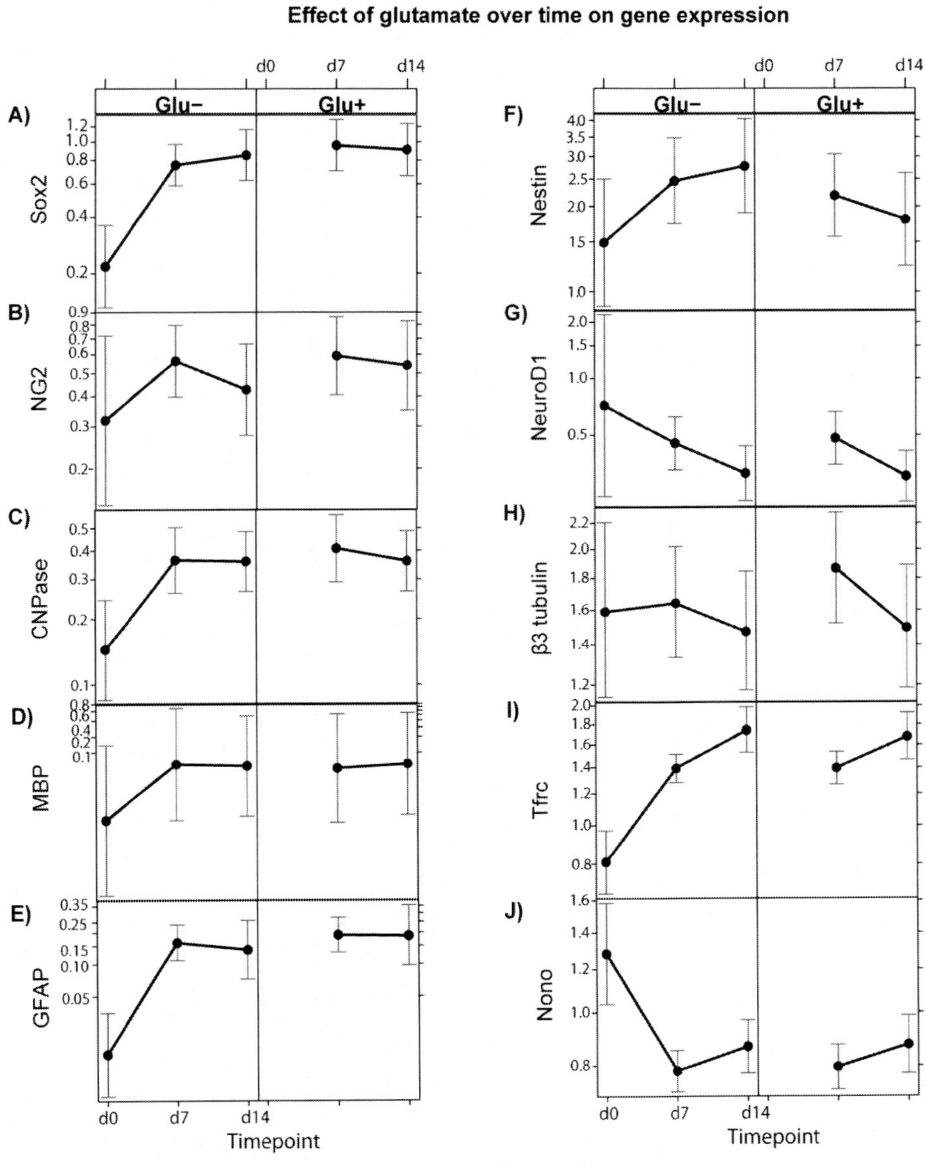

Figure 2. Effect plots of glutamate over time on neural cell marker gene expressions from differentiating NSPCs cultures. Plots represent the overall effect of 200μM glutamate, and its interaction with time based on mean estimates of calibrated normalized relative quantities and 95% confidence intervals derived from a fitted generalized linear model (glm) with a gamma distribution (CNRQ ~ Timepoint * FBS + FPN + Glutamate). Y-axis depicts mRNA abundance (log2). On day 0, floating neurospheres containing neural stem and progenitor cells (NSPCs) were plated on Matrigel coated dishes with or without FBS or 200μM glutamate and cultured for 14 days. At day 7 and 14, RNA was collected for RT-QPCR that used primers for the following cell markers: A) Sox2 and F) Nestin (immature cells), B) NG2 (oligodendrocyte precursor cells), C) CNPase (immature oligodendrocyte (OL)), D) MBP (mature OL), E) GFAP (astrocytes), G) NeuroD1 (neural progenitor cells), H) β3 tubulin (mature neurons), and two reference genes, I) Tfrc and J) Nono.

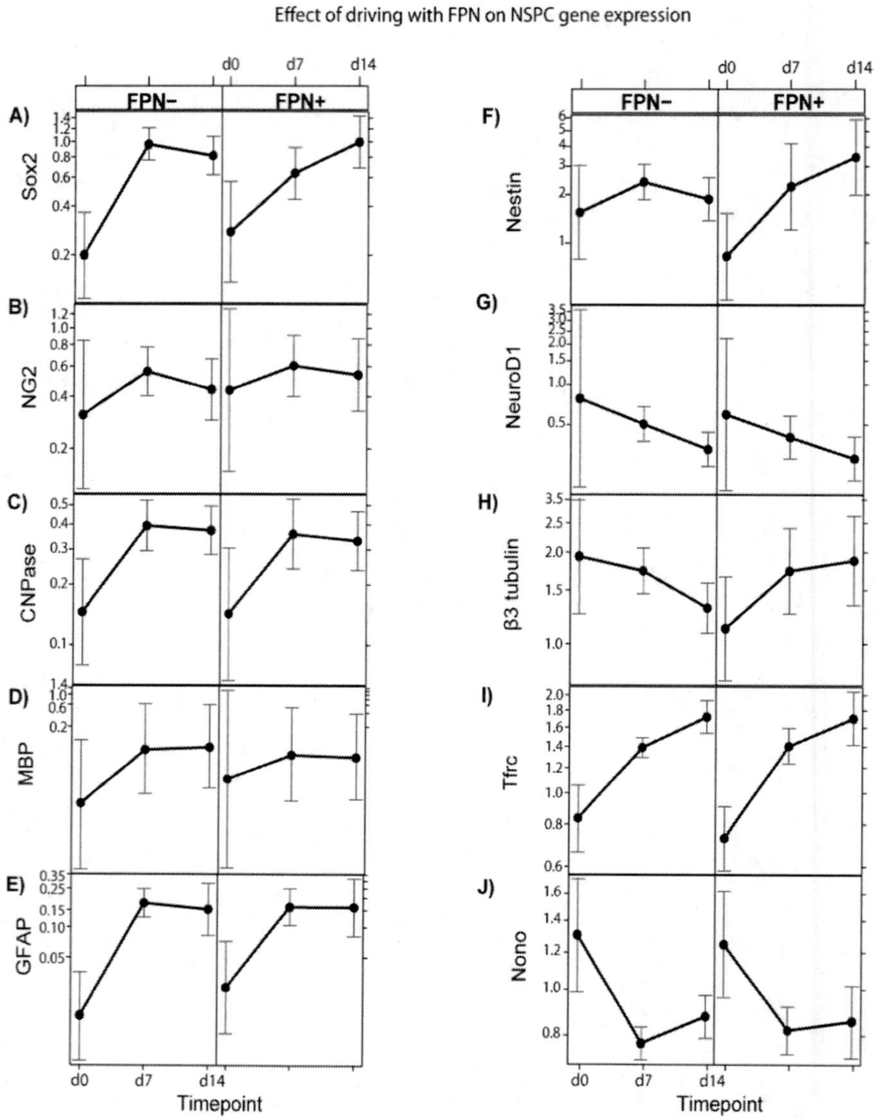

Figure 3. Effect plots of FPN driven cultures over time on neural cell marker gene expressions from differentiating NSPCs cultures. Plots represent the overall effect of driving NSPCs towards the oligodendrocyte lineage for 48h before plating with FPN media and these cultures subsequent interaction with time based on mean estimates of calibrated normalized relative quantities and 95% confidence intervals derived from a fitted generalized linear model (glm) with a gamma distribution (CNRQ ~ Timepoint * FBS + FPN + Glutamate). Y-axis depicts mRNA abundance (log2). On day 0, floating neurospheres containing FPN+ or FPN- NSPCS were plated on Matrigel coated dishes with or without FBS, and 200μM glutamate. At day 7 and 14, RNA was collected for RT-QPCR that used primers for the following cell markers: A) Sox2 and F) Nestin B) NG2 C) CNPase D) MBP E) GFAP G) NeuroD1 H) β3 tubulin and two reference genes, I) Tfrc and J) Nono. FPN only had an effect on nestin ($p = 0.07$) and significantly β3 tubulin ($p = 0.02$) causing a decrease in expression for both markers. A significant positive interaction between time and FPN was also observed for nestin ($p < 0.001$) and β3 tubulin ($p = 0.004$).

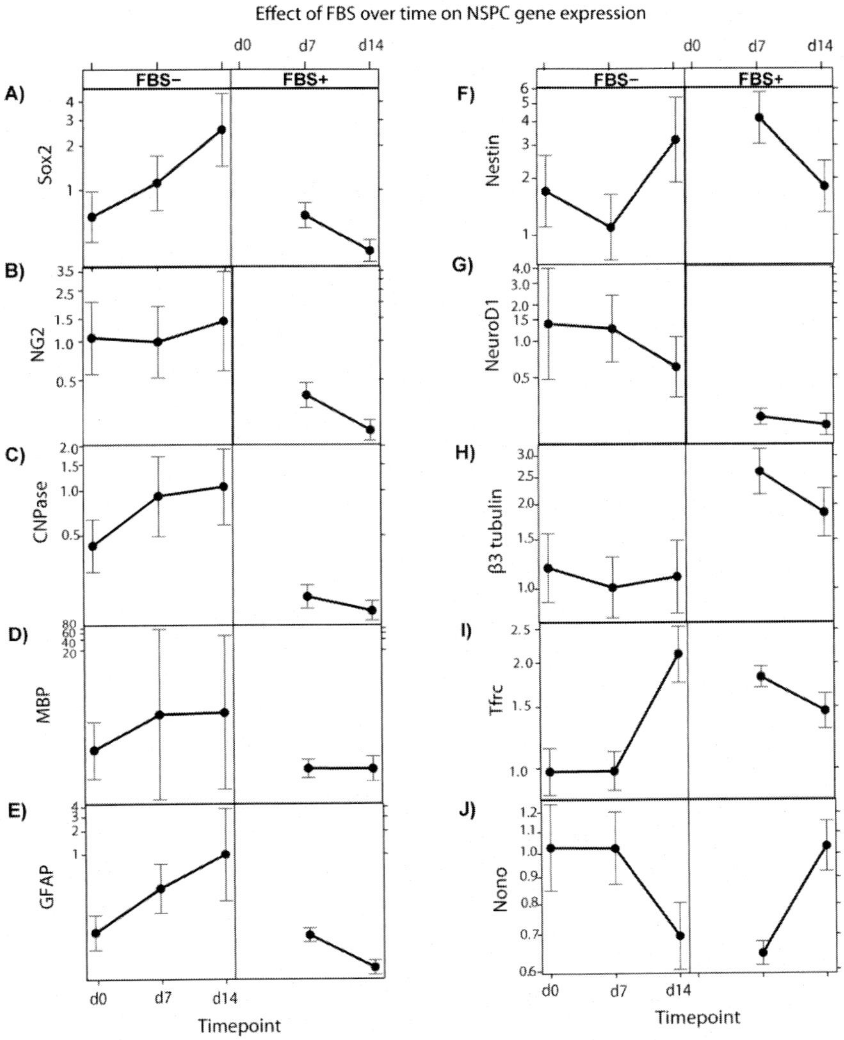

Figure 4. Effect plots of FBS and attachment to Matrigel over time on neural cell marker gene expressions from differentiating NSPCs cultures. Plots represent the overall effect of the differentiation cue, FBS, and its interaction with time based on mean estimates of calibrated normalized relative quantities and 95% confidence intervals derived from a fitted generalized linear model (glm) with a gamma distribution (CNRQ ~ Timepoint * FBS + FPN + Glutamate). Y-axis depicts mRNA abundance (log2). On day 0, floating neurospheres containing neural stem and progenitor cells (NSPCs) were plated on Matrigel coated dishes with or without FBS or 200μM glutamate and cultured for 14 days. Therefore, effects of attachment to Matrigel can be observed by comparing day 0 (unattached) to day 7 (attached) samples. At day 7 and 14, RNA was collected for RT-QPCR that used primers for the following cell markers: A) Sox2 and F) Nestin B) NG2 C) CNPase D) MBP E) GFAP G) NeuroD1 H) β3 tubulin and two reference genes, I) Tfrc and J) Nono. All markers except, nestin ($p = 0.07$) and MBP, were significantly affected by FBS ($p < 0.001$; Tfrc < 0.01) with β3 tubulin and Nono being the only markers to have increased expression versus decreased with FBS+. Time in culture without FBS had significant positive effects on Sox2, GFAP, and CNPase ($p < 0.001$, $p < 0.01$, $p < 0.05$) as seen as increased expression values at day14. Significant negative (Sox2, nestin $p < 0.001$; Gfap, Tfrc $p < 0.05$; NG2, β3 tubulin $p < 0.1$) and positive (Nono $p < 0.001$) interactions were observed between FBS and time (day7 to day14). All genes tested were present in the neurospheres at day0, with GFAP, Sox2, and CNPase ($p < 0.01$, $p < 0.05$, $p = 0.06$) increasing and nestin (nestin d7 $p < 0.05$) decreasing in expression upon attachment at day7.

Table 2. Summary of all significant GLM parameter estimates for all cell marker and factors tested on differentiating NSPCs

Parameter Estimates for
CNRQ ~ Timepoint + FBS + FPN + Glutamate + Timepoint:FBS + Timepoint:FPN + Timepoint:Glutamate

Cell Marker	Factor	Log(CNRQ) Mean Estimate ± SE	t_{obs}	p value
Sox2	Day 7[b]	0.71 ± 0.32	2.24	0.029
	Day 14	1.41 ± 0.38	3.75	< 0.001
	FBS	-1.91 ± 0.30	-6.27	< 0.001
	d7 : FBS	1.40 ± 0.39	3.59	< 0.001
Nestin	Day 7 [b]	-0.77 ± 0.33	-2.36	0.022
	FBS	-0.57 ± 0.31	-1.83	0.072
	FPN	-0.63 ± 0.35	-1.82	0.073
	d7 : FBS	1.90 ± 0.40	4.79	< 0.001
	d7 : FPN	1.24 ± 0.47-	2.65	0.010
NG2	FBS	-1.97 ± 0.46	-4.32	< 0.001
	d7 : FBS	1.01 ± 0.58	1.75	0.085
CNPase	Day 14	0.94 ± 0.3	2.47	0.016
	FBS	-1.92 ± 0.31	-6.22	< 0.001
MBP	FBS	-3.53 ± 2.44	-1.44	0.154
GFAP[a]	Day 7[b]	1.59 ± 0.49	3.23	0.002
	Day 14	2.48 ± 0.75	3.28	0.002
	FBS	-3.31 ± 0.69	-4.81	< 0.001
	d7 : FBS	1.95 ± 0.79	2.48	0.016
NeuroD1	FBS	-1.15 ± 0.32	-3.63	< 0.001
β3 tubulin	Day 7 [b]	-0.40 ± 0.22	-1.78	0.081
	FBS	0.53 ± 0.19	2.83	0.006
	FPN	-0.54 ± 0.23	-2.39	0.020
	d7 : FBS	0.43 ± 0.25	1.73	0.088
	d7: FPN	0.55 ± 0.30	1.82	0.074
	d14 : FPN	0.90 ± 0.30	3.00	0.004
Nono	Day 14	-0.40 ± 0.14	-2.79	0.007
	FBS	0.40 ± 0.10	2.97	< 0.001
	d7 : FBS	-0.86 ± 0.13	-6.68	< 0.001
Tfrc	Day 14	0.72 ± 0.13	5.52	< 0.001
	FBS	-0.37 ± 0.11	-3.28	0.002
	d7 : FBS	0.98 ± 0.13	7.31	<0.001

Summary of the parameter estimates for the main effects of the differentiation cue, FBS, on the relative mRNA levels of neural stem and progenitor NSPCs derived from a fitted generalized linear model (glm). The model with the best fit included a gamma distribution with a log-link function, all factors' full effects and interactions with time, and standard error (SE) weighted to the inverse proportion of the propagated SE: with a gamma distribution (CNRQ ~ Timepoint * FBS + FPN + Glutamate). At the full effects level, each factor is tested with the other factors held constant; therefore, data presented here represents the overall effect FBS had on the NSPCs cultures. On day 0, NSPCs were plated on Matrigel coated dishes with or without 5 % FBS or 200 μM glutamate and cultured for 14 days. On day 0, 7 and 14, RNA was collected for RT-QPCR that used primers for the following cell markers: Sox2 and Nestin, NG2, CNPase and MBP, GFAP, NeuroD1, β3 tubulin, and two reference genes, Tfrc and Nono. All markers except, nestin (p = 0.07) and MBP, were significantly affected by FBS with β3 tubulin and Nono being the only markers to have increased expression versus decreased with FBS+. Statistical analysis was performed in R Studio

[a] One outlier value removed from the GFAP data set without any changes to the trends observed.

[b] Effects observed at Day 7 include attachment from d 0 to d 7

Interestingly, the driving of NSPCs with FPN media showed no significant effect on cell marker mRNA levels, except nestin and β3 tubulin (Figure 3), which are markers for immature cells and mature neurons, respectively. In floating spheres, driving with FPN media 48 h beforehand caused a decrease in expression of nestin (FPN+ = -0.63, $t = -1.82$, $p = 0.07$) and β3 tubulin (FPN+ = -0.54, $t = -2.39$, $p = 0.02$) at day 0. By day 14, both nestin and β3 tubulin expression increased past levels in FPN-cultures at the same time point, showing a significant interaction between driving and culture time for these genes (FPN: d14 = 1.24, $t = 2.65$, $p = 0.01$ and FPN:d14 = 0.90, $t = 3.00$, $p = 0.004$, respectively) (Figure 3 and Table 2).

Not surprisingly, both FBS and culture duration had significant effects alone, and/or in synergy on all genes tested, except that of MBP (Figure 4). Over the course of the experiment, FBS significantly decreased mRNA levels of all gene markers ($p < 0.001$; Tfrc $p < 0.01$ and nestin $p = 0.07$) except for β3 tubulin and the reference gene, Nono, which significantly increased ($p < 0.001$) and MBP, which decreased non-significantly (Figure 4 and Table 2). In the presence of FBS, most genes had the highest expression levels at day 7 followed by a decrease in expression by day 14, except for Nono, which showed the opposite effect, implying a significant relationship between FBS and time (Sox 2, Nestin $p < 0.001$; GFAP, Tfrc $p < 0.05$; NG2 $p = 0.08$; β3 tubulin $p = 0.09$) (Figure 4 and Table 2). Other markers, CNPase, MBP, and neuroD1, showed no interactions between time and FBS. Without FBS present, time in culture had a significant positive effect on Sox2, GFAP, CNPase and Tfrc ($p < 0.001$, $p < 0.01$, $p < 0.05$, $p < 0.001$, respectively, (Table 2), with increased expression observed at day 14.

We also analyzed several traditional reference genes as part of our studies (Figure 2, 3, 4). We found that several of these were not stably expressed in our experimental conditions. It was observed that as NSPC started to express other non-stem cell genes, there was a tendency for significant drift in gene expression (e.g., Figure 3). Thus reference genes were not used as part of our overall analysis of gene expression in our experimental studies.

Effect of Attachment on NSPCs Expression Profile

We next sought to determine whether NSPCs that spontaneously attached to the substrate had any alterations in gene expression. Spontaneous attachment significantly decreased the immature marker nestin by 2.5 fold, and increased the immature neuronal marker, dcx, 3.3-fold from control ($p < 0.05$) (Figure 5). Two dcx assays were used to cover all possible transcript variants of the gene with the results for each being nearly identical. Although not significant, mRNA for the NPC marker, neuroD1, and mature oligodendrocyte marker, MBP both increased 2.0 fold upon attachment. The remainder of genes tested had < 1.5 fold changes in expression compared to control (Figure 5).

Therefore, the overall gene expression profile tended towards the neuronal and oligodendrocyte lineage upon spontaneous attachment.

The effect of attaching to Matrigel was also examined over the 14-day culture period. All genes tested were present in the neurospheres at day 0, with GFAP, Sox2, and CNPase showing increased mRNA amounts upon attachment at day 7 and further increasing at day 14 (d7/14 $p < 0.01$; d7 $p < 0.05$, d14 $p < 0.001$; d7 $p = 0.06$, d14 $p < 0.05$, respectively) (Figure 4). Neither reference gene was affected by attachment over the initial 7 days, but by day 14 mRNA levels had significantly increased and decreased for tfrc and nono, respectively ($p < 0.001$; $p < 0.01$). Nestin was the only transcript to have a decrease in levels upon attachment (d7 $p < 0.05$) with the rest of the genes tested unaffected attachment to Matrigel. MBP had one of the largest increases in mRNA abundance upon attachment, but due to large variance in the data set this was determined to be nonsignificant (Figure 4); therefore, MBP seems to be an inherently variable transcript and/or have an unexplained confounding factor associated with its expression within these experiments.

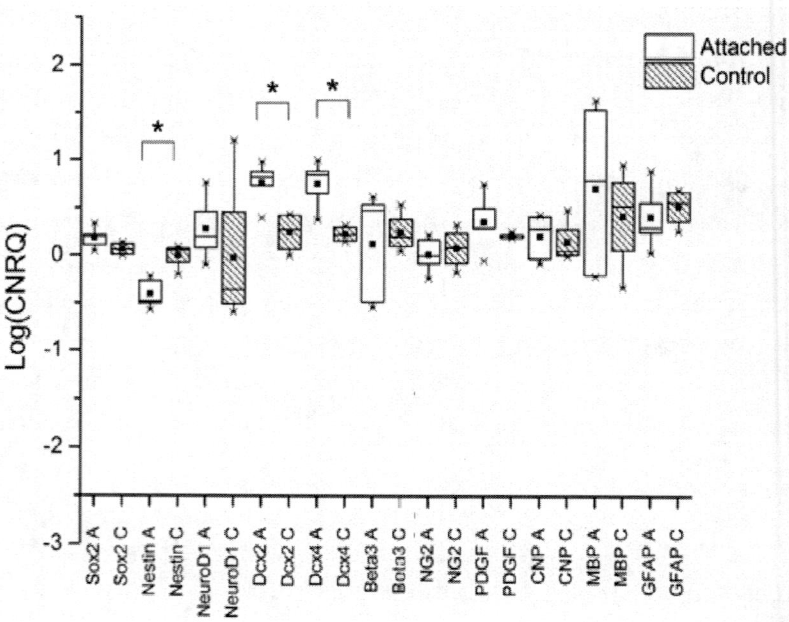

Figure 5. Effect of spontaneous attachment on NSPCs. Box plots consist of calibrated normalized relative quantities (CNRQs) of attached samples (white) that were log transformed and scaled against control samples of floating neurospheres cultures (hatched). Spontaneous attachment only significantly affected nestin and dcx with their expression decreasing 2.5 and increasing 3.3 fold, respectively, from control ($p < 0.05$). Although not significant, neuroD1and MBP both tended to increase 2.0 fold in expression upon attachment. The remainder of genes tested had <1.5 fold changes in expression compared to control. Therefore, the overall gene expression profile tended towards the neuronal and oligodendrocyte lineage upon attachment. (A = attached cultures, n = 5; C = Control, neurosphere cultures).

DISCUSSION

The effect of glutamate on the survival and proliferative capability of the population of NSPCs cells are largely unknown [27-31]. Many CNS differentiation studies have tended to focus on stem cell niches other than those obtained from the mature subventricular zone of the brain. In our study, we observed that the glutamate at the dose of 200μM had several effects on the expression of genes in NSPCs. More specifically, there was a shift towards cells of the oligodendroglial lineage and a decrease in gene expression involved in other cell types (e.g., stem cells or neurons) (Figure 2). Furthermore, we found that several traditional reference genes were not stably expressed under our experimental conditions, thus requiring the use of poisson-log normal GLM to analyze changes in target gene expression. It is also possible that other effects downstream were not detected by this study (e.g., changes in protein levels) as we solely focused on gene transcript levels and is part of our future studies. In contrast to glutamate stimulation, we found that exposure to FBS or mitogen withdraw, leading to cells shifting towards a more neuronal lineage.

Our findings in NSPCs mirror some of the effects observed in certain pathologies. For example, myelin regeneration can occur during the remission phase of multiple sclerosis (MS). Furthermore, NSPCs and oligodendrocyte progenitor cells (OPCs) express glutamatergic receptors [35-37]. It is widely accepted that there is continuous cross-talk between glial cells and neurons. For example, blocking AMPA receptors in demylinated lesions, inhibits oligodendroglial genesis [38]. In other studies, it is observed that glutamate released from neuronal endings can also simulate changes in OPCs [36, 37]. Thus our findings that glutamate guides cells down an oligodendroglial fate, support both the events in oligodendroglial genesis and certain pathologies.

In contrast, many earlier studies found no effect of glutamate on gene regulation. For example, Brazel et al., (2005) [30] found glutamate in combination with a NMDA receptor inhibitor to be ineffective at increasing protein levels of the cell marker proteins CNPase, GFAP, β3 tubulin or nestin, despite the observed increase in cells, likely neuronal precursors, proliferations in the NSC culture. The impact of glutamate on oligodendrogenesis from NSCs was also studied by Vernon et al., (2011) [39] who used an immortalized fetal human NSC line and found specifically that mGluR7 decreases oligodendrocyte and increases astrocyte differentiation. However, mGluR7 has never been shown to be expressed in adult NSPCs [27]. More recent work (2016) [28] demonstrated that the addition of glutamate up to 500 μM for 96 h significantly increases NSPCs proliferation and number, however, it does not significantly alter overall cell phenotype. Furthermore, 10h glutamate treatment also did not increase the number of NSPCs compared to controls. A possible explanation for some of these discrepancies in these earlier studies could be due to variance in reference gene/protein expression. In our study, we found that many reference genes were variably expressed in response to treatment. This variability would result in the masking of changes in gene expression. In our study, we found significant variability in gene expression, and because of this, could not rely on them as standard controls and strongly urge other studies to take this variability into consideration.

While a number of *in vitro* reports have suggested the additive role of individual or combinations of the growth factors in stem cell survival and neural differentiation [21-26], the cellular *responses* to individual *growth factor varies greatly* [40-43]. Moreover, most of these growth factors exhibit overt dose dependent effects on the differentiation state of the neural stem cells [43]. For example, it is well established that 10 ng/mL of FGF promotes the proliferation of undifferentiated stem cells, however, at 25 ng/mL the cell proliferation is not evident and instead an increase in neurons and oligodendrocytes are observed. Similarly, it has been shown that low doses of PDGFα promotes the oligodendrocyte differentiation, while at higher doses it reduces the astrocyte formation [43]. Interestingly, earlier reports have also indicated that the combination of PDGFα and FGF with other growth factors only produced the neurons and oligodendrocytes similar to the levels when no other growth factors were added [43]. Nevertheless, it is generally accepted that the combination of growth factors would have an additive effect on NSPCs differentiation.

In our study, the gene expression profile given by levels of cell marker transcripts of NSPCs cultures appears to primarily be affected by exposure to serum and GF withdrawal, with little effect observed by a combination of various growth factors (FGF, PDGF, NT3) in the FPN driving media (Figure 3). While we observed that the immature cell marker, nestin, and mature neuronal marker, β3 tubulin, were affected, however, we did not observe any increase in the OL lineage markers (NG2, CNP, MBP). Using primarily immunocytochemistry techniques, Neri et al., (2010) [23] found priming human NSPCs with FPN media for 7 days before differentiation increases the proportion of OPCs, pre-myelinating OL and neurons, while decreasing the proportion of astrocytes in cultures although they did not observe subsequent differentiation of OL lineage cells to fully mature MBP+ oligodendrocytes. Our results for driving the NSPCs are contrary to Neri et al., which may relate to driving time, or differences inherent to the species or age of NSPCs used. Neri et al., used human embryonic NSPCs that were primed with FPN media as neurospheres for 7 days prior to differentiation for 10 days with FBS. Thus, the length of time in FPN media is the greatest discrepancy, as in our study the incubation time was for 48 hours, and possibly that is an insufficient duration to dramatically affect the NSPCs differentiation. Further, it is well established that there can inherently be differences in responses to growth factors for NSPCs from rodents versus humans [40-42]. Furthermore, the expression profiles of receptors, including for growth factors, can also differ between NSPCs from embryonic versus adult origin, which can result in cells behaving differently to similar treatments [44, 45]. Therefore, the adult murine NSPCs could potentially require different concentrations or combinations of growth factors to optimally drive NSPCs towards the OL lineage compared to the embryonic human NSPCs used by Neri et al., (2010) [23]. We also examined the effect of growth factors withdrawal on NSPCs after FBS treatment that resulted in the reduction of immature (sox2, nestin) and precursor cells (OPC: NG2, NPC: neuroD1) expression during a 14-day differentiation period (Figure 4). However, the only mature cell marker transcript to increase was β3 tubulin, which increased with FBS+ by day 7 and subsequently, decreased by day 14. These *observations* are consistent with the Cavaliere et al., (2012) [46] who found that GF- differentiation of driven NSPCs towards O4+ OL cells increase from 50 to 72 % over 1 to 7 days, respectively, however, an increase in cell death observed after 10 days of differentiation. Thus, it can be inferred that the applied differentiation conditions used in the present study promoted the increase of the neuronal population from the preceding precursor population in an early seven-day period, however, that may have been followed by a cell death event by day 14.

It appears that the cell culturing substrate can have an impact on NSPC differentiation fate. We observed that when neurosphere cultures spontaneously attached to their culture dishes, the gene expression profile of the culture tended towards the neuronal and oligodendrocyte lineage. The significant decrease in the nestin transcript coinciding with an increased presence of neuroD1 (non-significant) and dcx ($p < 0.05$), suggesting that NSPCs were specifically differentiating into immature neurons upon spontaneous attachment (Figure 5). Less clear lineage progression was observed for oligodendrocyte cells as only MBP was significantly affected, suggesting an increased proportion of mature oligodendrocytes without impact on preceding pre-cursors. In contrast, attachment to the complex extra-cellular matrix (ECM) substrate, Matrigel, affected different cell markers as compared to spontaneous attachment. Matrigel-attached cultures with regular growth media (FBS/GF+) had significant increases in NSCs (Sox2), immature OL and astrocytes (GFAP) after seven days, and further increases at day 14. The mature OL marker, MBP, showed one of the largest increases in expression upon attachment at day 7, but due to large variance for this particular assay, the effect was not found to be significant. Therefore, Matrigel promoted the development of glial lineages, while not affecting, or potentially inhibiting, the attachment effect on neuronal lineage as observed with spontaneous attachment. Nevertheless, *further studies need* to be performed to confirm and reproduce these *results*.

CONCLUSION

In the present study, we demonstrated that glutamate (200μM) and combination of growth factors had several modulating effects on the gene expression profile of differentiated NSPCs culture. These changes were differentiation towards the oligodendroglial cell line. In contrast, stimulation with both FBS and GF withdrawal promoted the immature cells to develop towards the neuronal lineage and decrease proportions of glial cells. Interestingly, Matrigel-attached cultures with regular growth media, demonstrated significant increase in glial markers, with possible inhibition of the neuronal differentiation as observed with spontaneous attachment. Taken together, the current study suggests that the further optimization of OL driving protocols may redirect the NSPCs differentiation to an increased proportion of OL. As such, the ability to increase proportions of OL/neurons from NSPCs remain a necessary aspect of neurogenesis research and the current differentiation protocols should be further investigated with this goal in mind.

Acknowledgments

We would like to thank David Teece and Max Karnitsky for their technical expertise. Manuscript was modified from a thesis submitted by Katherine Ludlow as part of her MSc requirements at the University of Regina.

Ethical Compliance

The authors have stated all possible conflicts of interest within this work. The authors have stated all sources of funding for this work. If this work involved human participants, informed consent was received from each individual. If this work involved human participants, it was conducted in accordance with the 1964 Declaration of Helsinki. If this work involved experiments with humans or animals, it was conducted in accordance with the related institutions' research ethics guidelines.

References

[1] Rakic P (1985) Limits of neurogenesis in primates. *Science* 227:1054–1056.

[2] McTigue DM, Tripathi RB (2008) The life, death, and replacement of oligodendrocytes in the adult CNS. *J Neurochem* 107:1–19.

[3] Crawford AH, Chambers C, Franklin RJM (2013) Remyelination: the true regeneration of the central nervous system. *J Comp Pathol* 149:242–254.

[4] Maki T, Liang AC, Miyamoto N, Lo EH, Arai K (2013) Mechanisms of oligodendrocyte regeneration from ventricular-subventricular zone-derived progenitor cells in white matter diseases. *Front Cell Neurosci* 7:275.

[5] Altman J (1962) Are new neurons formed in the brains of adult mammals? *Science* 135:1127–1128.

[6] Temple S (1989) Division and differentiation of isolated CNS blast cells in microculture. *Nature* 340:471–473.

[7] Davis AA, Temple S (1994) A self-renewing multi-potential stem cell in embryonic rat cerebral cortex. *Nature* 372:263–266.

[8] Richards LJ, Kilpatrick TJ, Bartlett PF (1992) De novo generation of neuronal cells from the adult mouse brain. *Proc Natl Acad Sci USA* 89:8591–8595.

[9] Clelland C, Barker RA, Watts C (2008) Cell therapy in Huntington disease. *Neurosurg Focus* 24:1–12.

[10] Benraiss A, Toner MJ, Xu Q, Bruel-Jungerman E, Rogers EH, Wang F, Economides AN, Davidson BL, Kageyama R, Nedergaard M, Goldman SA (2013) Sustained mobilization of endogenous neural progen-itors delays disease progression in a transgenic model of huntington's disease. *Cell Stem Cell* 12:787–799.

[11] Madhavan L (2010) Transplantation of subventricular zone neural precursors induces an endogenous precursor cell response in a rat model of Parkinson's disease. *J Comp Neurol* 515: 102– 115.

[12] L'Episcopo F, Tirolo C, Testa N, Caniglia S, Morale MC, Impagnatiello F, Pluchino S, Marchetti B (2013) Aging-induced Nrf2-ARE pathway disruption in the subventricular zone drives neurogenic impairment in parkinsonian mice via PI3KWnt/β-catenin dysregu-lation. *J Neurosci 33*:1462–1485.

[13] Huang JK, Franklin RJM (2011) Regenerative medicine in multiple sclerosis: Identifying pharmacological targets of adult neural stem cell differentiation. *Neuro-chem Int* 59:329–332.

[14] Moyon S, Dubessy AL, Aigrot MS, Trotter M, Huang JK, Dauphinot L, Potier MC, Kerninon C, Melik Parsadaniantz S, Franklin RJM, Lubetzki C (2015) Demyelination Causes Adult CNS Progenitors to Revert to an Immature State and Express Immune Cues That Support Their Migration. *J Neurosci* 35:4–20.

[15] Haughey NJ, Nath A, Chan SL, Borchard AC, Rao MS, Mattson MP (2002) Disruption of neurogenesis by amyloid b -peptide, and perturbed neural progenitor cell homeostasis, in models of Alzheimer's disease. *J Neurochem* 83:1509–1524.

[16] Mu Y, Gage FH (2011) Adult hippocampal neuro-genesis and its role in Alzheimer's disease. *Mol Neurodegener* 6:85.

[17] Mothe AJ, Tam RY, Zahir T, Tator CH, Shoichet MS (2013) Repair of the injured spinal cord by transplan-tation of neural stem cells in a hyaluronanbased hydrogel. *Biomaterials* 34:3775-3783.

[18] Mothe AJ, Kulbatski I, Parr A, Mohareb M, Tator CH (2008) Adult spinal cord stem/progenitor cells trans-planted as neurospheres preferentially differentiate into oligodendrocytes in the adult rat spinal cord. *Cell Transplant* 17:735-751.

[19] Hernandez J, Torres-Espin A, Navarro X (2011) Adult stem cell transplants for spinal cord injury repair: current state in preclinical research. *Curr Stem Cell Res Ther* 6:273-87.

[20] Reynolds BA, Weiss S (1992) Generation of neurons and astrocytes from isolated cells of the adult mamm-alian central nervous system. *Science* 255:1707–1710.

[21] Mudò G, Bonomo A, Di Liberto V, Frinchi M, Fuxe K, Belluardo N (2009) The FGF2/FGFRs neurotrophic system promotes neurogenesis in the adult brain. *J Neural Transm* 116:995–1005.

[22] Hill RA, Patel KD, Medved J, Reiss AM, Nishiyama A (2013) NG2 cells in white matter but not gray matter proliferate in response to PDGF. *J Neurosci* 33:14558–14566.

[23] Neri M, Maderna C, Ferrari D, Cavazzin C, Vescovi AL, Gritti A (2010) Robust generation of oligo-dendrocyte progenitors from human neural stem cells and engraftment in experimental demyelination models in mice. *PLoS One* 5:e10145.

[24] Jackson EL, Garcia-Verdugo JM, Gil-Perotin S, Roy M, Quinones-Hinojosa A, VandenBerg S, Alvarez-Buylla A (2006) PDGFR alpha-positive B cells are neural stem cells in the adult SVZ that form glioma-like growths in response to increased PDGF signaling. *Neuron* 51:187–199.

[25] Mitew S, Hay CM, Peckham H, Xiao J, Koenning M, Emery B (2013) Mechanisms regulating the devel-opment of oligodendrocytes and central nervous system myelin. *Neuroscience* 276:29–47.

[26] Barres BA, Raff MC, Gaese F, Bartke I, Dechant G, Barde YA (1994) A crucial role for neurotrophin-3 in oligodendrocyte development. *Nature* 367:371–375.

[27] Jansson LC, Akerman KE (2014) The role of glutamate and its receptors in the proliferation, migration, differentiationand survival of neural progenitor cells. *J Neural Transm* 121:819-836.

[28] Hachem LD, Mothe AJ, Tator CH (2016) Glutamate increases invitro survival and proliferation and attenuates oxidative stress-induced cell death in adult spinal cord-derived neural stem/progenitor cells via on-NMDA ionotropic glutamate receptors. *Stem Cells Dev* 25:1223-1233.

[29] Haydar TF, Wang F, Schwartz ML, Rakic P (2000) Differential modulation of proliferation in the neo-cortical ventricular and subventricular zones. *J Neurosci* 20:5764-5774.

[30] Brazel CY, Nunez JL, Yang Z, Levison SW (2005) Glutamate enhances survival and proliferation of neural progenitors derived from the subventricular zone. *Neuroscience* 131:55-65.

[31] Jansson LC, Louhivuori L, Wigren HK, Nordstrom T, Louhivuori V, Castren ML, Akerman KE (2013) Effect of glutamate receptor antagonists on migrating neural progenitor cells. *Eur J Neurosci* 37:1369-1382.

[32] Matz MV, Wright RM, Scott JG (2013) No control genes required: Bayesian analysis of qRT-PCR data. *PLoS One* 8:e71448.

[33] Buttigieg J, Eftekharpour E, Karimi-Abdolrezaee S, Fehlings MG (2011) Molecular and electrophysiological evidence for the expression of BK channels in oligodendroglial precursor cells. *Eur J Neurosci* 34:538–547.

[34] Wu Y, Satkunendrarajah K, Teng Y, Chow DS-L, Buttigieg J, Fehlings MG (2013) Delayed post-injury administration of riluzole is neuroprotective in a pre-clinical rodent model of cervical spinal cord injury. *J Neurotrauma* 30: 441–452.

[35] Kukley M, Nishiyama A, Dietrich D (2010) The fate of synaptic input to NG2 glial cells: neurons specifically downregulate transmitter release onto differentiating oligodendroglial cells. *J Neurosci* 30: 8320–8331.

[36] Karadottir R, Hamilton NB, Bakiri Y, Attwell D (2008) Spiking and nonspiking classes of oligodendrocyte precursor glia in CNS white matter. *Nat Neurosci* 11: 450–456.

[37] Xiao L, Hu C, Yang W, Guo D, Li C, Shen W, Liu X, Aijun H, Dan W, He C (2013) NMDA receptor couples Rac1-GEF Tiam1 to direct oligodendrocyte precursor cell migration. *Glia* 61: 2078–2099.

[38] Gautier HOB, Evans KA, Volbracht K, James R, Sitnikov S, Lundgaard I, James F, Lao-Peregrin C, Reynolds R, Franklin RJ, Káradóttir RT (2015) Neuronal activity regulates remyelination via glutamate signalling to oligodendrocyte progenitors. *Nat Commun* 6:8518.

[39] Vernon AC, Smith EJ, Stevanato L, Modo M (2011) Selective activation of metabotropic glutamate receptor 7 induces inhibition of cellular proliferation and promotes astrocyte differentiation of ventral mesencephalon human neural stem/progenitor cells. *Neurochem Int* 59:421–431.

[40] Zhang SC, Ge B, Duncan ID (2000) Tracing human oligodendroglial development *in vitro*. *J Neurosci Res* 59:421–429.

[41] Chandran S, Compston A, Jauniaux E, Gilson J, Blakemore W, Svendsen C (2004) Differential generation of oligodendrocytes from human and rodent embryonic spinal cord neural precursors. *Glia* 47:314–324.

[42] Barateiro A, Fernandes A (2014) Temporal oligodendrocyte lineage progression: *In vitro* models of proliferation, differentiation and myelination. *Biochim Biophys Acta* 1843:1917-1929.

[43] Willerth SM, Faxel TE, Gottlieb DI, Sakiyama-Elbert SE (2007) The Effects of Soluble Growth Factors on Embryonic Stem Cell Differentiation Inside of Fibrin Scaffolds. *Stem Cells* 25:2235-2244.

[44] Maisel M, Herr A, Milosevic J, Hermann A, Habisch H-J, Schwarz S, Kirsch M, Antoniadis G, Brenner R, Hallmeyer-Elgner S, Lerche H, Schwarz J, Storch A (2007) Transcription profiling of adult and fetal human neuroprogenitors identifies

divergent paths to maintain the neuroprogenitor cell state. *Stem Cells* 25:1231–1240.

[45] McGinn MJ, Colello RJ, Sun D (2012) Age-related proteomic changes in the subventricular zone and their association with neural stem/progenitor cell proliferation. *J Neurosci Res* 90:1159–1168.

[46] Cavaliere F, Urra O, Alberdi E, Matute C (2012) Oligodendrocyte differentiation from adult multipotent stem cells is modulated by glutamate. *Cell Death Dis* 3:e268.

In: Manipulation of Stem Cells for Disease Benefits
Editor: Prasad Koka
ISBN: 978-1-53615-468-9

Chapter 9

COMPARING THE STEMNESS PROPERTIES OF DENTAL PULP CELLS (DPSCS), COLLECTED, PROCESSED, AND CRYOPRESERVED UNDER DIFFERENT CONDITIONS

***Nermeen El-Moataz Bellah Ahmed*[1,2,*], *Riham Mohamed Aly*[2,3], *Phoebe Magdy Abd El-Massieh*[1] and *Ahmad Farouk Abd El Azeem*[1,2]**

[1]Department of Oro-dental Genetics, Center of Medical Excellency, National Research Centre, Cairo, Egypt

[2]Stem Cell Laboratory, Center of Excellence for Advanced Sciences, National Research Centre, Cairo, Egypt

[3]Department of Basic Dental Science, National Research Center, Cairo, Egypt

ABSTRACT

This present study aims at the evaluation of different transportation, isolation, and cryopreservation conditions on the stemness properties of dental pulp stem cells (DPSCs), in an attempt to optimize those conditions to obtain high-quality cells for the needs of regenerative therapy. DPSCs were isolated from canine teeth that were placed in one of six different collection/transport solutions: phosphate buffered saline (PBS); PBS containing fetal bovine serum (FBS); Dulbecco modified Eagles' medium (DMEM); DMEM containing FBS; Hank's solution; or saline. Collected teeth were either processed after 3, 12, 24, 36, or 48 hours and using one of two different enzymes. The stemness properties of the isolated cells were evaluated in terms of proliferation, migration, and expression of stem cell markers. Moreover, DPSCs cryopreserved in one of two different

* Corresponding Author's E-mail: nermeenkandel@gmail.com.

cryopreservants and stored at -80°C then transferred to liquid nitrogen after either 1,12,24,48 hours or 1 week. After thawing, the cells were evaluated for viability using trypan blue test. The results indicate that dental pulp cells can be isolated from dental pulp up to 48 hours after tooth extraction, which implies that processing immediately after extraction may not be required for successful isolation. However, the stemness properties of the isolated cells were significantly affected by the transportation media and the isolation time. This study also indicates that the shorter the time elapsed between transferring the cryopreserved cells from -80°C to liquid nitrogen was, the higher the viability of the thawed cells was.

Keywords: stem cells, culture techniques, stemness

INTRODUCTION

Dental stem cells present a promising modality for cell therapy in dentistry as well as in other disciplines of medicine. This is owed to their self-renewal properties and their multipotency [1–5]. Dental pulp particularly has been recognized as a valuable source of stem cells. This is mainly due to its ease of accessibility as it can be feasibly collected from extracted third molars that are usually discarded. Previous studies have reported the ability of dental pulp stem cells (DPSCs) to differentiate into dentin and pulp like tissues in addition to their ability to differentiate into osteogenic, adipogenic, and chondrogenic lineages, which demonstrates their versatile regenerative properties [6–10]. These properties have generated a great deal of interest into the potential regenerative therapeutic applications of DPSCs. However, several challenges still exist in regards to the quality and safety in clinical applications, and a number of these challenges relate to the processing and the banking of these cells ex-vivo.

Isolation of DPSCs was originally reported in the year 2000. Since that time, a wide range of literature has been directed towards improving the isolation methods and the expansion methods in pursuance of generating a larger number of cells for use in clinical applications [1, 11–15]. However, to date, there has been little published that addresses the practical aspect of manipulating the pulp tissue immediately after tooth extraction [1, 16]. If DPSCs are to be used for regenerative purposes, it is important that clinicians are provided with practical pre-isolation conditions that would ensure the maximum viability of the cells isolated while maintaining their stemness. One of the challenges experienced during working with DPSCs is the determination of how soon the isolation procedures can start, especially if the place where extraction occurred is not at the same facility. There has always been a concern about the pulp tissue being degraded between the time of extraction and the time of initiation of stem cells isolation. Previous reports have shown that teeth that have been stored overnight yielded the same number of cells as those that were processed immediately, while another report has determined that cells could remain viable for up to five days [1, 17]. It is therefore important to determine the appropriate duration of time that would allow the cells to remain viable while identifying a suitable and feasible medium for storage and transportation.

Another challenge that affects the number of the isolated cells and the quality of the isolated cells is the tissue dissociation enzyme that is used during processing of the pulp tissues. Most of the published protocols for the isolation of DPSCs reported the use of collagenase; however, there have been reports of lot-to-lot variability among some collagenase products, and there have been some debates against its effect on cell phenotype and properties [18, 19]. Moreover, it is the FDA's consideration that cells that have been exposed to collagenase are "more than minimally manipulated," and the agency recommends the use of higher grade enzymes, which are also usually higher in cost [12, 20, 21].

Similar to cell isolation and processing techniques, the cryopreservation methods and the cryo-preservants that are used need to be thoroughly investigated for their effects on the viability and the proliferation of the isolated DPSCs. Storage of the cryopreserved DPSCs over various periods of time offers unique opportunities for the banking of teeth in anticipation for their future regenerative applications.

Here, we investigate a set of different conditions for transportation, isolation, and cryopreservation as well as their effects on the stemness properties of the isolated DPSCs. We studied how soon after extraction the isolation procedures can be initiated, without affecting the properties of the isolated cells. We also examined the effect of using some different transportation and storage media and digestive enzymes on the stemness of the isolated cells in terms of morphology, proliferation, migration, and expression of stem cell markers. Finally, we investigated the viability of cells under different cryopreservation conditions.

MATERIALS AND METHODS

Extraction and Preservation of Teeth

All of the experimental protocols were performed in accordance with the guidelines of the National Research Centre. All of the animals involved in this study were treated in accordance with the ethical standards set forth by the institution at which the study was conducted. Adult healthy mongrel dogs were used in this study, with an average body weight of 20-30 kg, and of ages ranging from 1-1.5 years. A mixture of anesthetic agents; Xylazine HCl (1mg/kg) and Ketamine HCl (5 mg/kg) was injected through each dog's cephalic vein. Teeth were aseptically and atraumatically extracted at the veterinary clinic of the Faculty of Veterinary Medicine at Cairo University in Egypt.

After the teeth were extracted, they were immediately placed in one of six different collection/transportation solutions: phosphate buffered saline (PBS; GIBCO, Invitrogen,

USA); PBS containing 10% fetal bovine serum (FBS; Invitrogen, Carlsbad, CA, USA); Dulbecco modified Eagles' medium (DMEM; Sigma-Aldrich, USA); DMEM containing 10% FBS, saline; or Hank's balanced salt solution (HBSS; Sigma, USA). All of the media that was used were supplemented with Penicillin/streptomycin (Invitrogen Co., USA).

Cell Isolation and Culture

The collected teeth were either processed after 3, 12, 24, 36 or 48 hours of extraction. For each tooth, the pulp was gently removed using a sterile dental probe and the collected pulp tissue was dissected and digested in 0.2% of either collagenase type II (Worthington Biochemical, Lakewood, NJ, USA) or Liberase MNP-S (Roche, Germany). The isolated dental pulp cells (DPCs) were cultured in Dulbecco modified eagle's medium (DMEM) supplemented with 10% FBS, 100 units/mL of penicillin, 100 µg/mL of streptomycin, and 0.25 µg/mL of Fungizone. Cells were selected on the basis of their ability to adhere to the tissue culture dish; non-adherent cells were removed during medium replacement after 5 days in culture. DPSCs isolated from up to 4 teeth were used to conduct the various assays for each group.

Viability and Morphological Assessment

At each isolation time point, the cells were evaluated for viability using trypan blue test. All isolated cells were regularly monitored using an inverted light microscope (Leica, 6000B-4) using Suite V3 (Leica) to asses and compare any morphological changes. Multiple representative fields of cells were photographed and the captured images were analyzed using Image J software (version 1.49r15) to determine the number of spindle-shaped cells. Four different areas were analyzed for each image.

Flow Cytometric Analysis

Evaluation of the stem cell markers expression was necessary to compare the ability of DPSCs to keep their stemness properties under different isolation conditions. 1×10^5 cells at the fifth passage of culture were detached from flasks using Accutase (Sigma-Aldrich). For blocking and reducing the non-specific binding receptors, the cells were incubated with FCR blocking reagent for twenty minutes at 4°C. The cells were further incubated with, CD105 (FITC, mouse, Abcam, Cambridge, UK), CD90 (FITC, mouse, R&D, USA), CD44 (FITC, mouse, R&D systems, USA), CD73 (FITC, mouse, Abcam,

Cambridge, UK), IgG1 isotype control (FITC, mouse, Biolegend, USA), and IgG2a isotype control (FITC, mouse, Santa Cruz, USA) for one hour, at 4°C. The cells were then washed with PBS supplemented with 20% FBS and then centrifuged at 1300 rpm for one minute at 4°C. The supernatant was discarded and the cells were re-suspended in Hank's solution (Invitrogen), which was supplemented with FBS, and 4-(2-hydroxyethyl)-1-piperazineethanesulf onic acid buffer solution (HEPS) (Invitrogen), to which 2 μg/ml of propidium iodide (PI) stain (Sigma) was added in order to stain dead cells. Labeled cells were analyzed using the FACSAria II flow cytometer (Becton Dickinson, USA). Only viable cells as determined by propidium iodide (PI) (Sigma-Aldrich) exclusion were gated and were analyzed.

Proliferation Assay

The extent of cell growth was assessed using a cell counting cell kit-8 (CCK-8) assay (Dojindo Laboratories, Kumamoto, Japan) according to the manufacturer's instructions. Briefly, DPSCs were plated at a density of $1x10^4$ cells per well and a volume of 100μL in 96 well plates. Cells were cultured for 24 hours with DMEM supplemented with 10% FBS at 37°C in a humidified 5% atmosphere before the test. At each time point (12, 24, 36 and 48h after cells seeding), 10 μL of CCK-8 solution was added to each well, followed by incubation for 4h at 37°C. The absorbance at a wavelength of 450 nm was determined by a multi-plate reader (Thermo Scientific, AppliskanMultimode).

Cell Migration Assay

At the fifth passage of culture, the ability of the cells isolated under different conditions to migrate towards FBS was compared by a horizontal chemotaxis assay using TAXIScan-FL (Effector Cell Institute, Tokyo, Japan). The TAXIScan-FL consists of an etched silicon substrate and a flat glass plate, both of which form two compartments with a 6-mm deep micro-channel. Each cell fraction (1×10^5cells/ml) was injected into a single hole in a serum-free media, while 1 mL of DMEM containing 10% FBS was injected in the contra hole. Images of cell migration were taken for twenty-four hours, and the number of migrating cells was counted.

Assessment of Viability of Cells Cryopreserved under Different Conditions

The viability of the cells has been tested after having been cryopreserved in either CP-1™ (Kyokuto Pharmaceutical Industrial, Tokyo Japan), or CELL-BANKER® (AMS

Biotechnology, UK), as follows: The cells were counted and centrifuged for three to five minutes at 2,000rpm and at 4°C. The supernatant was then discarded, and the cells were gently suspended with one of the two cryopreservation media (1 ml for 5 x 10^6 cells). The cell suspension was dispensed in 1ml aliquots to cryopreservation vials, then stored first at -80°C then transferred to the vapor phase of a liquid nitrogen freezer after 1 hour, 12 hours, 24 hours, 48 hours, and 1 week. After 24 hours in liquid nitrogen, the vials were thawed and the cells were evaluated for viability using trypan blue test.

Statistical Analysis

Data are reported as mean ± standard deviation (SD). Analysis of data was performed using SPSS 18 (Statistical Package for Scientific Studies) for Windows. Data were explored for normality using Shapiro-Wilk test of normality. Comparisons between groups for quantitative variables were carried out with the ANOVA test to detect the difference between groups. If any significance were detected by the ANOVA it was followed by the Tukey's Post hoc test to determine the group(s) responsible for the significance. Results were expressed in the form of P-values and differences were considered to be significant at $P \leq 0.05$.

RESULTS

Effect of Different Transportation/Isolation Conditions on Morphology and Viability of DPSCs

Primary cells were successfully isolated from the dental pulp of all teeth. Isolated DPSCs exhibited small, spindle-shaped morphology which was not changed through the passages. Neither the different transportation media nor the different isolation time affected the morphology of the isolated DPSCs (Figure 1). Further analysis of the captured images of the cells showed that the least number of spindle-shaped cells was found in the saline group when compared to the other groups, however, without significance (Figure 2).

There was no significant difference in the number of viable cells in DMEM, DMEM + FBS, PBS, PBS + FBS and Hank's solution groups, isolated at 3,12 and 24 hours. However, at 36 and 48 hours, the number of viable cells started to decrease significantly in the PBS and Hank's solution groups when compared to other groups. On the other hand, the saline group showed a significant decrease in the number of viable cells compared to other groups at all isolation times (Table 1). Cells isolated using different enzymes showed no significant difference in the number of the viable cells obtained (Figure 3.A).

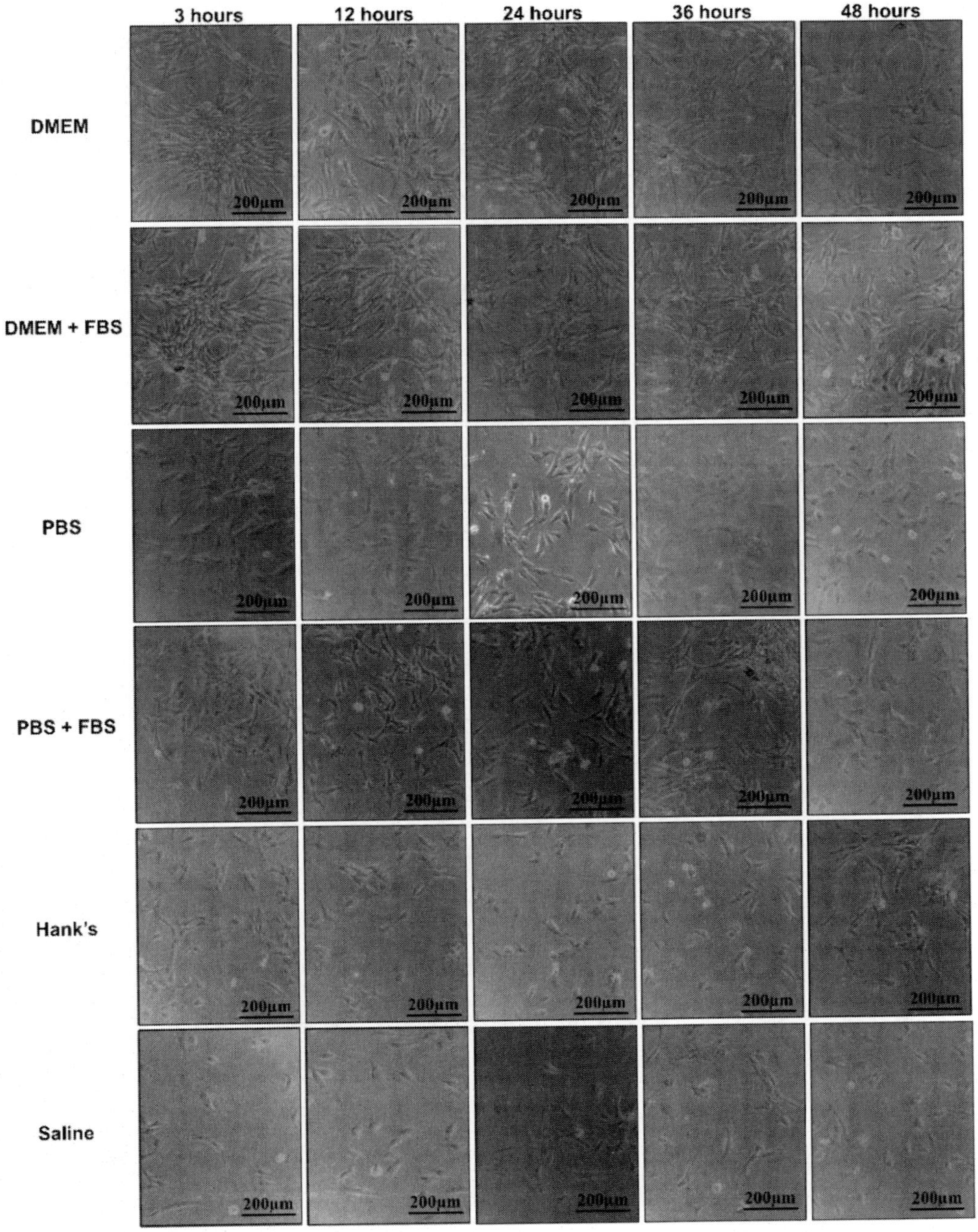

Figure 1. Morphology of DPSCs isolated under different transportation/isolation methods. Neither the different transportation media nor the different isolation time affected the morphology of the isolated cells.

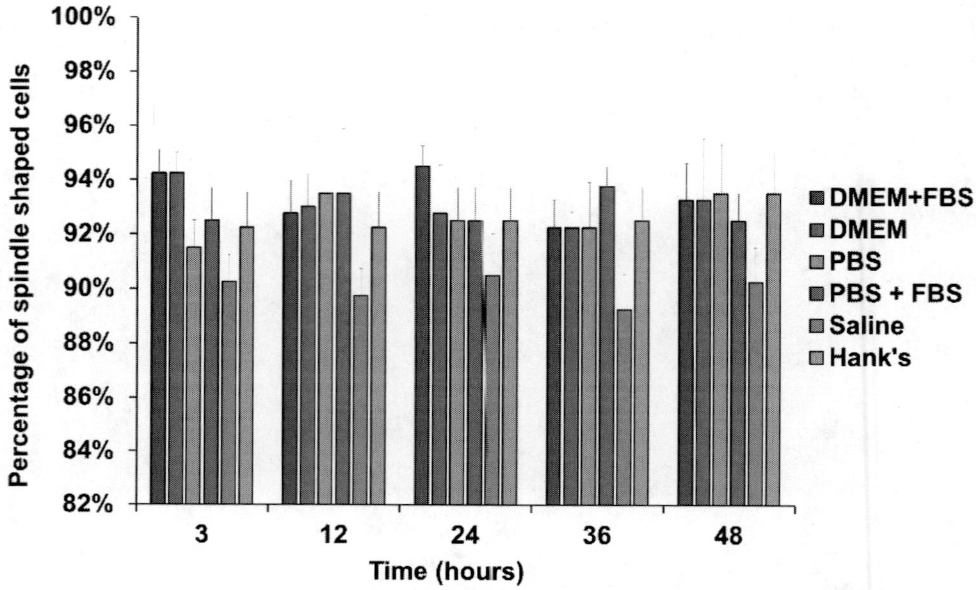

Figure 2. Percentage of the spindle-shaped cells in cells isolated under different transportation media/ isolation time. Although the percentage of spindle-shaped cells was decreased in the saline group compared to other groups, it was without significance.

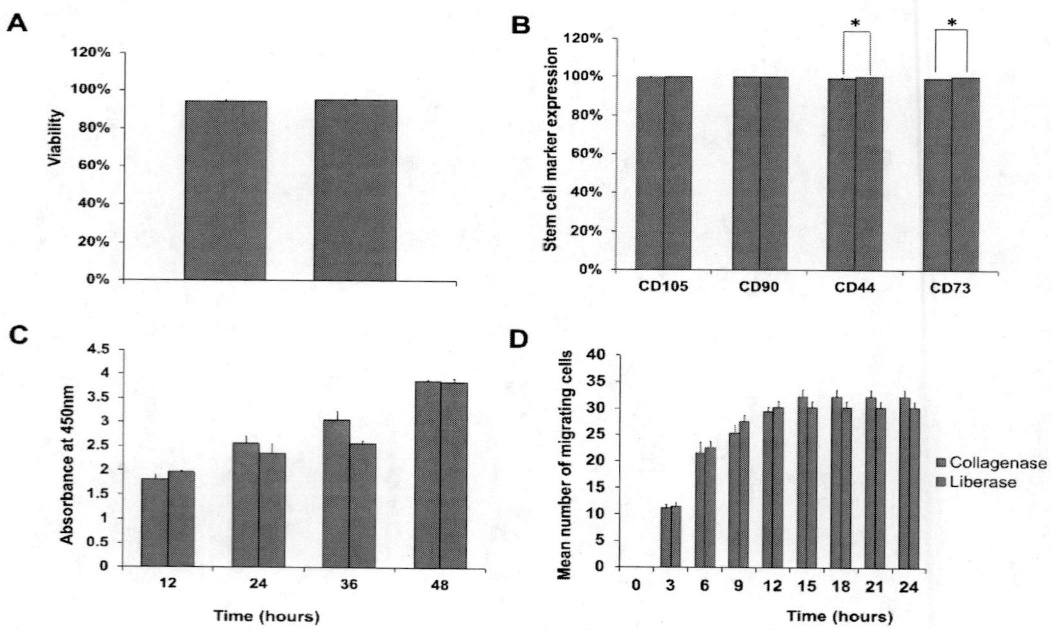

Figure 3. Stemness properties of DPSCs isolated with different digestion enzymes. (A) Viability. There was no significant difference between the two groups. (B) Stem cell markers expression. Cells isolated by Liberase enzyme exhibited significantly higher expression of CD73 and CD44 (mean ± S.D., n = 4. $*p < 0.05$). (C) Cell proliferation was detected at 450 nm absorbance. No significant difference was detected between the two groups (D) Migration of cells towards FBS. There was no significant difference between the two groups.

Table 1. Viability of cells isolated under different transportation/isolation conditions

	DMEM	DMEM + FBS	PBS	PBS + FBS	Saline	Hank's	p-value
3 hours	94.25 ± 1.5^{a}	94.25 ± 0.96^{a}	91.25 ± 2.06^{a}	92.5 ± 2.08^{a}	83 ± 2.16^{b}	90.75 ± 1.71^{a}	<0.001*
12 hours	85.5 ± 4.04^{a}	87.5 ± 1.73^{a}	87.25 ± 1.71^{a}	88.75 ± 1.5^{a}	71.75 ± 2.75^{b}	87.5 ± 2.08^{a}	<0.001*
24 hours	83.5 ± 1.29^{a}	82.75 ± 2.06^{a}	79 ± 3.37^{a}	82.5 ± 2.08^{a}	56.5 ± 2.65^{b}	79.5 ± 3.42^{a}	<0.001*
36 hours	77.25 ± 2.52^{ad}	80.05 ± 2.22^{a}	62.25 ± 2.87^{b}	76.5 ± 1.29^{ad}	39.25 ± 2.22^{c}	74.25 ± 3.30^{d}	<0.001*
48 hours	53.25 ± 5.38^{a}	68.25 ± 2.36^{b}	60 ± 4.55^{ad}	67.75 ± 2.22^{bd}	32.5 ± 2.08^{c}	71.75 ± 2.75^{b}	<0.001*

*statistically significant p-value < 0.05.

$^{a, b, c, \& d}$ different small letters indicate significant differences.

Effect of Different Transportation/Isolation Conditions on the Expression of Stem Cell Markers

Table 2. Stem cell markers expression in cells isolated under different transportation/isolation conditions

	DMEM	DMEM + FBS	PBS	PBS + FBS	Saline	Hank's	p-value
3 hours							
CD105	99.85 ± 0.19^{a}	99.78 ± 0.27^{a}	97.90 ± 1.54^{ac}	99.70 ± 0.47^{a}	91.21 ± 2.30^{b}	96.54 ± 0.88^{c}	<0.001*
CD90	99.43 ± 0.50^{a}	99.35 ± 0.51^{a}	97.13 ± 1.22^{a}	97.94 ± 0.35^{a}	86.31 ± 2.99^{b}	97.18 ± 0.95^{a}	<0.001*
CD44	98.63 ± 0.75^{a}	99.68 ± 0.23^{a}	97.32 ± 1.70^{a}	99.13 ± 0.33^{a}	83.48 ± 2.63^{b}	97.46 ± 1.90^{a}	<0.001*
CD73	98.87 ± 0.34^{ad}	99.48 ± 0.83^{a}	97.25 ± 0.50^{b}	99.29 ± 0.72^{a}	88.85 ± 1.03^{c}	97.76 ± 0.29^{bd}	<0.001*
12 hours							
CD105	99.65 ± 0.47^{a}	99.70 ± 0.35^{a}	97.14 ± 2.39^{a}	99.75 ± 0.50^{a}	85.96 ± 5.17^{b}	95.44 ± 0.80^{a}	<0.001*
CD90	99.90 ± 0.20^{a}	99.68 ± 0.32^{a}	96.38 ± 1.37^{b}	97.31 ± 0.64^{b}	83.81 ± 1.20^{c}	95.68 ± 0.57^{b}	<0.001*
CD44	98.93 ± 0.74^{a}	99.76 ± 0.28^{a}	96.82 ± 1.27^{ac}	98.92 ± 0.73^{a}	83.56 ± 2.64^{b}	93.71 ± 2.33^{c}	<0.001*
CD73	98.87 ± 0.34^{a}	99.76 ± 0.30^{a}	97.44 ± 1.2^{a}	99.29 ± 0.72^{a}	86.60 ± 3.09^{b}	92.98 ± 2.32^{c}	<0.001*
24 hours							
CD105	99.70 ± 0.36^{a}	99.86 ± 0.15^{a}	97.68 ± 1.62^{a}	99.25 ± 0.59^{a}	83.03 ± 4.58^{b}	82.86 ± 2.62^{b}	<0.001*
CD90	99.33 ± 0.51^{a}	99.35 ± 0.51^{a}	95.88 ± 0.45^{a}	97.93 ± 0.35^{a}	83.81 ± 3.45^{b}	87.41 ± 1.26^{c}	<0.001*
CD44	97.88 ± 0.96^{a}	99.68 ± 0.23^{a}	97.57 ± 1.68^{a}	97.88 ± 1.03^{a}	80.97 ± 1.82^{b}	89.60 ± 1.01^{c}	<0.001*
CD73	97.47 ± 0.71^{ab}	99.48 ± 0.83^{b}	95.00 ± 1.14^{ad}	98.45 ± 0.68^{ab}	82.18 ± 3.00^{c}	91.56 ± 3.16^{d}	<0.001*
36 hours							
CD105	99.83 ± 0.20^{a}	99.93 ± 0.08^{a}	96.65 ± 1.28^{bc}	99.38 ± 0.32^{ac}	86.17 ± 2.65^{d}	95.63 ± 0.99^{bc}	<0.001*
CD90	99.18 ± 0.34^{a}	99.53 ± 0.58^{a}	96.63 ± 1.01^{a}	97.94 ± 0.35^{a}	80.31 ± 2.27^{b}	93.27 ± 2.04^{c}	<0.001*
CD44	98.38 ± 0.54^{ab}	99.42 ± 0.32^{a}	97.08 ± 1.42^{bd}	99.13 ± 0.33^{ab}	81.67 ± 1.52^{c}	95.07 ± 1.22^{d}	<0.001*
CD73	98.87 ± 0.34^{a}	99.54 ± 0.13^{a}	97.25 ± 0.50^{ac}	99.29 ± 0.72^{a}	85.05 ± 2.19^{b}	95.76 ± 1.12^{c}	<0.001*
48 hours							
CD105	97.27 ± 0.89^{a}	97.18 ± 1.46^{a}	95.40 ± 1.15^{a}	95.58 ± 1.65^{a}	86.17 ± 2.65^{b}	95.63 ± 0.99^{a}	<0.001*
CD90	95.60 ± 1.84^{a}	97.13 ± 1.34^{a}	95.38 ± 0.91^{a}	96.94 ± 0.77^{a}	71.59 ± 5.76^{b}	93.27 ± 2.04^{a}	<0.001*
CD44	98.38 ± 0.54^{a}	96.47 ± 0.69^{a}	95.83 ± 1.17^{a}	96.94 ± 1.64^{a}	77.77 ± 5.46^{b}	95.07 ± 1.22^{a}	<0.001*
CD73	97.03 ± 1.49^{a}	97.63 ± 2.24^{a}	95.95 ± 0.83^{a}	97.54 ± 0.78^{a}	85.05 ± 2.19^{b}	95.76 ± 1.12^{a}	<0.001*

*statistically significant p-value < 0.05.

$^{a,b,c \& d}$ different small letters indicate significant differences.

All cultures at the fifth passage expressed mesenchymal stem cell markers; CD105, CD90, CD44, and CD73 when analyzed by flow cytometry (Table 2). However, the expression of those stem cell markers was significantly the least in the saline group when compared to other groups, at all isolation times. DPSCs that were isolated for three hours in Hank's solution group showed no significant difference in expressing stem cell markers when compared to other groups. However, cells isolated for twelve hours showed significantly decreased markers expression when compared to other groups except for the PBS group. DPSCs in Hank's solution group isolated at 24, 36, and 48 hours expressed stem cell markers at the lowest rate following those in the saline group. On the other hand, there was no significant difference between DPSCs isolated from teeth transported in DMEM, DMEM+FBS, PBS, and PBS+FBS at all isolation times.

When comparing cells isolated using different enzymes, no significant difference in the level of the expression of all stem cell markers was found, except for CD73 and CD44, which were significantly higher in cells isolated with Liberase (Figure 3 B).

Effect of Different Transportation/Isolation Conditions on DPSCs Proliferation Rate

Cell proliferation rate was evaluated at the 3rd culture passage. DMEM+FBS group exhibited the highest proliferation rate at all isolation times and all measured time points while the saline group showed the lowest. There was no significant difference between the proliferation rates of cells in DMEM and DMEM+FBS groups at all isolation times and all measured time points. At 3 hours isolation, although cells in saline and Hank's solution groups showed no significant difference in their proliferation rates compared to each other, they exhibited the lowest proliferation rates when compared to cells in other groups at all measured time points. At 12 hours isolation, cells in the PBS group began to show a signif-icant decrease in proliferation rate when compared to cells in DMEM, DMEM+FBS and PBS+FBS groups. However, still the proliferation rate of cells in Hank's solution and saline groups is significantly the lowest. At 24 hours isolation, cells in the saline group showed a significant decrease in proliferation rate when com-pared to all groups, while cells in PBS and Hank's solution groups showed no significant difference in their proliferation rates when compared to each other but showed a significant difference when compared to cells in DMEM, DMEM+FBS and PBS+FBS groups. At 36 hours, cells in PBS+FBS started to show a significant decrease in proliferation rate when com-pared to cells in DMEM and DMEM+FBS groups, and no significant difference when compared to cells in the PBS group. At 48 hours, the proliferation rate of cells in PBS+FBS group continued to significantly decrease and became closer to that of cells in Hank's solution and PBS groups (Table 3). DPSCs isolated using different enzymes showed no significant difference in their proliferation rates at all measured time points (Figure 3.C)

Effect of Different Transportation/Isolation Conditions on DPSCs Migration Capability

The migration ability towards FBS was examined in all cell cultures at the 5th passage. In general, the migration ability towards FBS was the highest in the cells isolated at 3 hours from teeth transported in DMEM and DMEM+FBS. A significant decrease in the migration ability was noticed in cells isolated at 36 and 48 hours, in all media groups. Cells in the saline group showed the least migration ability at all isolation times followed by cells in Hank's solution group (Table 4). On the other hand, cells isolated using different enzymes showed no significant difference in their migration ability towards FBS (Figure 3.D).

Effect of Different Cryopreservation Media /Method on DPSC Viability

Table 3. Proliferation of cells isolated under different transport/isolation conditions

	DMEM	DMEM+FBS	PBS	PBS+FBS	Saline	Hank's	p-value
3 hours							
12 hours	1.61 ± 0.14^a	1.96 ± 0.04^a	1.29 ± 0.30^a	1.44 ± 0.14^a	0.48 ± 0.12^b	0.63 ± 0.03^b	<0.001*
24 hours	1.59 ± 0.08^a	2.38 ± 0.17^a	0.78 ± 0.15^a	1.29 ± 0.08^a	0.10 ± 0.14^b	0.41 ± 0.03^b	<0.001*
36 hours	1.76 ± 0.26^a	2.66 ± 0.33^a	0.94 ± 0.26^a	1.65 ± 0.11^a	0.19 ± 0.10^b	0.39 ± 0.07^b	<0.001*
48 hours	2.87 ± 0.19^a	3.50 ± 0.08^a	2.25 ± 0.18^a	2.29 ± 0.57^a	0.42 ± 0.08^b	1.02 ± 0.12^b	<0.001*
12 hours							
12 hours	1.41 ± 0.14^a	1.74 ± 0.12^a	0.69 ± 0.06^b	1.24 ± 0.14^a	0.33 ± 0.05^c	0.53 ± 0.09^c	<0.001*
24 hours	1.38 ± 0.12^a	2.18 ± 0.16^a	1.18 ± 0.12^b	1.29 ± 0.08^a	0.35 ± 0.06^c	0.61 ± 0.26^c	<0.001*
36 hours	1.70 ± 0.16^a	2.46 ± 0.17^a	1.14 ± 0.07^b	1.42 ± 0.13^a	0.30 ± 0.06^c	0.53 ± 0.07^c	<0.001*
48 hours	2.61 ± 0.06^a	3.54 ± 0.00^a	1.90 ± 0.34^b	2.12 ± 0.58^a	0.40 ± 0.07^c	1.02 ± 0.12^c	<0.001*
24 hours							
12 hours	1.22 ± 0.14^a	1.55 ± 0.11^a	0.56 ± 0.09^b	1.09 ± 0.12^c	0.21 ± 0.08^d	0.31 ± 0.05^b	<0.001*
24 hours	1.18 ± 0.12^a	1.98 ± 0.26^a	0.98 ± 0.07^b	1.14 ± 0.08^c	0.20 ± 0.07^d	0.58 ± 0.21^b	<0.001*
36 hours	1.57 ± 0.09^a	2.31 ± 0.25^a	0.97 ± 0.05^b	1.29 ± 0.15^c	0.13 ± 0.09^d	0.53 ± 0.21^b	<0.001*
48 hours	2.53 ± 0.12^a	3.48 ± 0.12^a	1.60 ± 0.11^b	2.22 ± 0.31^c	0.32 ± 0.04^d	0.97 ± 0.09^b	<0.001*
36 hours							
12 hours	1.09 ± 0.11^a	1.45 ± 0.11^a	0.46 ± 0.09^b	1.02 ± 0.03^b	0.13 ± 0.06^c	0.23 ± 0.08^d	<0.001*
24 hours	1.11 ± 0.06^a	1.78 ± 0.22^a	0.88 ± 0.07^b	1.07 ± 0.12^b	0.15 ± 0.12^c	0.63 ± 0.14^d	<0.001*
36 hours	1.52 ± 0.10^a	2.16 ± 0.31^a	0.82 ± 0.06^b	1.09 ± 0.10^b	0.10 ± 0.07^c	0.56 ± 0.27^d	<0.001*
48 hours	2.31 ± 0.23^a	3.39 ± 0.11^a	1.36 ± 0.22^b	2.02 ± 0.25^b	0.15 ± 0.08^c	0.94 ± 0.06^d	<0.001*
48 hours							
12 hours	0.92 ± 0.12^a	1.25 ± 0.11^a	0.41 ± 0.13^b	0.99 ± 0.03^b	0.08 ± 0.04^c	0.18 ± 0.03^b	<0.001*
24 hours	1.04 ± 0.11^a	1.52 ± 0.15^a	0.78 ± 0.14^b	0.89 ± 0.09^b	0.08 ± 0.07^c	0.48 ± 0.16^b	<0.001*
36 hours	1.42 ± 0.13^a	1.74 ± 0.19^a	0.69 ± 0.11^b	0.99 ± 0.07^b	0.05 ± 0.07^c	0.41 ± 0.05^b	<0.001*
48 hours	2.22 ± 0.14^a	3.26 ± 0.06^a	1.33 ± 0.09^b	1.87 ± 0.06^b	0.17 ± 0.07^c	0.84 ± 0.06^b	<0.001*

*statistically significant p-value < 0.05.

[a, b, c, & d] different small letters indicate significant differences.

Table 4. Number of migrating cells isolated under transportation/isolation methods towards FBS

	DMEM	DMEM + FBS	PBS	PBS+FBS	Saline	Hank's	p-value
3 hours							
3 hours	8 ± 0.82^{a}	11.5 ± 1.29^{b}	5.5 ± 1.29^{ac}	8 ± 0.82^{a}	3.5 ± 1.29^{c}	6.25 ± 1.5^{a}	<0.001*
6 hours	15.25 ± 1.26^{a}	22.5 ± 2.08^{b}	8.25 ± 1.5^{c}	13.75 ± 2.63^{ae}	6.5 ± 1.73^{cd}	10 ± 2.16^{ce}	<0.001*
9 hours	19 ± 0.82^{a}	27.5 ± 2.08^{b}	12 ± 2.16^{c}	17.75 ± 3.30^{a}	10 ± 2.16^{cd}	11 ± 1.41^{ce}	<0.001*
12 hours	21.25 ± 1.5^{a}	30.25 ± 2.06^{b}	15 ± 2.16^{c}	20.25 ± 2.36^{a}	13 ± 2.45^{c}	14.5 ± 2.52^{c}	<0.001*
15 hours	22.75 ± 0.96^{a}	30.25 ± 2.06^{b}	16 ± 1.83^{cd}	20.25 ± 2.36^{ad}	13 ± 2.45^{c}	14.5 ± 2.52^{c}	<0.001*
18 hours	22.75 ± 0.96^{a}	30.25 ± 2.06^{b}	16 ± 1.83^{cd}	20.25 ± 2.36^{ad}	13 ± 2.45^{c}	14.5 ± 2.52^{c}	<0.001*
21 hours	22.75 ± 0.96^{a}	30.25 ± 2.06^{b}	16 ± 1.83^{cd}	20.25 ± 2.36^{ad}	13 ± 2.45^{c}	14.5 ± 2.52^{c}	<0.001*
24 hours	22.75 ± 0.96^{a}	30.25 ± 2.06^{b}	16 ± 1.83^{cd}	20.25 ± 2.36^{ad}	13 ± 2.45^{c}	14.5 ± 2.52^{c}	<0.001*
12 hours							
3 hours	7 ± 0.82^{a}	10.5 ± 1.29^{b}	5 ± 0.82^{ac}	7.25 ± 0.96^{a}	2.75 ± 0.5^{c}	5.25 ± 1.5^{a}	<0.001*
6 hours	14 ± 0.82^{a}	16.5 ± 2.38^{a}	7.25 ± 1.5^{b}	12.75 ± 2.63^{a}	5.75 ± 1.5^{b}	8.25 ± 0.96^{b}	<0.001*
9 hours	17 ± 1.41^{a}	22 ± 2.45^{b}	10.25 ± 1.5^{c}	16.25 ± 2.99^{a}	8.25 ± 1.5^{c}	10.5 ± 1.29^{c}	<0.001*
12 hours	19 ± 0.82^{a}	25.75 ± 2.63^{b}	13.25 ± 1.71^{c}	18 ± 2^{a}	11 ± 1.41^{c}	12.75 ± 0.96^{c}	<0.001*
15 hours	21 ± 1.15^{a}	25.75 ± 2.63^{b}	15.25 ± 1.5^{cd}	18 ± 2^{ad}	11 ± 1.41^{e}	12.75 ± 0.96^{ce}	<0.001*
18 hours	21 ± 1.15^{a}	25.75 ± 2.63^{b}	16 ± 1.83^{cd}	18 ± 2^{ad}	11 ± 1.41^{e}	12.75 ± 0.96^{ce}	<0.001*
21 hours	21 ± 1.15^{a}	25.75 ± 2.63^{b}	16 ± 1.83^{cd}	18 ± 2^{ad}	11 ± 1.41^{e}	12.75 ± 0.96^{ce}	<0.001*
24 hours	21 ± 1.15^{a}	25.75 ± 2.63^{b}	16 ± 1.83^{cd}	18 ± 2^{ad}	11 ± 1.41^{e}	12.75 ± 0.96^{ce}	<0.001*
24 hours							
3 hours	6 ± 0.82^{ac}	10.25 ± 0.96^{b}	4 ± 0.82^{cd}	6.25 ± 0.96^{a}	2.5 ± 0.58^{d}	5.25 ± 1.5^{ac}	<0.001*
6 hours	12 ± 0.82^{ac}	14.5 ± 0.58^{a}	6.25 ± 1.5^{bd}	11 ± 2.16^{ce}	4.5 ± 0.58^{d}	8.25 ± 0.96^{be}	<0.001*
9 hours	14.25 ± 0.96^{ac}	16.5 ± 3.87^{a}	9.25 ± 1.5^{be}	13.75 ± 1.89^{ace}	6.75 ± 0.96^{b}	10.5 ± 1.29^{bc}	<0.001*
12 hours	16.25 ± 0.96^{ab}	17.75 ± 3.86^{ac}	12.25 ± 1.71^{bd}	15.5 ± 1.91^{bc}	9 ± 1.41^{d}	10.5 ± 1.29^{d}	<0.001*
15 hours	18 ± 0.82^{ab}	19.25 ± 2.22^{a}	13.75 ± 0.96^{ce}	15.5 ± 1.91^{bc}	9 ± 1.41^{d}	10.5 ± 1.29^{de}	<0.001*
18 hours	18 ± 0.82^{ab}	19.25 ± 2.22^{a}	13.75 ± 0.96^{ce}	15.5 ± 1.91^{bc}	9 ± 1.41^{d}	10.5 ± 1.29^{de}	<0.001*
21 hours	18 ± 0.82^{ab}	19.25 ± 2.22^{a}	13.75 ± 0.96^{ce}	15.5 ± 1.91^{bc}	9 ± 1.41^{d}	10.5 ± 1.29^{de}	<0.001*
24 hours	18 ± 0.82^{ab}	19.25 ± 2.22^{a}	13.75 ± 0.96^{ce}	15.5 ± 1.91^{bc}	9 ± 1.41^{d}	10.5 ± 1.29^{de}	<0.001*

*statistically significant p-value < 0.05.

$^{a, b, c, d \& e}$ different small letters indicate significant differences.

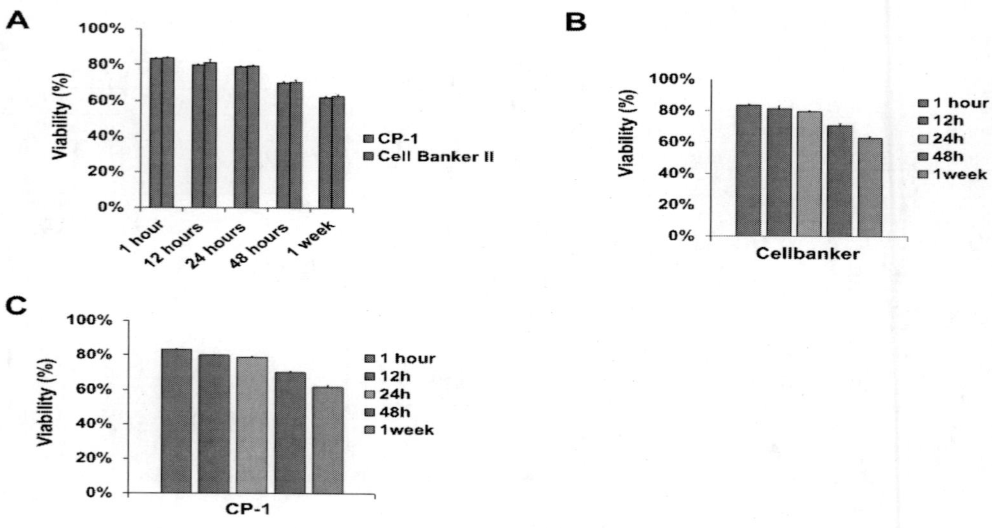

Figure 4. Effect of different cryopreservation media/method on DPSC viability. (A) There was no significant difference in the number of viable cells between cells cryopreserved in CP-1 and Cellbanker. (B) and (C) The number of viable cells cryopreserved in Cellbanker and CP-1 respectively decreased as the time elapsed between transferring the cryopreserved cells from -80°C to liquid nitrogen increased.

There was no significant difference in the number of viable cells when DPSCs were cryopreserved in either CP-1 or Cellbanker under all cryopreserving conditions (Figure 4.A). However, the longer the time elapsed between transferring the cryopreserved cells from -80°C to liquid nitrogen, the less the viable cells retrieved after thawing (Figure 4.B and C).

DISCUSSION

Over the course of the last decade, various methods of isolation and expansion of DPSCs have been extensively investigated given the promising role these cells can potentially play in cell-based therapies and regenerative medicine. However, most of the reports lacked homogeneity where loss of stemness and genomic instability of the isolated cells were described in some cases [22–24]. This has led to the growing demand for establishing optimized experimental procedures that would lead to safe expansion and preservation of the isolated cells. In our present study, we investigated the effect of several conditions that would promote the efficiency of DPSCs isolation through analyzing several parameters.

In the first part of the present study, the role of different transportation media was investigated as a crucial factor that helps protect the tissues from undergoing degradation during the time elapsed between tooth extraction and initiation of isolation procedures. Similarly, the time at which the isolation start after extraction was investigated as another significant factor that may affect the properties of the isolated cells. DPSCs were successfully isolated up to 48 hours from teeth transported in different media. Interestingly, neither the different transportation media nor the different isolation time affected the morphology of the isolated DPSCs. However, the saline group showed less number of spindle-shaped cells compared to other groups but without significance. These two observations indicate that neither the presence of serum nor the instant isolation is critical for successful isolation of DPSCs. Other studies have reported similar results but on other MSCs [25-27].

On the other hand, viability proliferation rate, and migration ability were affected by different transportation/isolation conditions. In general, cells in the saline group showed the least viability, proliferation rate and migration ability among all other groups. Our results coincide with a recent study that reported successful isolation of DPSCs isolated from teeth preserved in saline supplemented with Gentamicin [28]. However, our study shows that saline cannot be considered the best transportation media when it comes to preserving the stemness properties of the isolated cells. Alternatively, cells in the DMEM+FBS group demonstrated the highest viability and proliferation rate with successful cell migration capability compared to all other tested groups. However, without significance when compared to DMEM and with slight significance when compared to PBS + FBS group. Cells in the PBS and Hank's solution groups behaved almost the same, however, cells in the PBS group were significantly better in terms of proliferation rate and migration ability. It seemed that the addition of serum to PBS improved the properties of the isolated cells, indicating the important role of serum for obtaining high-quality cells with good stemness properties. On the contrary, some studies found cell survival was not affected when the sample was transported in different media with or without the addition of serum [16, 25].

The expression of mesenchymal cell markers CD105, CD90, CD44, and CD73 were also analyzed as these markers are routinely used for the definition of human MSCs [29, 30]. DPSCs isolated from teeth stored in DMEM, DMEM+FBS, PBS, and PBS+FBS at all isolation times expressed those mesenchymal markers. Still, coinciding with the previous pattern of results, the level of expression of the previously mentioned markers were the least in the saline group followed by Hank's solution group which, again, implies that both saline and Hank's solution alter the stemness properties of the isolated cells.

In the second part of the present study, we examined using two enzymes; collagenase type II and Liberase for isolating stem cells via the digestion method. Our results indicate that dental pulp tissue can be successfully processed using different enzymes which previous studies have also found possible [20]. Many studies successfully used Liberase enzyme for the isolation of stem cells from various tissue sources, like; skin and pancreas and dental pulp [31-33]. However, to our knowledge, none has compared its effect on stemness properties of the isolated cells to the commonly used collagenase enzyme. Interestingly, our results showed that there was no significant impact of the type of enzyme used on any of the parameters tested except for significantly higher expressions of CD73 and CD44 in the cells isolated using Liberase enzyme.

Finally, we assessed the effect of different cryopreservation media/method on DPSC viability. CP-1 and Cell banker cryopreservant are now being widely used as a safe and low-cost substitute to DMSO which has been reported to elicit cytotoxic effects on cells as well to induce differentiation of neural-like cells [34, 35]. In general, the viability of the post-thawed cells was not affected by the type of the cryopreservant used yet was affected by the time elapsed between transferring the cryopreserved cells from -80°C to liquid nitrogen as the longer the time interval of the transfer the less the viable cells retrieved after thawing.

Conclusion

Transport media and isolation time seem to be critical factors potentially influencing DPSCs quality. The type of the enzyme used and the method of cryopreservation are also important for obtaining viable and good quality DPSCs for future clinical applications.

ETHICAL COMPLIANCE

The authors have stated all possible conflicts of interest within this work. The authors have stated all sources of funding for this work. If this work involved human participants, informed consent was received from each individual. If this work involved human participants, it was conducted in accordance with the 1964 Declaration of Helsinki. If this work involved experiments with humans or animals, it was conducted in accordance with the related institutions' research ethics guidelines.

REFERENCES

[1] Eubanks EJ, Tarle SA, Kaigler D. Tooth storage, dental pulp stem cell isolation, and clinical scale expansion without animal serum. *J Endod.* 2014;40(5):652–657.

[2] Huang GTJ, Gronthos S, Shi S. Mesenchymal stem cells derived from dental tissues *vs.* those from other sources: Their biology and role in regenerative medicine. *J Dent Res.* 2009;88(9):792–806.

[3] Hynes K, Menicanin D, Gronthos S, Bartold PM. Clinical utility of stem cells for periodontal regen-eration. *Periodontol* 2000. 2012;59(1):203–227.

[4] Hosoya A, Nakamura H, Ninomiya T, Hoshi K, Yoshiba K, Yoshiba N, Takahashi M, Okabe T, Sahara N, Yamada H, Kasahara E, Ozawa H. Hard tissue formation in subcutaneously transplanted rat dental pulp. *J Dent Res.* 2007;86(5):469–474.

[5] Park JY, Jeon SH, Choung PH. Efficacy of periodontal stem cell transplantation in the treatment of advanced periodontitis. *Cell Transpl.* 2011;20(2):271–285.

[6] d'Aquino R, De Rosa A, Lanza V, Tirino V, Laino L, Graziano A, Desiderio V, Laino G, Papaccio G. Human mandible bone defect repair by the grafting of dental pulp stem/progenitor cells and collagen sponge biocomplexes. *Eur Cell Mater.* 2009;18:75–83.

[7] Kerkis I, Caplan AI. Stem cells in dental pulp of deciduous teeth. *Tissue Eng Part B Rev.* 2012;18(2): 129–138.

[8] Saito A, Saito E, Handa R, Honma Y, Kawanami M. Influence of residual bone on recombinant human bone morphogenetic protein-2 induced periodontal regeneration in experimental periodontitis in dogs. *J Periodontol.* 2009;80(6):961–968.

[9] Yamada Y, Ito K, Nakamura S, Ueda M, Nagasaka T. Promising cell-based therapy for bone regeneration using stem cells from deciduous teeth, dental pulp, and bone marrow. *Cell Transplant.* 2011;20(7):1003–1013.

[10] Zhang W, Ahluwalia IP, Literman R, Kaplan DL, Yelick PC. Human dental pulp progenitor cell behavior on aqueous and hexafluoroisopropanol based silk scaffolds. *J Biomed Mater Res Part A.* 2011;97A(4): 414–422.

[11] Chen Y-K, Huang AH-C, Chan AW-S, Shieh T-Y, Lin L-M. Human dental pulp stem cells derived from different cryopreservation methods of human dental pulp tissues of diseased teeth. *J Oral Pathol Med.* 2011;40(10):793–800.

[12] Ducret M, Fabre H, Degoul O, Atzeni G, McGuckin C, Forraz N, Alliot-Licht B, Mallein-Gerin F, Perrier-Groult E, Farges JC. Manufacturing of dental pulp cell-based products from human third molars: current strategies and future investigations. *Front Physiol.* 2015;6:213.

[13] Ferro F, Spelat R, Beltrami AP, Cesselli D, Curcio F. Isolation and characterization of human dental pulp-derived stem cells by using media containing low human serum percentage as clinical grade substitutes for bovine serum. *PLoS One.* 2012;7(11):1–9.

[14] Gronthos S, Mankani M, Brahim J, Robey PG, Shi S. Postnatal human dental pulp stem cells (DPSCs) *in vitro* and *in vivo*. *Proc Natl Acad Sci USA.* 2000;97 (25): 13625–13630.

[15] Karamzadeh R, Eslaminejad MB, Aflatoonian R. Isolation, characterization and comparative differe-ntiation of human dental pulp stem cells derived from permanent teeth by using two different methods. *J Vis Exp.* 2012;(69).

[16] Perry BC, Zhou D, Wu X, Yang FC, Byers MA, Chu TM, Hockema JJ, Woods EJ, Goebel WS. Collection, cryopreservation, and characterization of human dental pulp-derived mesenchymal stem cells for banking and clinical use. *Tissue Eng Part C Methods.* 2008;14(2): 149–156.

[17] Woods EJ, Perry BC, Hockema JJ, Larson L, Zhou D, Goebel WS. Optimized cryopreservation method for human dental pulp-derived stem cells and their tissues of origin for banking and clinical use. *Cryobiology* 2009;59(2):150–157.

[18] Busser H, De Bruyn C, Urbain F, Najar M, Pieters K, Raicevic G, Meuleman N, Bron D, Lagneaux L. Isolation of adipose-derived stromal cells without enzymatic treatment: expansion, phenotypical, and functional characterization. *Stem Cells Dev.* 2014;23 (19):2390–2400.

[19] Ohnuma K, Fujiki A, Yanagihara K, Tachikawa S, Hayashi Y, Ito Y, Onuma Y, Chan T, Michiue T, Furue MK, Asashima M. Enzyme-free passage of human pluripotent stem cells by controlling divalent cations. *Sci Rep.* 2014;4:4646.

[20] Carvalho PP, Gimble JM, Dias IR, Gomes ME, Reis RL. Xenofree enzymatic products for the isolation of human adipose-derived stromal/stem cells. *Tissue Eng Part C Methods.* 2013;19(6):473–478.

[21] Halme DG, Kessler DA. FDA Regulation of stem-cell based therapies. *N Engl J Med.* 2006;355(16):1730–1735.

[22] Yu J, He H, Tang C, Zhang G, Li Y, Wang R, Shi J, Jin Y. Differentiation potential of STRO-1+ dental pulp stem cells changes during cell passaging. *BMC Cell Biol.* 2010;11(1):32.

[23] Martin-Piedra MA, Garzon I, Oliveira AC, Alfonso-Rodriguez CA, Carriel V, Scionti G, Alaminos M. Cell viability and proliferation capability of long-term human dental pulp stem cell cultures. *Cytotherapy.* 2014;16(2):266–277.

[24] Duailibi MT, Kulikowski LD, Duailibi SE, Lipay MV, Melaragno MI, Ferreira LM, Vacanti JP, Yelick PC. Cytogenetic instability of dental pulp stem cell lines. *J Mol Histol.* 2012;43(1):89–94.

[25] Bronzini I, Patruno M, Iacopetti I, Martinello T. Influence of temperature, time and different media on mesenchymal stromal cells shipped for clinical application. *Vet J.* 2012;194:121-123.

[26] Mercati F, Pascucci L, Curina G, Scocco P, Tardella FM, Dall'Aglio C, Marini C, Ceccarelli P. Evaluation of storage conditions on equine adipose tissue-derived multipotent mesenchymal stromal cells. *Vet J.* 2014; 200:339-342.

[27] Garvican ER, Cree S, Bull L, Smith RK, Dudhia J. Viability of equine mesenchymal stem cells during transport and implantation. *Stem Cell Res Ther.* 2014; 5:1.

[28] Huynh NC-N, Le SH, Doan VN, Ngo LTQ, Tran HLB. Simplified conditions for storing and cryopreservation of dental pulp stem cells. *Arch Oral Biol.* 2017;84: 74–81.

[29] d'Aquino R, De Rosa A, Laino G, Caruso F, Guida L, Rullo R, Checchi V, Laino L, Tirino V, Papaccio G. Human dental pulp stem cells: from biology to clinical applications. *J Exp Zool B Mol Dev Evol.* 2009;312B (5):408–415.

[30] Dominici M, Le Blanc K, Mueller I, Slaper-Cortenbach I, Marini F, Krause D, Deans R, Keating A, Prockop Dj, Horwitz E. Minimal criteria for defining multipotent mesenchymal stromal cells. The international society for cellular therapy position statement. *Cytotherapy.* 2006;8:315–7.

[31] Forni MF, Ramos A, Pereira AH, Sogayar MC. Simultaneous isolation of three different stem cell populations from murine skin. *PloS one.* 2015;10(10): e0140143.

[32] Danner S, Petschnik AE, Jany C. Successful isolation of a proliferating cell population with stem cell-like properties from rat pancreas using Liberase TL research grade. *Cell Analysis.* 2010;1

[33] Ahmed NE-B, Murakami M, Kaneko S, Nakashima M. The effects of hypoxia on the stemness properties of human dental pulp stem cells (DPSCs). *Sci. Rep.* 2016; 6:35476.

[34] Oishi K, Noguchi H, Yukawa H, Miyazaki T, Kato R, Kitagawa Y, Ueda M, Hayashi S. Cryopreservation of mouse adipose tissue-derived stem/progenitor cells. *Cell Transplant.* 2008;17:35–41.

[35] Miyagi-Shiohira C, Kobayashi N, Saitoh I, Watanabe M, Noguchi Y, Matsushita M, Noguchi H. Evaluation of serum-free, xeno-free cryopreservation solutions for human adipose-derived mesenchymal stem cells. *Cell Med* 2016;9(1–2):15–20.

In: Manipulation of Stem Cells for Disease Benefits
Editor: Prasad Koka
ISBN: 978-1-53615-468-9

Chapter 10

SAFE AND ACCELERATED EXPANSION OF DENTAL PULP STEM CELLS CULTURED IN PLATELET-RICH-PLASMA-SUPPLEMENTED MEDIA

Heba Shawky[1], Mohamed Gad[2], Dina Sabry[3], Ahmed W. Abou Zeid[1], Mona El Batran[1] and Riham M. Aly[1,4,*]

[1]Basic Dental Science Department, Oral and Dental Research Division, National Research Centre, Cairo, Egypt

[2]Department of Oral Biology, Faculty of Dentistry, Cairo University, Cairo, Egypt

[3]Department of Medical Biochemistry and Molecular Biology, Faculty of Medicine, Cairo University, Cairo, Egypt

[4]Stem Cell Laboratory, Centre of Excellence for Advanced Sciences, National Research Centre, Cairo, Egypt

ABSTRACT

Background: Dental pulp stem cells (DPSCs) are considered an easily accessible source of mesenchymal stem cells holding great promise for use in tissue repair and regenerative medicine. In order for DPSCs to be used in therapeutic clinical applications, issues like safely enhancing culture expansion need to be addressed.

Objective: In this research, we aimed to assess the safety of platelet-rich plasma (PRP) as a promoter of proliferation in comparison to routinely used animal derived supplements.

Methods: The effect of PRP on the proliferation of DPSCs was assessed by MTT assay. Expression of stemness-related genes *OCT4 & INTGRIN1* was analyzed by real-time quantitative PCR. DNA sequencing was performed for *OCT4 & INTGRIN1* genes to

* Corresponding Author's E-mail: riham.aly@gmail.com.

ensure that the isolated DPSCs stem cell properties were not altered by the PRP supplemented media.

Results: At a concentration of 1% with platelet count of 1.5 x $10^6/cm^3$, PRP was able to significantly increase the proliferation rate while maintaining the viability of DPSCs in comparison to routinely used 15% FBS. Mesenchymal stem cell surface markers expression (CD29, CD105) were not altered by PRP supplementation. Moreover, PRP in cultures significantly promoted expression of stemness markers *OCT4 & INTGRIN1* compared with 10% FBS. The results were confirmed by DNA sequencing for *OCT4 & INTGRIN1* genes where DPSCs cultured in PRP demonstrated 100% matching with the control group indicating that PRP supplementation didn't alter the nucleotide sequence of stem cell genes.

Conclusions: Taken together, our results indicate that PRP is a safe and efficient promoter of proliferation and can readily substitute traditional animal derived supplements like FBS.

Keywords: platelet-rich plasma, dental pulp stem cells, proliferation, stemness

INTRODUCTION

Over the past decade, an increasing amount of research has been directed towards the translation of stem cells to repair and regenerate body organs and tissues to clinical applications [1–5]. The success of tissue engineering applications can be dramatically improved by the addition of adjuncts that can increase the proliferation and differentiation of stem cells. This can be achieved through the implementation of growth factors in order to recruit stem cells to tissue defects and to subsequently stimulate them to achieve regeneration [6–8]. However, when clinical application is considered, issues like safely increasing cell number, the use of non xenogenic supplements and possible immune rejection need to be addressed [9].

One representative modality that uses growth factor delivery to achieve tissue regeneration is the addition of natural supplements to increase the proliferation and differentiation of stem cells. Platelet-rich plasma could be considered as such a valuable and safe adjunct that can promote healing in many procedures in dental and oral surgery. Platelet-rich plasma contains proteins that are responsible for cell adhesion, namely fibrin, fibronectin, and vitronectin. It plays an important role in tissue regeneration processes by stimulating fibroblasts to produce structural proteins responsible for formation of new collagen and elastin. Also, it supports remodeling and angiogenesis, in addition to activation of mesenchymal stem cells [10].

As stem cell based therapies are heading towards clinical use, it is therefore essential to modify culture media to allow for maximum cell expansion *in vitro*. Thus, the present work aims to assess the role of PRP as a promoter of proliferation of human dental pulp stem cells.

MATERIAL AND METHODS

Sample Collection

Seven impacted third molars indicated for extraction were collected from healthy patients whose age ranged from 16–26 years. Extraction was performed at the National Research Centre clinics after acquiring the approval of the Centre's ethical committee. Dental pulp stem cells isolation followed the protocol described by Gronthos et al. 2002 [11]. Prior to extraction patients received chlorhexidine mouth rinse to reduce oral microbial flora. The freshly extracted molar was then grooved using a diamond stone at nearly the level of the cemento- enamel junction using sterile saline coolant to facilitate later splitting. The samples were immediately placed in a sterile tube containing phosphate buffer solution (PBS) and transferred to the laboratory in less than 2 hours. Using a sterile cement spatula under a safety cabinet, the crown was split and the pulp was gently removed in sterilized conditions using sterile tweezers, a small excavator and K- files and then immediately placed in (PBS).

Isolation and Culture of DPSCs

The extirpated pulp tissues were washed in phosphate buffer solution (PBS) three times and minced into small pieces 1 mm^3 using sterile scissors and surgical blades. The minced pieces were then collected in sterile labeled 15 ml falcon tubes to which, a digesting solution consisting of 0.02 mg/ml collagenase type I, was added for 20 minutes at 37°C. The digestive reaction was stopped by the addition of culture media. The culture media consisted of Dulbeco modified Eagle's medium (DMEM) with L-glutamine, (Gibco, Invitrogen Life Technologies, USA) supplemented with 15% fetal bovine serum, (Gibco, Invitrogen Life Technologies, USA), antibiotics; penicillin/streptomycin (Penicillin G100 unit/ml and Streptomycin 100 µg/ml) and finally antimycotic agent (Fungizone, 0.25 µg/ml). The tubes were centrifuged at room temperature to obtain a cell pellet of pulp derived cells. The supernatant was discarded, and then the cells in the pellet were re-suspended in complete culture media through successive pipetting. Single cell suspensions were obtained by passing the digested tissues through a 70µm cell strainer (Becton/Dickinson, USA). Passaging was performed when primary cell culture of adherent cells reached 70% confluence.

Flow Cytometry Analysis for Identification and Characterization of Isolated DPSCs

Flow cytometric analysis for CD29, CD105, CD34 and CD45 was performed to confirm the existence of mesenchymal stem cells in the isolated cells and to rule out the existence of any non-mesenchymal stem cells. Cell analysis was performed using cytomics FC 500 flow cytometer (Beckman coulter, USA) and CXP software version 2.2 the expression of MSC markers was quantified as the following steps: Adherent cells (at the end of 3rd passage) were trypsinized and adjusted to $1x10^6$ cells/ml. Then 1×10^6 cells were incubated with 10 ml of monocolonal antibodies against: CD34 and CD 45 to show their negativity and CD29 and CD 105 to show their positivity (Beckman coulter, USA) at 4^0C in the dark. The same species of isotypes served as negative control. After 20 minutes incubation, 2 ml of PBS containing 2% FBS solution were added to each tube of monocolonal treated cells. The mixtures were then centrifuged for 5 minutes at 2500 rpm followed by discarding the supernatant and re-suspending cells in 500 ml PBS containing 2%FBS.

PRP Preparation and Grouping of DPSCs

Ten milliliters of venous blood were drawn from a donor and transferred into two test tubes containing Ethylene Diamine Tetra Acetic Acid (EDTA) as an anticoagulant. The drawn blood was then centrifuged at 5000 rpm for 15 minutes. The blood and plasma formed two layers; the supernatant being plasma. The plasma was then aspirated with a micropipette and transferred to a sterile test tube without an anticoagulant. The samples of plasma were subjected to a second centrifugation at 2000 rpm for 10 minutes, which allowed the precipitation of the platelets (0.8 to 1.2 ml) to fall onto the bottom, while the surface Platelet Poor Plasma was discarded using a micropipette. The platelet-rich plasma was transferred to a dish and stored at room temperature until further use. According to the media used the previously isolated dental pulp stem cells were allocated into two groups; (Control group) where DPSCs were cultured in regular culture media and (PRP group) where DPSCs were cultured in the above mentioned culture media supplemented with 1% and 5% platelet-rich plasma with platelet count of $1.5 \times 10^6/cmm^3$. PRP concentrations were calculated as volume percentage of added PRP to the total volume of culture media [9, 12].

Assessing Proliferation Capacity of DPSCs via MTT Assay

Daily follow up of stem cells was performed to ensure cell viability. Cultures from DPSCs were monitored using inverted light microscope (Olympus, USA) with digital camera for taking images (Nikon, Japan). MTT assay was performed to compare proliferation of all tested concentrations. This assay is based on the cellular conversion of a tetrazolium salt to formazon. Control and treated cells were incubated with MTT (0.2 mg/ml) diluted in the appropriate media for 60 min at 37°C in 96-well plates. Culture medium was removed and formazon was solubilized. The extent of reduction of MTT to formazon within cells was quantified with a spectrophotometer at a wavelength of 450 nm. Absorbance is considered as directly proportional to the number of living cells in culture. Cell proliferation was measured on days 3, 7, 10 and 14 according the cell proliferation kit protocol (Vybrant, Invitrogen). Viability of cells at day 14 was calculated thusly: *cell viability (%) = measurement of day 14 / measurement of day 3 x 100* [13].

Real-Time Quantitative PCR Analysis

RT-PCR was performed to analyze the level of expression of 2 stemness-related genes namely, *OCT4* and INTEGRIN1 in both groups at the third passage. The mRNA expression level was quantified by real-time quantitative PCR. 1000 ng of the total RNA from each sample was used for cDNA synthesis by reverse transcription using High capacity cDNA Reverse Transcriptase kit (Applied Biosystem, USA). The cDNA was subsequently amplified with the Syber Green I PCR Master Kit in a 48-well plate using the Step One instrument (Applied Biosystem, USA) as follows: 10 minutes at 95^0C for enzyme activation followed by 40 cycles of 15 seconds at 95^0C, 20 seconds at 55^0C and 30 second at 72^0C for the amplification step. Changes in the expression of each target gene (Integrin and Oct 4) were normalized relative to the mean critical threshold (CT) values of GAPDH housekeeping gene by the **ΔΔ Ct** method. We used 1μM of both primers specific for each target gene (***OCT4*****;** FWD: 5`-GAC AAC AAT GAC AAC CTT CAG GAG A-3`, REV: 5`-CTG GCG CCG GTT ACA GAA CCA-3`. ***INTGRIN1*****;** FWD: 5`-GTGAGTCAACCCCAACTACACT-3`, REV: 5`-AAGGCTCTGCACTG AACACATTC-3`).

DNA Sequencing

To ensure that the isolated DPSCs stem cell properties were not altered by the PRP supplemented media. DNA sequencing was performed for *OCT4* and *INTEGRIN1* genes and compared the results with the control group**.** PCR products samples were sequenced with forward primer using a Big Dye Terminator 3.1 Cycle Sequencing Kit (Applied Biosystems, Foster City, CA, USA), according to the manufacturer's instructions. Briefly; PCR sequencing cycling reaction with final total volume 20 μl which was included 8μl big dye terminator, 3.2 μl of 1 M mole diluted forward primer, 1μl PCR product and 7.8 μl nuclease free water. The thermal profile conditions will be 94^0C for 4 minutes and 95^0C for 15 sec, 55^0C for 30 sec and finally 60^0C for 4 minutes for 25 cycles. The sequencing cycling PCR products were purified with a centri-sep nucleic acid gel purified columns (Life technology, Invitrogen). Ten μl of Hi Di formamide were added to 10 μl of purified PCR products. The mix was denatured in PCR thermal cycler (Biometra, Germany) at 95^{0}C for 5 minutes. The reactions were performed in an automatic Sequencer ABI PRISM 310 Genetic Analyzer (Applied Biosystems, Foster City, Calif.). The sequences obtained were analyzed using the GenBank BLAST tool. Subsequently, the sequences were edited and aligned using the BioEdit Sequence Alignment.

Statistical Analysis

Data were coded and entered using the statistical package SPSS (Statistical Package for the Social Sciences) version 24. Data was summarized using mean and standard deviation in quantitative data. Comparisons between groups were done using unpaired t test. For comparison of serial measurements within each group repeated measures ANOVA was used. *P* values less than 0.05 were considered as statistically significant.

RESULTS

Isolation and Characterization of DPSCs via Flow Cytometry

Dental stem cells isolated from human impacted third molars were successfully isolated. Following the isolation and culturing procedures, the stem cells began to attach to bottom of the culture plates. The cultured cells were observed on regular basis using an inverted light microscope. At the beginning of culture after enzymatic digestion and initial seeding, DPSC adapted an elongated shape and some cells started to become spindle in shape (Figure 1A). DPSCs continued to proliferate and propagate until reaching 80% confluence by day 12. Cells supplemented with 1% PRP appeared to be more in number and showed more morphological diversity (elongated, spindle, stellate shaped) than DPSCs in control group. DPSCs cultured in 1% PRP reached 80% confluence by day 10 and were successfully maintained for 10 passages. Flow cytometric analysis of isolated DPSCs demonstrated positive expression of putative mesenchymal stem cell markers; CD29 and CD105. The percentages of those two markers illustrated positive expression after multiple passaging in 1% PRP (Figure 1B and 1C).

Assessment of Proliferation by MTT Assay

On days 3, 7, 10, 14 the number of viable cells cultured in 1% PRP was found to be significantly higher than the control group ($p < 0.05$). When 5% PRP concentration was applied, a significant decrease in proliferation of DPSCs over the time course studied was noticed (Supplementary Figure 1).

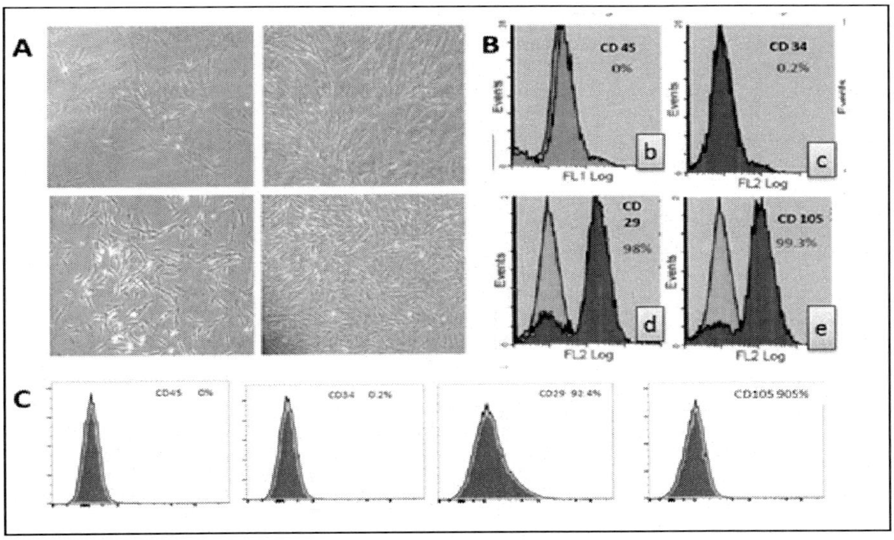

Figure 1. (A) Phase contrast microscopic observation of human dental pulp-derived MSCs (DPSCs) at the first passage either cultured in complete culture media (Upper photo) or in PRP supplemented media (lower photo), arrows indicate colony formation. Scale Bar 200 μm (B) Flow cytometric characterization analysis of isolated DPSCs, cells illustrated negative expression of CD34 and CD45 (b & c) and were uniformly positive for CD29 and CD105 (d & e). (C) Flow cytometric characterization analysis of DPSCs after multiple passaging in 1% PRP supplemented media.

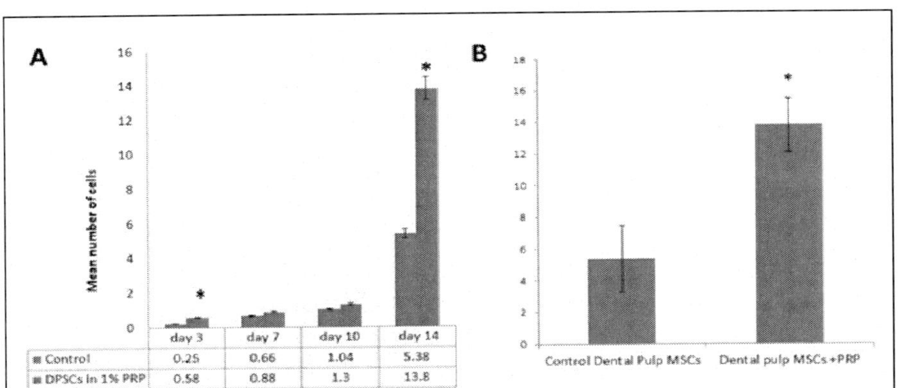

Figure 2. (A) MTT assay of DPSCs in control group and 1% PRP group on days 3, 7, 10 and 14 days. Proliferation of DPSCs was significantly higher in PRP group on days 3 and 14. Results are presented as mean ± SEM of three independent experiments (n = 3). (B) Cell viability of DPSCs cultured in both groups at 450 absorbance (* $P < 0.05$).

DPSCs cultured in 1% PRP exhibited higher proliferation rate starting from day 10 to day 14 after initial slow growth from day 3 to day 10 with the PRP group being significantly higher. It was also evident that the proliferation of 1% PRP group increased compared to that of control group from day 3 to day 14 collectively with the highest increase on the day 14 (Figure2A). On day 14, viability of the cells was assessed; the results revealed that the number of viable cells cultured in 1% PRP supplemented culture media was significantly higher (Figure2B).

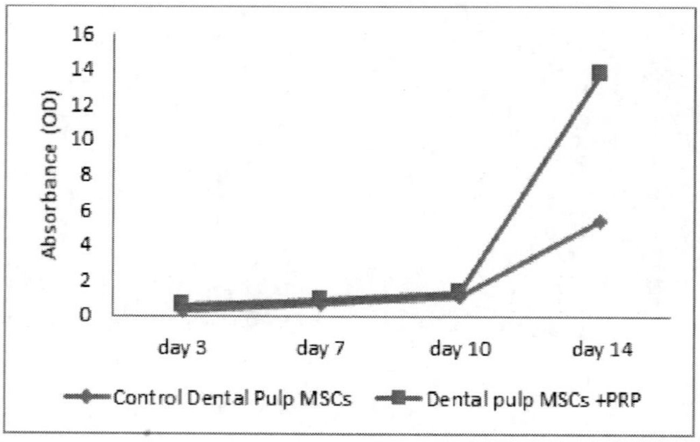

Figure 3. Growth curve illustrating proliferation of DPSCs in control group and 1% PRP group as detected by MTT assay at optical density 450 nm. PRP group illustrated a significantly higher value compared with the control group at every time point tested starting from day 3. Results are presented as mean ± SEM of three independent experiments (n = 3); *P < 0.05.

Molecular Assessment of OCT4 and INTEGRIN1 Gene Expression by Real-Time Quantitative PCR

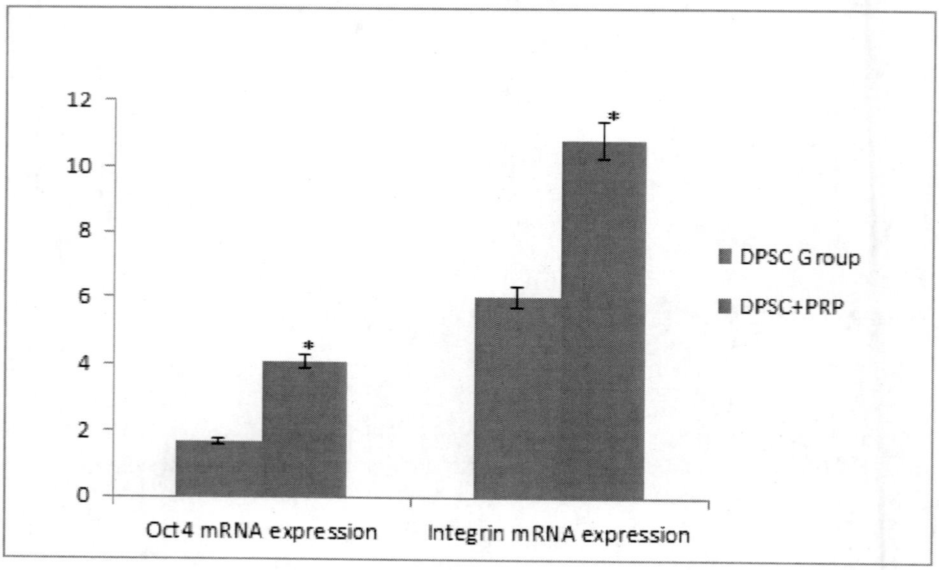

Figure 4. RT- PCR of OCT4 and INTGRIN1 gene expression of DPSCs in control group and 1% PRP. Both OCT4 and INTGRIN1gene expression were significantly higher in PRP group (P < 0.001). Results are presented as mean ± SEM of three independent experiments (n = 3). * P < 0.05.

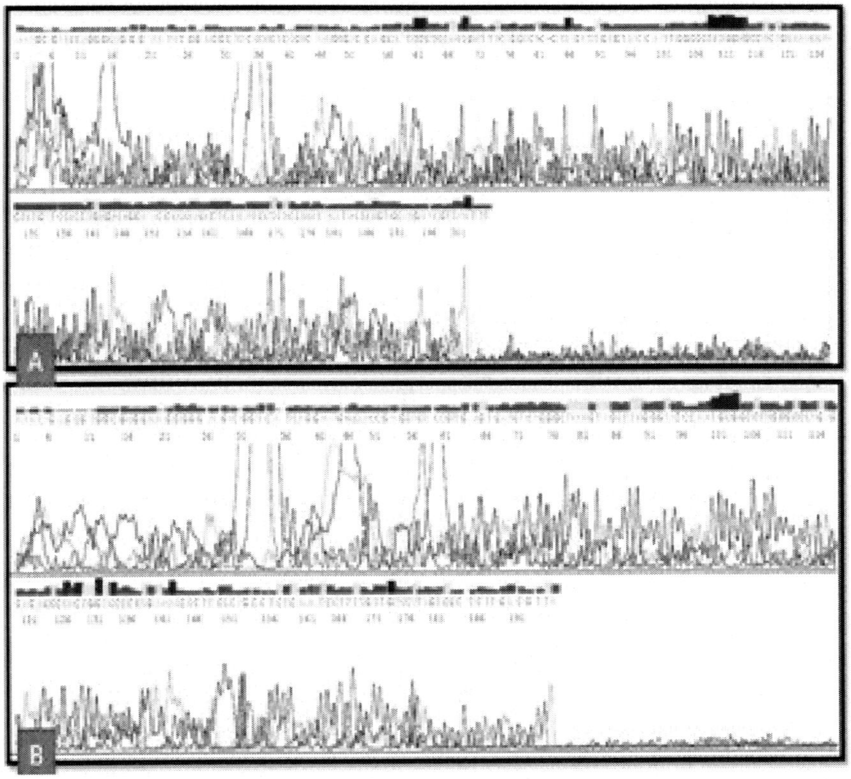

Figure 5. DNA sequence of homo sapiens transcript variant of OCT4B2 mRNA, complete cds in (A) Control (DPSCs without PRP supplementation) (B) DPSCs with PRP supplementation. Gene bank accession number is kj700311.1.

The proliferation results were further confirmed by a molecular assessment of *OCT4* and *INTGRIN1* genes' expression. The corresponding results showed that the expression of *OCT4* and the expression of *INTGRIN1* were both significantly higher in PRP cultures (Figure 4).

DNA Sequencing

To ensure that the isolated DPSC stem cell properties were not altered by the PRP supplemented media. DNA sequencing was performed for *OCT4* and *INTEGRIN1* genes and the results were compared with the control group. The results showed that the DNA sequencing for *OCT4* & *INTGRIN1* genes of DPSCs cultured in PRP were 100% matching with that of DPSCs in control group which indicated that the PRP supplementation didn't change the nucleotide sequence of stem cell genes (Figures 5 and 6).

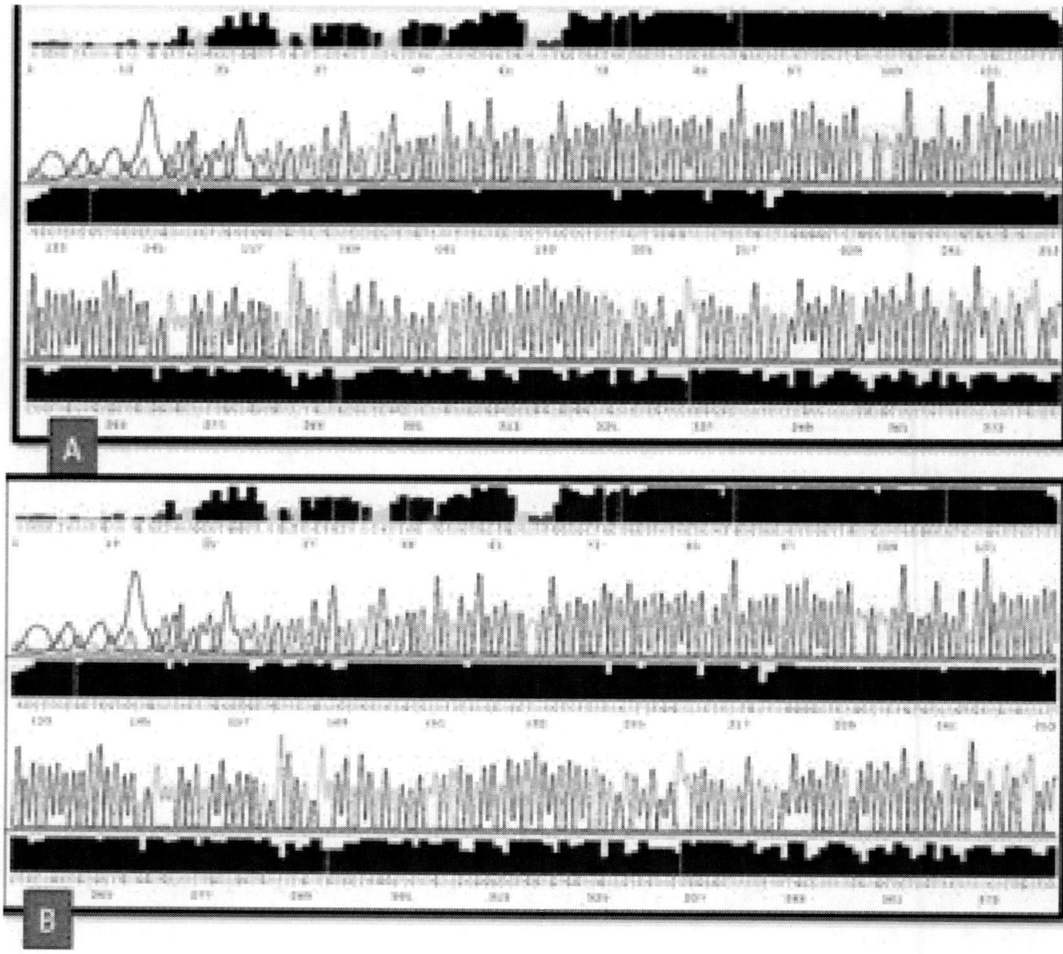

Figure 6. DNA sequence of homo sapiens transcript variant of INTGRIN1 mRNA, complete cds in (A) Control DPSCs without PRP supplementation) (B) DPSCs with PRP supplementation. Gene bank accession number is NM 000212.2.

Discussion

Stem cell research in dentistry has recently grown rapidly with endless possible applications in oral and maxillofacial tissue regeneration [14]. Dental pulp, in particular, presents a promising source of adult stem cells that can be isolated in a minimally invasive procedure as opposed to other tissues that require surgical intervention [1, 15–18]. However, due to the small size of the dental pulp tissue, the yielded population of stem cells is insufficient for large scale clinical application and multiple passaging is usually required in order to acquire sufficient number of cells, a process which reduces the potency of cultured cells [19]. In the present study, in order to promote DPSCs proliferation and to increase the yielded cell number, platelet-rich plasma was applied as a potent enhancer of proliferation. Platelet-rich plasma has been widely used in various surgical fields and was reported to induce tissue repair and regeneration effectively [10]. PRP can be easily prepared from autologous peripheral blood in large quantities and with minimal donor site morbidity. It consists of autologous platelets concentrated in small volume of plasma, with abundant content of naturally inherent growth factors and matrix elements that are otherwise expensive to obtain [7]. PRP can thus act as an easily acquired proliferative enhancer that doesn`t cost much. Past studies have investigated the effect of PRP on proliferation of different types of mesenchymal stem cells (MSCs); [8, 12, 20]; however the effect of PRP on human dental pulp stem cells was the least tested.

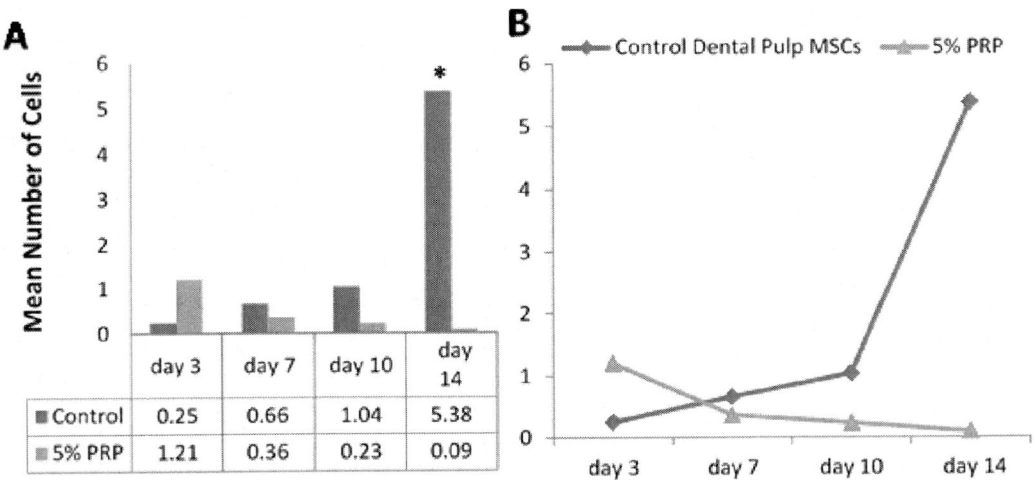

Supplementary Figure 1. (A) MTT assay of DPSCs in control group and 5% PRP group on days 3, 7, 10 and 14 days. Proliferation of DPSCs was significantly reduced in 5% PRP group from days 7 to 14. Results are presented as mean ± SEM of three independent experiments (n = 3). (B) Growth curve illustrating proliferation of DPSCs in control group and 5% PRP group as detected by MTT assay at optical density 450 nm. 5%PRP group illustrated significantly reduced values compared with the control group starting from day 7. Results are presented as mean ± SEM of three independent experiments (n = 3); (* $P < 0.05$).

In the present study DPSCs were isolated from dental pulp of impacted third molar according to Gronthos et al., 2000 [16]. Mesenchymal stem cell identity of the isolated cells was characterized guided by their ability to adhere to culture plated. Addition-ally, isolated cells expressed MSCs specific cell surface markers; CD 29, CD105 and lack of CD 45, CD 34 expression, the same pattern was illustrated after several passages in PRP supplemented culture media indicating that this supplementation at the indicated percentage did not alter the stem cell iden-tity of the cultured cells. Cell morphology analysis of both groups demonstrated diverse morphological appearances ranging from spindle to stellate shaped cells consistently through several passages. DPSCs cultured in PRP reached confluence earlier than those cultured without PRP which is mainly attributed to the rich content of growth factors found in PRP. In order to demonstrate the difference in the proliferation pattern between DPSCs cultured in PRP and DPSCs cultured without PRP; MTT assay was performed. MTT enables simple and reliable counting of metabolically active cells while indicating their viability and proliferation rate. Its main advantages are its rapidity and precision, and the lack of any radio-isotope [22]. Our results demonstrated that DPSCs cultured in 1% PRP proliferated faster than DPSCs cultured without PRP. These results were generally in agreement with previous studies that also revealed that DPSCs supplemented with 1% PRP exhibited a higher proliferation rate compared to DPSCs without PRP based on the results of MTT and colony forming ability [6]. Our results were also in accordance with previous studies on human adipose stem cells who reported that treatment with PRP resulted in a statistically significant increase in cell proliferation [20]. However, our findings revealed that PRP at a concentration of 5% significantly reduced the proliferation of DPSCs which was in consistence with Lee et al. who attributed this decrease to the negative feedback caused by the increased growth factors at higher concentrations of PRP [9].

To confirm that the proliferative effect achieved by PRP did not affect the stemness of the isolated DPSCs, molecular assessment of *OCT4* expression and *INTGRIN1* expression in both experimental conditions was performed. *INTGRIN1* is a member of the integrin family, which are heterodimeric proteins made up of alpha and beta subunits. Integrin family members are membrane receptors involved in cell adhesion and recognition in a variety of processes including embryogenesis, hemostasis, tissue repair, immune response and metastatic diffusion of tumor cells. Its expression indicates human MSC [17, 23]. Expression of *OCT4* was also analyzed since it is considered an indicative marker of stemness [24]. In accordance with previous studies, both OCT4 & INTGRIN1 demonstrated a significantly higher expression in PRP group [25, 26]. It has been reported that some gross chromosomal changes tend to occur in stem cells culture especially when the culture conditions are manipulated [27, 28]. Comparing genomes in the starting and in manipulated cultures provide adequate evaluation of these changes. DNA sequencing was reported to serve as a powerful tool for identifying any alterations in cell populations, especially those of stem cells [29]. In the present study, DNA sequencing confirmed that PRP supplementation didn't alter the nucleotide sequence of stem cell genes. Taken together, our results indicated that PRP is a safe and efficient natural promoter of proliferation and can readily substitute traditional animal derived supplements like FBS. Finally, in an era where there is an increasing demand for safe and ethically accepted alternatives for application in future regenerative medicine and cell based therapies; PRP can be considered a powerful and promising runner-up.

ACKNOWLEDGMENTS

This research did not receive any specific grant from funding agencies in the public, commercial, or not-for-profit sectors.

Conflict of Interest

The authors declare that they have no conflict of interest.

Ethical Compliance

The authors have stated all possible conflicts of interest within this work. The authors have stated all sources of funding for this work. If this work involved human participants, informed consent was received from each individual. If this work involved human participants, it was conducted in accordance with the 1964 Declaration of Helsinki. If this work involved experiments with humans or animals, it was conducted in accordance with the related institutions' research ethics guidelines.

References

[1] Laino G, Graziano A, D'Aquino R, Pirozzi G, Lanza V, Valiante S, et al. An approachable human adult stem cell source for hard-tissue engineering. *J Cell Physiol*. 2006.

[2] d'Aquino R, De Rosa A, Laino G, Caruso F, Guida L, Rullo R, et al. Human dental pulp stem cells: from biology to clinical applications. *J Exp Zool B Mol Dev* Evol. 2009;312B(5):408–15.

[3] Meirelles Lda S, Nardi NB. Methodology, biology and clinical applications of mesenchymal stem cells. *Front Biosci* (Landmark Ed. 2009).

[4] Estrela C, de Alencar AHG c alves, Kitten GT, Vencio EF, Gava E, C E, et al. Mesenchymal stem cells in the dental tissues: perspectives for tissue regeneration. *Braz Dent J*. 2011.

[5] Anitua E, Troya M, Zalduendo M. Progress in the use of dental pulp stem cells in regenerative medicine. *Cytotherapy* [Internet]. 2018 Apr 1 [cited 2018 Jul 22]; 20(4):479–98. Available from: https://www.sciencedirect.com/science/article/pii/S1465324918300033.

[6] Jo Y, Lee H, Lee U, Seo B, Choung P. *The Effect of Platelet-Rich Plasma on Proliferation of Dental Stem Cells Derived from Human Tooth*. 2006;3(4):440–4.

[7] Intini G. The use of platelet-rich plasma in bone reconstruction therapy. *Biomaterials*. 2009.

[8] Egusa H, Sonoyama W, Nishimura M, Atsuta I, Akiyama K. Stem cells in dentistry - Part I: Stem cell sources. *J Prosthodont Res*. 2012;56(3):151–65.

[9] Lee UL, Jeon SH, Park JY, Choung PH. Effect of platelet-rich plasma on dental stem cells derived from human impacted third molars. *Regen Med*. 2011;6(1): 67–79.

[10] Albanese A, Licata ME, Polizzi B, Campisi G. Platelet-rich plasma (PRP) in dental and oral surgery: from the wound healing to bone regeneration. *Immun Ageing*. 2013;10(1):23.

[11] Gronthos S, Brahim J, Li W, Fisher LW, Cherman N, Boyde A, et al. Stem Cell Properties of Human Dental Pulp Stem Cells. *J Dent Res*. 2002;81(8):531–5.

[12] Xu F, Li H, Yin Q, Liang Z, Huang M, Chi G, et al. Effect of activated autologous platelet-rich plasma on proliferation and osteogenic differentiation of human adipose-derived stem cells in vitro. *Am J Transl Res* 2015;7(2):257–70.

[13] Guan Z, Shi S, Kamolmatyakul S. Proliferation and mineralization ability of dental pulp cells derived from primary and permanent teeth. *Songklanakarin J Sci Technol*. 2011;33(2):129–34.

[14] Lee S-M, Zhang Q, Le AD. Dental Stem Cells: Sources and Potential Applications. *Curr Oral Heal Reports*. 2014;1(1):34–42.

[15] V. T, F. P, A. DR, Tirino V, Paino F, De Rosa A, et al. Identification, isolation, characterization, and banking of human dental pulp stem cells. *Methods in Molecular Biology*. 2012.

[16] Gronthos S, Mankani M, Brahim J, Robey PG, Shi S. Postnatal human dental pulp stem cells (DPSCs) in vitro and in vivo. *Proc Natl Acad Sci USA*. 2000; 97(25): 13625–30.

[17] Marchionni C, Bonsi L, Alviano F, Lanzoni G, Di Tullio A, Costa R, et al. Angiogenic potential of human Dental Pulp Stromal (STEM) Cells. *Int J Immunopathol Pharmacol*. 2009.

[18] Yasui T, Mabuchi Y, Morikawa S, Onizawa K, Akazawa C, Nakagawa T, et al. Isolation of dental pulp stem cells with high osteogenic potential. *Inflamm Regen* [Internet]. 2017 Dec 10 [cited 2018 Jul 22];37(1): 8. Available from: http://inflammregen.biomedcentral.com/articles/10.1186/s41232-017-0039-4.

[19] Lizier NF, Kerkis A, Gomes CM, Hebling J, Oliveira CF, Caplan AI, et al. Scaling-up of dental pulp stem cells isolated from multiple niches. *PLoS One*. 2012.

[20] Tavakolinejad S, Khosravi M, Mashkani B, Bideskan AE, Mossavi NS, Parizadeh SMR, et al. The effect of Human platelet-rich plasma on adipose-derived stem cell proliferation and osteogenic differentiation. *Iran Biomed J*. 2014;18(3):150–6.

[21] Gronthos S, Mankani M, Brahim J, Robey PG, Shi S. Postnatal human dental pulp stem cells (DPSCs) *in vitro* and *in vivo*. *Proc Natl Acad Sci USA*. 2000; 97(25): 13625–30.

[22] Nedel F, Soki FN, Conde MCM, Zeitlin BD, Tarquinio SBC, Nör JE, et al. Comparative analysis of two colorimetric assays in dental pulp cell density. *Int Endod J*. 2011.

[23] You-Young J, Hee-Jung L, Sun-Young K, Choung H-W, Joo-Young P, Jong-Hoon C, et al. Isolation and Characterization of Postnatal Stem Cells from Human Dental Tissues. *Tissue Eng*. 2007.

[24] Zangrossi S, Marabese M, Broggini M, Giordano R, D'Erasmo M, Montelatici E, et al. Oct-4 expression in adult human differentiated cells challenges its role as a pure stem cell marker. *Stem Cells*. 2007;25(7):1675–80.

[25] Tai MH, Chang CC, Olson LK, Trosko JE. Oct4 expression in adult human stem cells: evidence in support of the stem cell theory of carcinogenesis. *Carcinogenesis*. 2004.

[26] MacHado E, Fernandes MH, De Sousa Gomes P. Dental stem cells for craniofacial tissue engineering. Vol. 113, *Oral Surgery, Oral Medicine, Oral Pathology and Oral Radiology*. 2012. p. 728–33.

[27] Teitell MA. How to assess a stem cell genome. *Nat Reports Stem Cells* [Internet]. 2008 Jul 10 [cited 2018 Sep 4]; Available from: http://www.nature.com/doi finder/10.1038/stemcells.2008.85.

[28] Ludtmann MHR, Arber C, Bartolome F, De Vicente M, Preza E, Carro E, et al. Mutations in valosin-containing protein (VCP) decrease ADP/ATP trans-location across the mitochondrial membrane and impair energy metabolism in human neurons. *Journal of Biological Chemistry*. 2017 [cited 2018 Sep 4]; Available from: http://www.jbc.org/cgi/doi/10. 1074/jbc.M116.762898.

[29] Wen L, Tang F. Single-cell sequencing in stem cell biology. *Genome Biol* [Internet]. 2016 Apr 15 [cited 2018 Sep 4];17:71. Available from: http://www.ncbi. nlm.nih.gov/pubmed/27083874.

In: Manipulation of Stem Cells for Disease Benefits
Editor: Prasad Koka
ISBN: 978-1-53615-468-9

Chapter 11

WHAT CAN I DO WHEN RUGER IS LIMPING?

Inger Birgitta Sundell*
Department of Anthropology, Wayne State University,
Detroit, MI, US

ABSTRACT

Domesticated animals or companion animals are pets that share a psychological bond with their owners. Today there are some 77 million dogs in the USA. The attitudes towards pets have changed and many pets are treated as family members. Dogs live longer lives than ever because preventive health care has become available for them by veterinarians in the health care field who devote much effort towards disease prevention, early detection, reduced invasiveness, and personalized therapies. Regular health exams and immunization programs help ensure that conditions are prevented or treated early. Millions of pets will develop diseases with close analogy to human diseases such as osteoarthritis. Pet owners will look for treatment options to help their beloved pets. Several major pet-insurance companies have recently added stem cell trans-plants to the lists of procedures for which they will pay.

Stem cell therapy for dogs is a decision for the owner, and it means considering both the best interest of the dog and the owners financial possibilities. Stem cell technology is a new branch of veterinary medicine but unfortunately there is not yet much information on possible adverse side effects available. Stem cells can be harvested from a variety of adult animal tissues then be injected and induced to grow into different mature cell types.

BACKGROUND

Dogs seem to have had a very special place among humans in ancient societies. At archaeological excavation sites many dog burials have been found, while burials of other

* Corresponding Author's Email: du2557 @wayne.edu.

animals are not often found. For example, 5,000 and 8,000 year old remains of buried dogs have been found at Lake Baikal, in Siberia. These dogs were buried alongside humans in cemeteries and this indicates that dogs were held in high esteem by humans and were treated like humans or family members. In support of this theory chemical analysis of dog bones have shown that the Lake Baikal dogs consumed same diet as humans ate (Losey et al. 2013). It is possible that the ancient dogs fed of discarded left-overs of human meals but it is also possible that they were fed by their human owners. This provide evidence that people had emotional bonds to their dogs. Humans allowed dogs within their dwellings and dogs were also kept as working companions. Dead dogs were buried by humans who sacrificed items such as collars and spoons for the dogs to use in afterlife. Dogs were the only domestic mammals among the Aboriginals of North America and Australia (Clutton-Brock 1995). Already Darwin speculated about the origins of dogs but he believed that dogs must have had more than one wild ancestor (*Darwin 1859*). Modern science have provided convincing morphological, behavioral and genetic evidence for an evolution of ancient wolfs (*Canis lupus*) to our domesticated dogs (*Canis familiaris*) (Savolainen et al. 2002, Pang et al. 2009, Lindblad-Toh et al. 2005, von Holdt et al. 2010, DeMello 2012). Anthropologists believe that domestication was a deliberately accomplished by human manipulation (Clutton-Brock J 1995). If wolves evolved into dogs via natural evolutionary processes including geographic space and chronological time this is a similar process to other mammalian taxa (Crockford SJ 2006, Dobney K& Larson G, 2006). The hypothesis that small stature wolves colonized areas close to human settlements in search of protection and easy food access is another possibility. These low ranking small wolves (omegas) had the lowest rank in the wild wolf packs, and could be driven from the pack. Omega wolves found an easier life scavenging around human settlements in their search of food and protection. In fact when humans became settled agriculturalists the interaction between humans and wolfs became more stable. Agriculture made it possible for humans to support themselves with food while remaining in the same location, human dwellings developed to more secure structures. The development also suggests a mutual need for connection between humans and dogs. Indeed dogs appear more frequently in the Old and New Worlds once agriculture develops and humans become stationary (Byers & Flannery 1967, Hassan & Gautier 2002, Blench, Spriggs & Higham 1998, Plug & Voigt 1985, Prates, Prevosti & Berón 2010). Dogs evolved and are still evolving through their association with people via natural adaptation, human selection, or genetic drift.

When humans made the transition from hunters and gatherers to agricultural societies, their lower limb strength and overall mobility decreased. Hunter and gatherers spent their days in search of food. They traveled long distances on foot. Human bones are flexible and adapt quickly to a reduction in physical activity. The leg bones of a male living near 5,300 BC compare to those of today's top-trained athletes, but bone from males living near 2000 BC are more similar to modern man. Results obtained by investigation of skeletal remains reveal reduced activity level among humans over the years. In hunter-gatherer societies, dogs were probably hunting partners and a food source. In agricultural societies dogs became companions. Mortality rates for dogs were high. Com-mon causes of death were malnutrition and attacks by other animals. Since dogs were working companions their lifestyle changed when human lifestyle changed. When humans settled as agriculturalists dogs were no longer needed to pull sleds, follow hunters, as a food source, or to herd livestock. Instead they became playmates for children and beloved companions.

Modern lifestyle may emphasize or strengthen the bonds between owner and pets (*Archer 1997*). Modern individuals have fewer extended family networks, family sizes are smaller, and more people are living alone in urban areas than in the past. Pets mean more to their owners that in the past.

MODERN LIFE INFLUENCED HEALTH

When human became able to conquer contagious disease, spoiled food, contaminated water, mal-nutrition, exposure, and injuries their life expectancy increased. Life expectancy doubled in the past 160 years or increased with about three months every year. Once humans lived longer they cared more for their pets by keeping pet animals healthy by treating and preventing illness when possible. The annual cost for veterinarian care for a dog is different and based on a variety of factors like the breed and size of the dog, to the quality of food and accessories to the person's ability and willingness to treat chronic health problems. Owning a healthy dog strengthen the pet-human relationships and it can become a longer-lasting positive experience.

Ethnographic research show that dog owners experience many positive feelings when interacting with their dog. In this study of committed pet owners, Belk (1996) found that owners described their relationship with pets similar to human family members it reduced stress, provide security and protection. Figure 1 and 2 show how couples pose with their dogs for a photographer. Dogs can fill many functions such as be an exercise partner and improve cardiovascular health, provide friendship, company, affection, and love. Dogs improve both physical and psychological well-being among owners (Podberscek 1997; Belk 1996). There are research studies on the human 'caregiver burden' or the response to physical and mental challenges caregivers experience while they care for a sick family member. However little is known about the impact of the caregiver burden on owners of animals with chronic or terminal diseases. Sptitznagel {2017} showed greater stress and symptoms of depression and anxiety among owners of animals who suffer from chronic or terminal disease. Given the deep connection that many dog owners develop with their pet more research on how owners cope with the loss of a pet is needed. Dogs are now used as therapy animals for vulnerable populations such as the blind, veterans with post-traumatic stress disorder, etc.

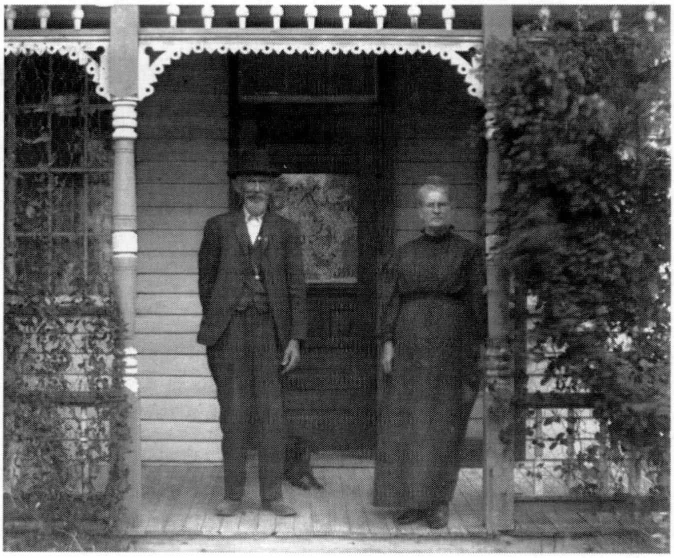

Figure 1. Photo is from New Knoxville, Ohio and were captured by a local photographer between 1850 and 1890. New Knoxville is located in southern Auglaize County, an area dominated by agriculture. The small dog on the porch is clearly a family member, not a hunting or herding dog. The dog stays on the porch by his human family without being restrained. Photo courtesy of New Knoxville Historic Society.

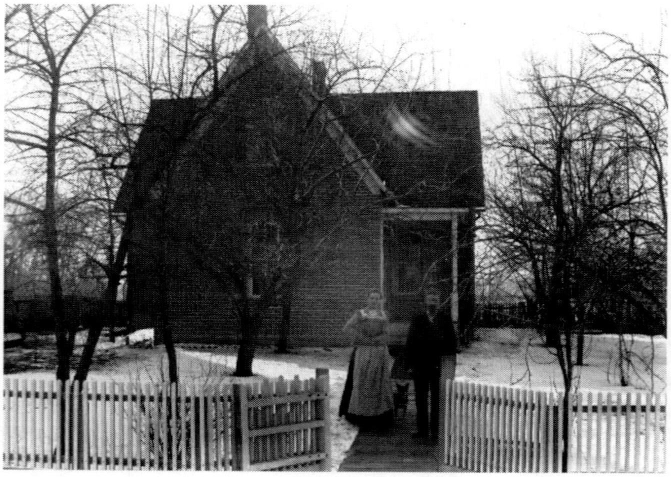

Figure 2. Photo is from New Knoxville, Ohio and were captured by a local photographer between 1850 and 1890. New Knoxville is a small village with less than 1,000 inhabitants, they were descending from immigrants from the German village of Ladbergen. The dog pose for a photo with the family. Photo courtesy of New Knoxville Historic Society.

One disease that has become more frequent among family pets is osteoarthritis (OA), a degeneration disease that affect the joint cartilage, it is caused by inflammation and cause serious pain (Fox SM, 2012). OA occurs in approximately 20% of all American dogs and is one of the most common conditions seen in middle-aged to senior pets. Younger dogs can also develop arthritis, but OA is more common in older dogs, large breed dogs and working dogs than in smaller breed dogs. The dog's quality of life becomes a serious concern with disease progression. The first line of treatment is long-term cyclo-oxygenase-inhibiting non-steroidal anti-inflammatory drug (NSAID) therapy, physical therapy, diet and weight management, and dietary supplements (Fox SM, 2012). NSAIDs needs to be administrated daily, require prescription refills, carry risks of possible gastrointestinal, renal, and hepatic complications. Orally distributed medications can be difficult to administer to pets and it usually means that owner's compliance is poor.

Stem Cell Therapy for Dogs

Mesenchymal stem cell (MSC) therapy relieves the owner of the burden of daily pain medication administration, may be associated with good tissue regeneration, and can be a good therapeutic solution (Fox SM, 2012). MSC therapy is currently considered a safe although costly procedure to treat bone, joint, and ligament problems. The main purpose is to reduce pain and improve function of the affected joints. Cells for injection can be derived from the dog's own adipose tissue, so immune reactions are rare. Harvesting the adipose tissue for stem cell isolation takes 30 to 60 minutes and is performed under general anesthesia. Adipose tissue is sent to a laboratory for processing, and the purified MSCs are returned for infusion. MSC can mature by multi-lineage differentiation to become adipogenic, osteogenic, and chondrogenic cells and also have the ability to self-renew (Vieira et al. 2010, Zuk et al. 2002). Instead of treating arthritis pain of the joints it with anti-inflammatory drugs to provide temporary pain reduction, allogenic stem cell transplant may reverse arthritis. However the treatment results with MSC transplant is not always completely successful, further studies are needed to show positive results. It is not unlikely that more veterinarians will offer stem cell therapies in the future to meet an increased demand.

MSC are released and activated by injury signals and can migrate through the bloodstream to distant sites of injury (Caplan & Dennis 2006, Hernigou 2015, Caplan & Correa 2011). Following infusion the purified, concentrated MSC will accumulate at the site of injury or at the sites of injury. Microenvironment at an injury site produce cytokines that attract MSCs, and this trigger injury-specific or adaptive responses to reduce the injury/ disease process (Murphy et al. 2013). MSC can be injected directly into the injured joint, ligament, where bone will begin to grow and replace the damaged tissue with new, healthy tissue. Long-term positive effects of stem cell therapy have not been researched sufficiently to document the progress of MSC therapy in pets yet.

Treatment costs, which include the surgery to retrieve stem cells, processing of the cells, and the initial injection, average $2,000 to $3,000 but may be worth it for adult dogs with long life expectancy. In a study of MSC treated dogs had lower veterinary score of pain on manipulation than age, weight, and sex age matched controls (92.76 versus 50.22%) and the veterinary global score (86.89 versus 30.75%) (Harman et al. 2016). Both male and female dogs of large and small breeds were included in the study. Global assessment and quality of life measurements are done through an interpretation by the owner and/or veterinarian. Both veterinarians and dog owners evaluated stem cell-treated dogs as improved as compared to placebo-treated dogs.

Caring for a Dog with Joint Disease

Evans-Pritchard (1950) and Geertz (1973) have described how animals become incorporated in the social environment. Humans give their pet dog a name just like children are given names. The names are used to call them, most dogs learn to listen to their name. Dogs become members of the human household and is care for by their owners. Dogs are kept and bred to provide emotional closeness to the family members (DeMello 2012). Franklin (1990) have said that "The relationship with pets is the closest and most humanized of human-animal relations" and that represents a drastic change in attitudes towards dog ownership. More people have become prepared to spend money on their pets, so pet industries have developed and produced more and more products and services for pets. Services and products include pet health products, pet psychologists, pet clothing, pet daycare, and even pet mortuary services. Pets are considered companions. The therapeutic values of keeping pets has received medical and scientific attention. The postmodern condition with high stress levels, mental and physical conditions can be improved by therapy dogs. The cultural and social significance of pet ownership can provide social benefits that society can no longer offer.

Therapy dogs and their owners work together as a team to improve the lives of other people but these dogs are not covered or protected under the Federal Housing Act or Americans with Disabilities act. A therapy dogs visits various facilities and locations such a nursing homes, classrooms, libraries, assisted living centers, hospices, funeral homes, schools, shelters even courtroom. Animal-assisted interventions to improve human health, have become increasingly popular in clinical settings. The dog's most common behaviors during visits to a children's' hospital were lip licking and tail wagging (McCullough et al. 2018). Service dogs on the other hand are dogs trained to perform a task or tasks to assist a person with a disability or impairment. A service dog must be with their person at all times and has special access privileges in public places. These dogs fulfill very important functions, and they have received many hours of specialized training.

The relationship between owner and dog makes caring for the ailing dog mentally difficult. Arthritis in dogs was not treated by veterinarians until the late 1960s. Over time, scientists and veterinarians have produced therapies and an abundance of information on how to treat the condition. An owner who sees the beloved dog suffer as their joints can no longer withstand the regular wear and tear of everyday life are willing to consider treatment options. When a dogs body shown signs of normal aging the dogs strong survival drive will prevent them from showing signs of distress early. Dogs do all they can to act happy so they may have experienced pain long before the owner notice. This is a remaining behavior from the time of the wild dogs, old and sick dogs can be left behind by a hunting pack. The period from birth to old age is much shorter for most domestic animals than for people, and death is a normal part of the life cycle. In some cases no budget can change the outcome. Because of the bonds between owner and pet stem cell therapy should be decided after serious consideration. Owning a healthy pet is a positive experience but losing a loved pet companion is just as stressful as losing a human partner.

CONCLUSION

Stem cell therapy for arthritic dogs have good potential for a pain free future. Health insurance for dogs will provide some financial support for stem cell therapy dog owners have to consider the economy versus the health benefits. To be a candidate for stem cell therapy the dog should to be between adult (2 to 7 years of age) and the owner should realize that this is not a one-shot treatment that will cure all pain. Treatment might have to be repeated. More studies is needed to determine outcome in dogs that receive stem cell injections or stem cell in combination with other medication. Joint replacement is an alternative and while it is more invasive it is an established and well documented alternative, or an option if MSC therapy fails.

ETHICAL COMPLIANCE

The authors have stated all possible conflicts of interest within this work. The authors have stated all sources of funding for this work. If this work involved human participants, informed consent was received from each individual. If this work involved human participants, it was conducted in accordance with the 1964 Declaration of Helsinki. If this work involved experiments with humans or animals, it was conducted in accordance with the related institutions' research ethics guidelines.

REFERENCES

[1] Archer, J. (1997). Why Do People Love Their Pets? *Evolution and Human Behaviour* 18, 237-259.

[2] Belk, RW. (1996). Metaphoric Relationships with Pets (Electronic version). *Society & Animals*, 4(2). Retrieved from http://www.psyeta.org/sa/sa4.2/belk.html.

[3] Blench R, Spriggs M, Bellwood P (1998) in Expansion of East and Southeast Asian Neolithic in Archaeology and Language II: Archaeological Data and Linguistic Hypotheses, *The archaeology of Papuan and Austronesian prehistory in the Northern Moluccas, Eastern Indonesia*, eds Blench R, Spriggs M (Routledge, New York), pp. 128–140.

[4] Blench R, Spriggs M, Higham CFW (1998) in Expansion of East and Southeast Asian Neolithic in Archaeology and Language II: Archaeological Data and Linguistic Hypotheses, *Archaeology, linguistics and the expansion of the East and Southeast Asian Neolithic*, eds Blench R, Spriggs M (Routledge, New York), pp. 103–114.

[5] Byers DS, Flannery KV (1967) in *The Prehistory of the Tehuacan Valley, Vertebrate fauna and hunting patterns,* ed Byers DS (Univ of Texas Press, Austin), pp. 132–177.

[6] Caplan AI, Correa D. The MSC: an injury drugstore. *Cell Stem Cell* (2011) 9(1):11–5.

[7] Caplan AI, Dennis JE. Mesenchymal stem cells as trophic mediators. *J Cell Biochem* (2006) 98(5):1076–84.

[8] Clutton-Brock J (1995) Origin of the dog: domestication and early history. In: Serpell J, editor. *The Domestic Dog: Its Evolution, Behaviour and Interaction with People*. Cambridge: Cambridge University Press. pp. 7–20.

[9] Crockford SJ (2006) *Rhythms of Life: Thyroid Hormone and the Origin of Species.* Victoria, B.C.: Trafford. 272 p.

[10] Darwin C (1859) *On the Origin of Species by Means of Natural Selection, or the Preservation of Favoured Races in the Struggle for Life* (John Murray, London).

[11] DeMello M (2012) Animals and Society. *An Introduction to Human-Animal Studies*. Columbia University Press.

[12] Dobney K, Larson G (2006) Genetics and animal domestication: new windows on an elusive process. *Journal of Zoology* 269: 261–271.

[13] Fox SM. Painful decisions for senior pets. *Vet Clin North Am Small Anim Pract* (2012) 42(4):727–48.

[14] Harman, R., Carlson, K., Gaynor, J., Gustafson, S., Dhupa, S., Clement, K., Adams, C. (2016). A Prospective, Randomized, Masked, and Placebo-Controlled Efficacy Study of Intraarticular Allogeneic Adipose Stem Cells for the Treatment of Osteoarthritis in Dogs. *Frontiers in Veterinary Science,* 3, 81.

[15] Hassan FA, Gautier A (2002) Droughts, Food and Culture: Ecological Change and Food Security in Africa's Later Prehistory, *The evidence for the earliest livestock in North Africa: Or adventures with large bovids, ovicaptrids, dogs and pigs*, ed Hassan FA (Kluwer Academic/Plenum, New York), pp. 195–207.

[16] Hernigou P. Bone transplantation and tissue engineering, part IV. Mesenchymal stem cells: history in orthopedic surgery from Cohnheim and Goujon to the Nobel Prize of Yamanaka. *Int Orthop* (2015) 39(4):807–17.

[17] Lindblad-Toh K, et al. (2005) Genome sequence, comparative analysis and haplotype structure of the domestic dog. *Nature* 438:803–819.

[18] Losey RJ, Garvie-Lok S, Leonard JA, Katzenberg MA, Germonpré M, Nomokonova T, et al. (2013) Burying Dogs in Ancient Cis-Baikal, Siberia: Temporal Trends and Relationships with Human Diet and Subsistence Practices. *PLoS ONE* 8(5): e63740.

[19] McCullough A, Jenkins MA, Ruehrdanz A, Gilmer MJ, Olson J, Pawar A, Holley L, Sierra-Rivera S, Linder DE, Pichette D. Grossman NJ, Hellman C, Guerin A, O'Haire ME (2018) Physiological and behavioral effects of animal-assisted interventions on therapy dogs in pediatric oncology settings. *Applied Animal Behaviour Science* 200; 86-95.

[20] Murphy MB, Moncivais K, Caplan AI. Mesenchymal stem cells: Environmentally responsive therapeutics for regenerative medicine. *Exp Mol Med* (2013).

[21] Pang JF, Kluetsch C, Zou XJ, Zhang A, Luo LY, et al. (2009) mtDNA data indicate a single origin for dogs south of Yangtze River, less than 16,300 years ago, from numerous wolves. *Molecular Biology and Evolution* 26: 2849–2864.

[22] Plug I, Voigt EA (1985) Archaeozoological studies of Iron Age communities in southern Africa. In: Wendorf, F & Close, A. (eds) *Advances in World Archaeology* 4:189–238. London: Academic Press.

[23] Podberscek, AL. (1997). Illuminating Issues of Companion Animal Welfare through Research into Human-Animal Interactions. *Animal Welfare,* 6, 365-72.

[24] Prates L, Prevosti FJ, Berón M (2010) First records of prehispanic dogs in southern South America (Pampa-Patagonia, Argentina). *Current Anthropology* 51:273–280.

[25] Savolainen P, Zhang YP, Luo J, Lundeberg J, Leitner T (2002) Genetic evidence for an East Asian origin of domestic dogs. *Science* 298: 1610–1613.

[26] Spitznagel MB, Jacobson DM, Cox MD, Carlson MD. Caregiver burden in owners of a sick companion animal: a cross-sectional observational study. *Veterinary Record*, 2017.

[27] Vieira NM, Brandalise V, Zucconi E, Secco M, Strauss BE, Zatz M. Isolation, characterization, and differentiation potential of canine adipose-derived stem cells. *Cell Transplant* (2010) 19(3):279–89.

[28] von Holdt BM, Pollinger JP, Lohmueller KE, Han E, Parker HG, et al. (2010) Genome-wide SNP and haplotype analyses reveal a rich history underlying dog domestication. *Nature* 464: 898–903.

[29] Zuk PA, Zhu M, Ashjian P, De Ugarte DA, Huang JI, Mizuno H, et al. Human adipose tissue is a source of multipotent stem cells. *Mol Biol Cell* (2002) 13: 4279–95.

In: Manipulation of Stem Cells for Disease Benefits
Editor: Prasad Koka
ISBN: 978-1-53615-468-9

Chapter 12

Bone Marrow Stromal Cells Improve the Formalin Tonic Pain and Feeding Behavior in the Complete Thoracic Spinal Cord Injury in Rats

***Suneel Kumar*[1,*], *Suman Jain*[1], *Sujata Mohanty*[2], *Thirumurthy Velpandian*[3] and *Rashmi Mathur*[1]**

[1]Department of Physiology, India Institute of Medical Sciences, Ansari Nagar, New Delhi, India
[2]Stem Cell Facility, India Institute of Medical Sciences, Ansari Nagar, New Delhi, India
[3]Ocular Pharmacy and Pharmacology, India Institute of Medical Sciences, Ansari Nagar, New Delhi, India

Abstract

Bone marrow stromal cells (BMSC) have been investigated in the central nervous system repair after injury. However, the effectiveness of these cells in the treatment of spinal cord injury (SCI) induced hyperalgesia, allodynia, and hypoalgesia is far from clear. In this study, we investigated the therapeutic effect of BMSC on formalin tonic pain and feeding behavior after thoracic complete SCI. Adult male rats underwent complete transection of the spinal cord and later at day 9 of SCI received a direct injection of pre-labeled BMSC cells around the injury site. Formalin pain behavior was studied once at the end of week 8 after SCI while feeding behavior was studied every day pre- and post-SCI. After the formalin pain study, rats were sacrificed for histological and neurochemical studies. Formalin pain behavior was decreased after SCI at week 8. This formalin pain behavior partially recovered in the BMSC transplanted rats. During the study period, feeding behavior was affected severely after SCI. However, it was

* Corresponding Author's E-mail: aiims.suneel@gmail.com.

improved in the BMSC group of rats. Neurochemicals such as serotonin and dopamine were affected after SCI in different brain regions which were restored partially by BMSC transplantation. Histological studies revealed the presence of pre-labeled BMSC that filled the lesion cavities in the transplanted group. Data suggest the beneficial effect of BMSC transplantation on supraspinal mediated feeding and formalin tonic pain behaviors that are associated with altered neurotransmitter levels in the SCI rats.

Keywords: spinal cord injury, bone marrow stromal cells, formalin pain, feeding behavior, serotonin, dopamine

INTRODUCTION

Traumatic complete spinal cord injury (SCI) leads to a cascade of secondary events in both spinal and supraspinal regions [1]. The former effects are widely studied while the latter effects, due to either post-incomplete or complete SCI, are lately identified and may involve sensorimotor cortex, thalamic nuclei, cerebellum, and arcuate nucleus (ARC) [2-4]. Alteration in sensory functions (hyperalgesia and allodynia), a significant reduction in feeding behavior, and body weight are possibly the supraspinal effects of SCI [1, 5]. Nevertheless, the management of SCI pain is far from satisfactory.

In the last decade, bone marrow stromal cells (BMSC) have been reported as possessing a great potential to repair the damage done to the central nervous system [6]. Several SCI studies have shown BMSC to survive, proliferate, and provide beneficial effects on locomotion, spinal reflexes of complete and incomplete SCI [6-7]. Formalin pain responses involve several brain areas including the cortex, brainstem (BS), and diencephalon [8] besides the final common pathway from the spinal cord for its exhibition [9]. However, only a few studies report the effect of SCI on formalin pain, suggesting both hyperalgesia and hypoalgesia, albeit in different models of SCI [10-12]. Feeding behavior is also controlled by mainly ventromedial hypothalamus (VMH), lateral hypothalamus (LH), and ARC amongst other regions of the brain, and their related neurotransmitters [13]. It is accepted widely that formalin pain and feeding behavior are controlled by supraspinal regions which were affected after the SCI. Our previous report on the decrease in the feeding behavior and on body weight loss after SCI is supported by other reports [5, 14-16]. Our recent report in the complete SCI rat model suggested a decrease in the formalin pain [17], which is also supported by other reports [11].

As we know that SCI affect the spinal and supra-spinal areas of the central nervous system and the formalin pain model is the tool to assess these affected regions at the same time [1, 18]. Therefore, we selected this model to study chronic pain post-SCI. To the best of our knowledge, there is no study regarding the effects of BMSC transplantation on formalin pain, feeding behavior, and associated neurotransmitter in the SCI rats.

Therefore, it was pertinent to study the therapeutic effect of BMSC on centrally mediated behaviors in the complete thoracic SCI rats.

METHODS

Isolation and Characterization of Rat BMSC Cells

Inbred group of adult male rats (200-220 g, n = 3) were used for BMSC cells isolation and culture [7]. Briefly, rats were aseptically sacrificed, femur and tibia isolated, stroma isolated, and then expanded accordingly [7, 19] using Dulbecco modified eagle media (DMEM, GIBCO) with low glucose. The medium was supplemented with 15% fetal bovine serum (FBS, Hyclone), 2 mM glutamax (Invitrogen) and 100 U/mL Pen-Strep (P/S, Invitrogen). The non-adherent cells were removed and replenished with fresh medium until cells reached ~90% confluency. Cells were then detached using trypsin-EDTA (Invitrogen) and characterized as per published protocol using primary (CD44, CD90, CD45, and HLAII), secondary antibodies, and appropriate isotype-matched controls [7].

Spinal Cord Injury and BMSC Cells Transplantation

All the experimental protocols were approved by the Institutional Ethics Committee for animal experimentation. Total 40 adult male Wistar rats (200-250 g) were used and SCI was performed under the mixture of ketamine (60 mg/kg) and xylazine (10 mg/kg) anesthesia using aseptic condition. In the Sham group of rats, only the laminectomy (T10-T12 vertebrae) was performed to expose the spinal cord while complete spinal cord transection at T11 vertebra was done using fine dura micro-scissor in the SCI group of rats [5]. The two ends of the spinal cord were lifted to make sure the completeness of injury under a microscope, and then the gap was filled with gel foam (AbGel, India) and wound stitched. All of the rats were then returned to their cages individually and they were maintained under standard conditions (24±2.0°C, light: dark cycle, 14:10 h, food, and water *ad libitum*). Immediately after SCI, the rats were injected with lactated Ringer's and antibiotics (gentamycin, 15-20 mg/kg; cefazolin, 25-50 mg/kg), and their body temperatures were maintained using a thermostat pad (CMA 150, USA). Their urinary bladders were manually evacuated daily twice per day. The rats were divided into Sham group (n = 15), SCI group (n = 10), and BMSC group (n = 12).

In the BMSC group, cells were injected on SCI day 9 for better survival [7]. Briefly, BMSC were pre-labeled (PKH26, Sigma-Aldrich), and then ~2.5 x 10^5 cells in 10 μL PBS were injected (2 μL/min x 5) into the injury site using Hamilton syringe stereotaxically. The needle was left for another 5 min to prevent the backflow of cells. In the SCI group, rats received only 10 μL of PBS without any cells. The PKH26-positive area (n = 3) was examined 1 day after transplantation to check for the injection reproducibility (data not shown).

Formalin Tonic Pain

At post-SCI week 8, the rats were pre-conditioned for 30 min in the clear plexiglass observation chamber (30 x 25 x 20 cm, 10 small holes of 0.5 cm diameter for ventilation. A large mirror (34 x 25 cm) fixed at a 45° angle below the chamber provided a complete view of the rat during pain-related behavior. Then, rats were injected 50 μL of 5% formalin (pH 7.4) into left dorsal hindpaw [17-18]. The formalin-induced nociceptive behavior was rated and recorded automatically as category T0 = when BW equally borne by all the limbs, T1 = when injected paw rested lightly on the floor, T2 = when injected paw elevated and specially cared for, and T3 = when injected paw licked, bitten or shaken. Average pain ratings (PR) of every block (5 min) and session (60 min) were obtained utilizing the Q-basic based program to determine the category of pain responses. Simultaneously, another observer who was blinded to the groups counted the number of behaviors (flinching, biting, and licking) in the 1st min of every block. Rats were then sacrificed (decapitate) for either neuro-transmitter estimation (Sham, n = 8, SCI, n = 6, BMSC, n = 8) or perfused for spinal cord histology.

Feeding Behavior

Rats were daily provided with fresh drinking water in leak-proof bottles and laboratory food pellets (Ashirwad Industries, India) in spill-proof food-container *ad libitum*. An observer daily (9:00 h) accurately weighed the food and water, and then provided to each animal irrespective to their group identity and leftover were measured at the same time the next day. The food and water intake were noted daily while the body weight of rats was recorded weekly [5].

5-HT and Dopamine (DA) Estimations in Different Brain Regions

All the standards (Sigma Aldrich, USA) were weighed accurately and were serially diluted to obtain working concentration for quantification by liquid chromatography-mass spectrometry with ion spray mode (LC-MS-ESI) as per our published protocol [17, 7]. API 4000Q Trap (Applied BioSystems, USA) equipped with ESI source that operated in the positive ion mode coupled with Thermo Finnegan ultra high-performance-LC was used for the quantification. The analyst version of 1.4.2 software (ABS Biosystems, USA) with its inbuilt algorithm was used to define a source and compound dependent parameters to reach maximum sensitivity for quantification. Singly charged Q1 mass for 5-HT (177.1), DA (154.1), and homatropine as an internal control (276.1, IS) were determined. A program of linear gradient reaching 40% of acetonitrile (with 0.1% formic acid, FA) at 8 min against 0.1% FA in milliQ water with the flow rate of 500 μL/min was used to separate the neurotransmitters using Supelco C18 column. These measures permitted the sensitivity of 2 ng/mL. On the estimation day, pre-weighed brain tissues (cortex, BS, remaining forebrain area; RFA) were thawed and chopped, and extracting solvent (200 μL of 70% acetonitrile in 0.1% FA+500 ng/mL IS) was added. It was subjected to vortex (1 minute), homogenization for 1 minute using Polytron (Polytron-Aggregate, PT-2100, Switzerland). To the above homogenate, extracting solvent (300 μL) was added to make 500 μL. This was sonicated for 6 minutes followed by centrifugation (7840 g) for 10 minutes. The supernatant (200 μL) was removed and subjected for quantification using LC-MS method [7].

Spinal Cord Histological Analysis

Rats were deeply anesthetized with a mixture of ketamine and xylazine before sacrificing for histological study. Briefly, rats were slowly perfused intracardially with fixative (4% paraformaldehyde, 0.1 M PB), the spinal cord was separated, immersed in the same fixative (4°C) for overnight then switched to a graded sucrose solution (15% to 30%). Longitudinal cryosections (20 μm) were cut (Microm HM 550, Thermo Scientific, USA) and adhered onto gelatin-pre-coated slides [5]. The sections were examined for the presence of transplanted labeled-BMSC under a fluorescent microscope (Nikon Eclipse 80i, Japan). For spinal cord lesion volume, 5-central sections were studied for each rat using software (NIS Elements AR 3.0, Japan).

Statistical Analysis

Data are presented as mean ± SD (standard deviation). The data of 5-HT and DA was log-transferred before analysis. The comparison between the groups was analyzed using one-way ANOVA followed by posthoc analysis using Bonferroni correction. The comparison within the group was analyzed using the generalized estimated equation with posthoc analysis using Bonferroni correction. A significant change was considered if $p < 0.05$.

RESULTS

The BMSC cells were positive for CD44 and CD90 while negative for CD45 and HLAII which represents the true phenotypes of BMSC in an un-differentiated state (Table 1).

Table 1. Flow cytometry analysis of surface antigen expression on BMSC after passage-3

Study No.	Cell Surface Antigen Markers (%)				
	CD44	CD45	CD34	HLA II	CD90
1	52.5	0.7	0	0	30.4
2	61.7	0.4	0	0	52.1
3	55.4	0.7	0	0	45

Formalin Tonic Pain

All the rats were tested for formalin tonic stimuli to hindpaw after 8 weeks of SCI (Figure 1). We found that time spent in category T2, T3 decreased significantly and T0, T1 increased in all the blocks of SCI group when compared to Sham group. However, in the BMSC group, time spent in the various categories was similar (except for block 10 min, $p = 0.027$ and 30 min, $p = 0.006$) to that observed in Sham group of rats, thereby resulting in partial restoration of eualgesia state (Figure 1Aa-c). The average pain rating analysis during 1 h also showed a decrease pain rating of SCI ($p < 0.001$) and BMSC group ($p < 0.05$) compared to Sham group. BMSC group of rats significantly improved the average pain rating ($p < 0.0001$) compared to SCI rats (Figure 1B). The number of pain behaviors did not vary during the early phase (5-10 min) amongst any group but it decreased ($p < 0.001$) during the late phase (block III-XII) in both SCI and BMSC ($p < 0.01$) groups as compared to Sham group (Table 2). However, a significant ($p < 0.001$) improvement was observed in the BMSC group compared to SCI over all the blocks (Table 3, Figure 1C), suggesting partial functional recovery by transplantation of BMSC.

Feeding Behavior

Similarly, these rats were also studied for their daily feeding behavior pre-and post-SCI. One-week data was averaged and compared between the groups at each time point.

Food Intake (FI)

The FI decreased significantly ($p < 0.001$) after SCI during 1 week in all the group of rats. However, in the Sham and BMSC groups, it increased ($p < 0.001$) gradually over the period of 8 weeks in comparison to pre-surgery week. The FI remained lower ($p < 0.006$) during the entire study period in the SCI group. However, BMSC transplanted rats were able to achieve comparable FI as Sham group after 4 weeks of SCI, suggesting the beneficial effect of BMSC transplantation (Figure 2a).

Table 2. Block and session-PR during formalin pain

Block (5 min)	Block-PR (Mean ± SD)			*P value*		
	Sham Group	SCI Group	BMSC Group	Sham vs. SCI	Sham vs. BMSC	BMSC vs. SCI
I	2.17 ± 0.23	1.54 ± 0.41	1.91 ± 0.13	0.003	0.315	0.107
II	1.93 ± 0.26	1.09 ± 0.01	1.65 ± 0.06*	0.0001	0.027	0.0001
III	2.09 ± 0.21	0.89 ± 0.13*	1.90 ± 0.06	0.0001	0.104	0.0001
IV	2.24 ± 0.20	1.24 ± 0.57	2.04 ± 0.04	0.0001	0.943	0.003
V	2.30 ± 0.29	1.76 ± 0.12	2.03 ± 0.05	0.0001	0.061	0.089
VI	2.24 ± 0.19	1.87 ± 0.09*	1.95 ± 0.08	0.001	0.006	0.995
VII	2.22 ± 0.25	1.56 ± 0.40	2.00 ± 0.06	0.002	0.531	0.039
VIII	2.14 ± 0.15	1.86 ± 0.17	2.01 ± 0.06	0.009	0.328	0.295
IX	2.05 ± 0.11	1.83 ± 0.36	2.02 ± 0.09*	0.309	1.000	0.504
X	2.07 ± 0.18	1.64 ± 0.43	1.88 ± 0.25	0.055	0.819	0.511
XI	1.90 ± 0.31	1.87 ± 0.15*	1.96 ± 0.09	1.000	1.000	1.000
XII	1.99 ± 0.09	1.65 ± 0.34	2.05 ± 0.11	0.026	1.000	0.014
Session-PR	2.11 ± 0.09	1.57 ± 0.13	1.95+0.04	0.0001	0.02	0.0001

*indicates comparison of the block I versus blocks II-XII in each group. * denotes $p < 0.004$.

Table 3. Formalin-induced pain behaviors (flinching/biting/licking)

1st min/ block	Pain Behavior (Mean ± SD)			*P value*		
	Sham Group	SCI Group	BMSC Group	Sham vs. SCI	Sham vs. BMSC	BMSC vs. SCI
I	20.0 ± 1.54	21.0 ± 2.60	20.5 ± 1.76	1.000	1.000	1.000
II	5.14 ± 0.69	5.83 ± 0.75	6.0 ± 1.41	0.684	0.418	1.000
III	2.57 ± 0.53	2.83 ± 0.98	5.83 ± 1.47	1.000	0.0001	0.0001
IV	7.85 ± 0.69	7.5 ± 1.045	11.33 ± 1.36	1.000	0.0001	0.0001
V	11.28 ± 1.11	8.83 ± 0.75	12.33 ± 1.21	0.002	0.274	0.0001
VI	12.43 ± 1.98	11.0 ± 0.89	13.33 ± 1.03	0.279	0.823	0.038
VII	16.85 ± 0.69	8.16 ± 1.33	13.83 ± 3.54	0.0001	0.068	0.001
VIII	20.0 ± 2.16	6.5 ± 0.84	12.5 ± 2.16	0.0001	0.0001	0.0001
IX	15.14 ± 1.57	4.83 ± 0.75	8.33 ± 1.03	0.0001	0.0001	0.0001
X	11.85 ± 1.46	4.33 ± 0.82	7.83 ± 0.98	0.0001	0.0001	0.0001
XI	7.14 ± 1.34	4.5 ± 1.37	5.33 ± 0.82	0.004	0.050	0.759
XII	4.28 ± 1.60	3.33 ± 1.50	3.66 ± 0.82	0.690	1.000	1.000

Water Intake (WI)

Similarly, a decrease in WI was observed ($p < 0.006$) in the SCI and BMSC group of rats as compared to their respective pre-surgery week intake. Though in the latter group, it increased gradually and became non-significant by post-SCI week 3 while in the SCI group, it remained at a lower level until the end (Figure 2b). In comparison to Sham group, BMSC group did not show any significant ($p > 0.05$) difference from post-SCI week 4, whereas, SCI group showed a decrease in the WI significantly ($p < 0.01$) till the observation period, suggesting a gradual recovery in the WI of BMSC transplanted rats.

Body Weight

Body weight of these rats gradually increased in the Sham group ($p < 0.006$) from pre-surgery to post-surgery week 8 while it remained lower ($p < 0.006$) during week 1-8 in the SCI and BMSC groups. A trend of improvement was observed in the latter group (Figure 2c).

5-HT and DA Estimations in Different Brain Regions

In these rats, we also measured the neuro-transmitter level after formalin test and we found that 5-HT decreased significantly in the SCI and BMSC groups of rats as compared to Sham group of rats in the cortex and RFA regions of the brain (Figure 3a), though the decrease was less in the latter group. The DA level increased (cortex) in the SCI group which was restored by BMSC transplantation (Figure 3b).

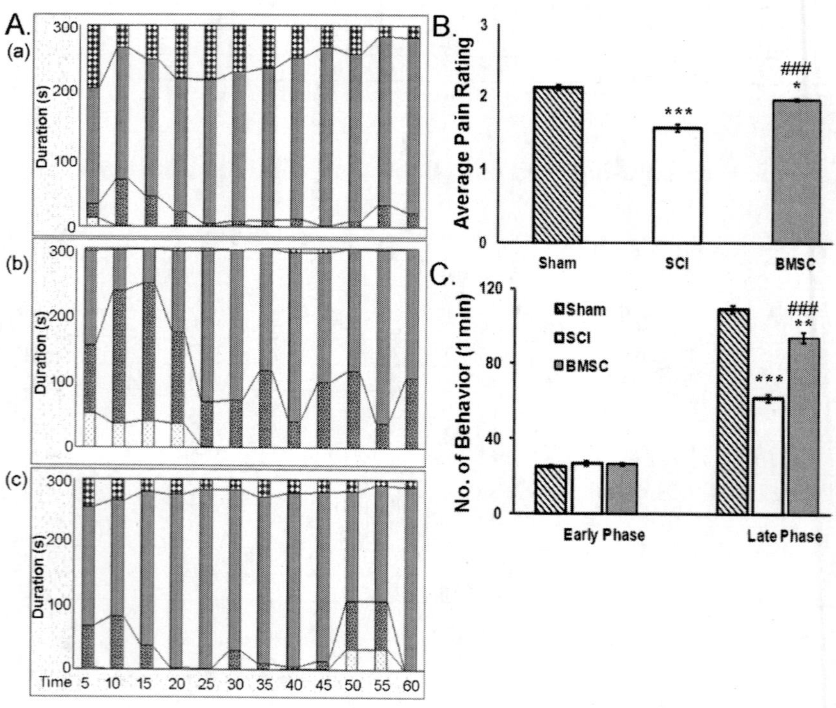

Figure 1. Effect of BMSC transplantation on formalin behavior after SCI in rats. It represents the duration of every category [T0 (□), T1 (▩), T2 (▥), T3 (◪)] in each block of Sham (a), SCI (b), and BMSC (c) group. Graph B depicts session-PR and C depicts total pain behaviors during formalin pain. * indicates comparison of Sham versus SCI/BMSC group while # indicates comparison of SCI versus BMSC group. *$p < 0.05$, **$p < 0.01$, and ***/###$p < 0.001$.

Spinal Cord Histological Analysis

In order to examine the beneficial effects of BMSC transplantation on spinal cord repair, the severity of trauma at the injury site was evaluated histopathologically. Microscopic examination of the spinal cord revealed differences between vehicle injected (Figure 4a) and BMSC transplanted rats (Figure 4b). Large lesion cavities were seen in former group while in the latter, cavities were loosely filled with cells that support a significant decrease in lesion volume ($p < 0.002$) in the BMSC group (Figure 4c). We found some pre-labeled BMSC around the lesion site (Figure 4d) that shows the survival of few transplanted cells.

DISCUSSION

In the present study, we found the beneficial role of rat BMSC on formalin tonic pain and feeding behavior after complete SCI in rats. Qualitative and quantitative analysis of formalin pain and feeding behavior were carried out. In addition, quantitative changes of 5-HT and DA level in different brain regions after injury and post-BMSC transplantation was tested. BMSC were selected based upon several beneficial characteristics amongst other cell type's namely autologous donor availability, rapid expansion, and migrating capacity, non-immunogenic, secrete different trophic factors, axonal sprouting, neovascularization, and immuno-modulation [6, 19-20].

We recently showed that these cells are capable of improving locomotion, sensorimotor, spinal reflexes when transplanted on SCI day 9 in the complete SCI rats [7]. The literature also supported our recent report on SCI [21, 22] as we used the suggested optimum window (post-SCI 1-2 weeks) of transplantation [23]. The outcome of sensorimotor behavior and SCI-size by BMSC transplantation appears to be dictated by the severity of the injury, the age of SCI and simultaneous release of trophic factors [21-22, 24-27]. We, therefore, transplanted these cells on SCI day 9 to provide the optimal micro-environment post-injury. BMSC are also having the capacity to differentiate into different cells types but this is still a debatable issue [25, 28-29].

The SCI per se affects several brain regions namely ARC, hindlimb area of somatosensory cortex (HL), parietal cortex (PAR) and thalamus as well as neuronal death in somatosensory cortex, and an immediate hyperexcitability and reorganization [2, 4, 30-31]. Besides, paraventricular nucleus (hypo-thalamus) neurons exhibit increased spontaneous activity, enlarged receptive fields, enhanced evoked activity, and abnormal burst firing pattern [32]. These alterations are suggested to contribute significantly to the development of agonizing pain after SCI. Formalin is widely reported to activate various brain regions for its elaboration [8]. In our SCI rats, pain behavior (lick, flinch, biting) was significantly reduced only during the late phase indicating a poor response to algogen. Further, they spent lesser time in categories representative of severe pain (T2/T3) and reciprocally more in categories representative of mild pain (T0/T1). The spatial pattern and intensity of neural substrate activation are reported to be a function of time following the formalin stimulus. During early and late phase of formalin pain, increase in the regional cerebral blood flow is seen in the HL, medial thalamus, retrosplenial cortex, and anterior dorsal nucleus of thalamus, habenular complex, interpeduncular nucleus, periaqueductal gray, PAR, and paraventricular nucleus [33]. It is clear that the regional cerebral blood flow increases especially in the limbic regions during the late phase. Amygdalar stimulation reduces the formalin pain while VMH lesion promoted hyperalgesia [34-35]. These reports possibly explain attenuation of formalin pain in our rats and indirectly indicate that the SCI involves limbic areas specifically the amygdala, hypothalamus, and thalamus.

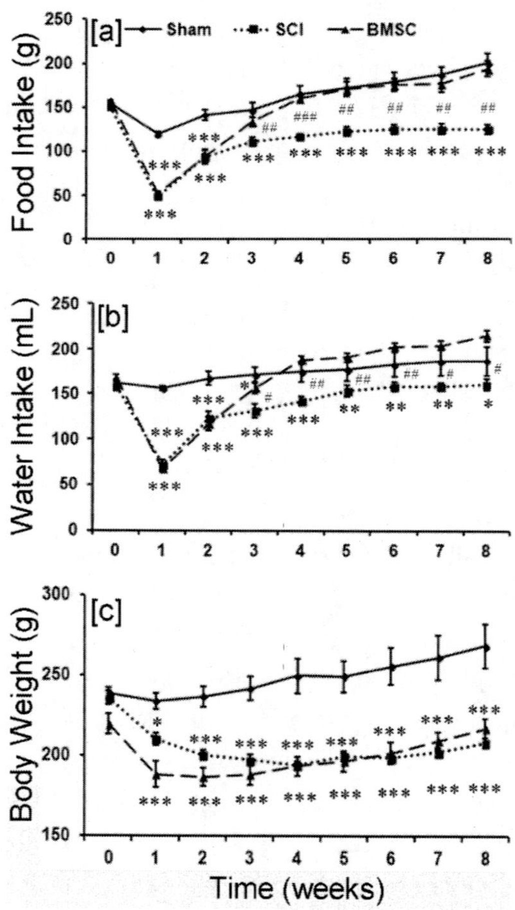

Figure 2. Effect of BMSC transplantation on feeding behavior after SCI in rats. FI (a), WI (b), and body weight (c) averaged for 1 week and compared between Sham (n = 15), SCI (n = 10), and BMSC transplanted SCI (BMSC, n = 12) group of rats. * indicates comparison of Sham versus SCI/BMSC group while # indicates comparison of SCI versus BMSC group. */#p < 0.05, **/##p < 0.01, and ***/###p < 0.001.

At the outset, it appears to be spinal segmental effect interfering with the common motor pathway although it does not restrict the other intact body parts to soothe the rat. Moreover, it has been reported that spinal transection and the transection through various brain regions did not diminish acute and tonic phase licking and flinching responses to hindpaw formalin injection [36]. Therefore, we were able to record flinching behavior at week 8 in all the groups. Sasaki and co-workers [37] reported that the transplantation of BMSC expressing brain-derived neurotrophic factors promote functional recovery, sprouting of the corticospinal tract, raphe spinal fibers, and protection of corticospinal tract neurons after SCI. We also observed the functional improvement in the BBB score by BMSC transplantation [7]. Although, we did not estimate the patterns of trophic factors in these rats [37].

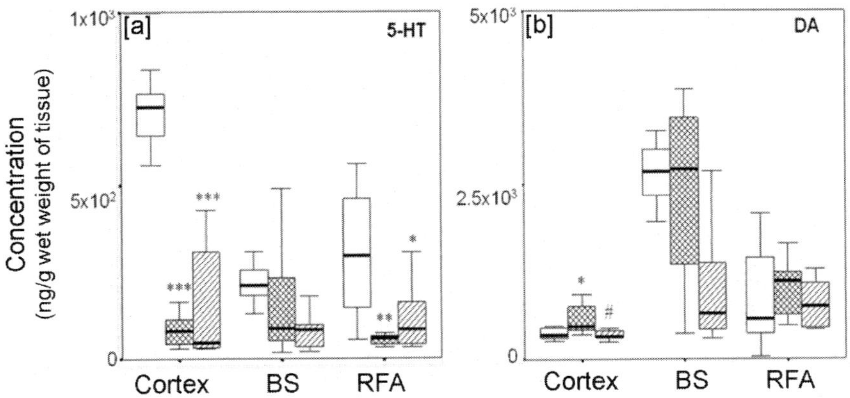

Figure 3. Figure shows the concentration of neurotransmitters in different brain regions of Sham (□, n = 8), SCI (▩, n = 6), and BMSC (▨, n = 8) groups. * indicates comparison of Sham versus SCI/BMSC group while # indicates comparison of SCI versus BMSC group. */#p < 0.05, **p < 0.01, and ***p < 0.001.

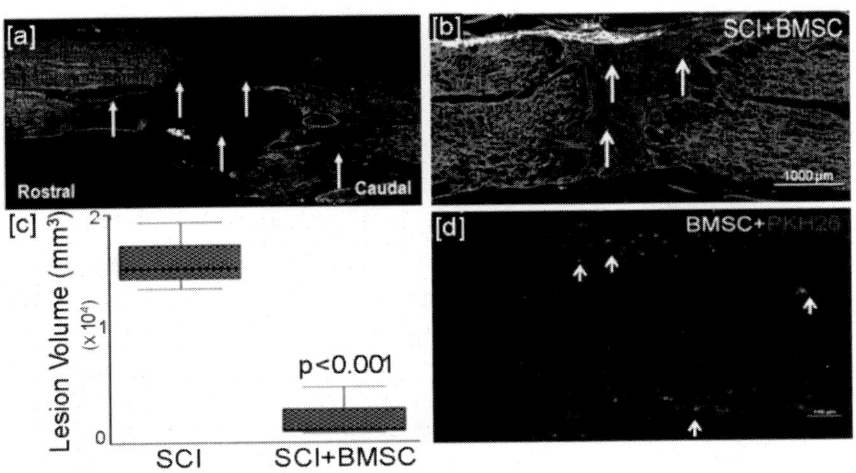

Figure 4. Figure shows photomicrographs of SCI (a, n = 4) and BMSC (b, n = 4) groups. Graph c shows the lesion volume while graph d shows the presence of BMSC in the transplanted group after 7 weeks.

Similarly, these rats were also studied for their daily feeding behavior which shows the decrease in the FI and WI, and body weight significantly after SCI during the study period. The above-mentioned evidence of alterations in the supraspinal mediated region associated with a change in formalin pain is further substantiated by the aberrations in yet another function such as feeding behavior after SCI as reported previously [5]. Primeaux and co-workers have also reported a loss of body weight involving fat mass, lean tissue mass ratio, area under the curve of glucose tolerance test and plasma insulin level, atrophy of muscles, gastrointestinal transit, and absorption [14] which is also probably mediated by the hypothalamus [38]. It is clear from the above that there is substantial evidence for the central effects of SCI, however, it can be further strengthened by estimation of the neurochemical profile associated with these functions such as central pain and feeding behavior processing. During formalin pain in the normal rat, there is evidence in favour of an increase in the 5-HT and its metabolites in the CA1 region of hippocampus [39], DA in basal ganglia [40-41], glutamate and arginine in the nucleus accumbens; glutamate, aspartate, and arginine in the basolateral nucleus of the amygdala [42]. In our SCI rats, the concentration of 5-HT attenuated in the cortex, BS, and RFA which further supports the decrease in formalin pain. On the contrary glutamate, glycine, and GABA release is showed to decrease in the PAG during formalin pain in intact rat [43-44]. Whereas, GABA, glutamate, and norepinephrine increased in our rats (data not shown) again support reduced formalin pain in them. Microdialysates from locus coeruleus contain almost 4-fold elevation in norepinephrine and its metabolite release in the early phase, which return to baseline in the late phase of the formalin pain [45].

On the other hand, primarily VMH, and LH control the feeding behavior amongst other brain regions [38] which is fine regulated by the concert of neurotransmitters. The magnitude of FI is dictated by the site of action and type of receptor activated. In normal rats, FI is reduced by a decrease in the concentration of 5-HT in LH [46] or increase in norepinephrine, GABA or DA in LH [47-48]. On the other hand, GABA acts on mGlu2 receptors of VMH to decrease FI [46, 49]. In the present study, the persistent decrease in the feeding behavior of SCI rats may also be due to a decrease in 5-HT and an increase in the DA concentrations.

In conclusion, BMSC transplantation in complete SCI rats restores the supraspinal mediated functions in addition to preventing the secondary tissue damage (Figure 4) as evident in the spinal cord histology and BMSC survival near the injury site. We suggest that transplantation of BMSC at the complete transection SCI site on day 9 limited the secondary injury processes in pari passu with the promotion of recovery processes which is also supported by our recent report on functional recovery after SCI [7]. Overall, data suggest a beneficial effect of BMSC transplantation in the recovery of supraspinal dysfunction induced by the complete transection of the spinal cord.

ACKNOWLEDGMENTS

Authors greatly acknowledge the financial support provided by Indian Council of Medical Research (I-552) to Professor Rashmi Mathur; New Delhi, India. We thank Mamta Sharma and Sanjeev Beniwal from the Department of Physiology; AIIMS; for technical assistance.

ETHICAL COMPLIANCE

The authors have stated all possible conflicts of interest within this work. The authors have stated all sources of funding for this work. If this work involved human participants, informed consent was received from each individual. If this work involved human participants, it was conducted in accordance with the 1964 Declaration of Helsinki. If this work involved experiments with humans or animals, it was conducted in accordance with the related institutions' research ethics guidelines.

REFERENCES

[1] Yezierski, RP. Spinal cord injury pain: spinal and supraspinal mechanisms. *J Rehabil Res Dev*, 2009, 46, 95-107.

[2] Aguilar, J; Valera, DH; Alonso-Calvino, E; Yague, JG; Moxon, KA; Oliviero, A; Foffani, G. Spinal cord injury immediately changes the state of the brain. *J Neurosci,* 2010, 30, 7528-37.

[3] Cramer, SC; Lastra, L; Lacourse, MG; Cohen, MJ. Brain motor system functions after chronic complete spinal cord injury. *Brain,* 2005, 128, 2941-50.

[4] Morrow, TJ; Paulson, PE; Brewer, KL; Yezierski, RP; Casey, KL. Chronic, selective forebrain responses to excitotoxic dorsal horn injury. *Exp Neurol*, 2000, 161, 220-6.

[5] Kumar, S; Jain, S; Behari, J; Avelev, VD; Mathur, R. Effect of magnetic field on food and water intake and body weight of spinal cord injured rats. *Indian J Exp Biol*, 2010, 48, 982-6.

[6] Tetzlaff, W; Okon, EB; Karimi-Abdolrezaee, S; Hill, CE; Sparling, JS; Plemel, JR; Plunet, WT; Tsai, EC; Baptiste, D; Smithson, LJ; et al. A systematic review of cellular transplantation therapies for spinal cord injury. *J Neurotrauma*, 2011, 28, 1611-82.

[7] Kumar, S; Jain, S; Mohanty, S; Velpandian, T; Sreenivas, V; Mathur, R. Rat bone marrow stromal cell transplantation ameliorates complete spinal cord injury

induced sensorimotor dysfunctions and associated neurotransmitters. *Indian J Exp Biol*, 2018, 56, 535-46.

[8] Baulmann, J; Spitznagel, H; Herdegen, T; Unger, T; Culman, J. Tachykinin receptor inhibition and c-fos expression in the rat brain following formalin-induced pain. *Neuroscience,* 2000, 95, 813-20.

[9] Hough, LB; Rice, FL. H3 receptors and pain modulation: Peripheral; spinal; and brain interactions. *J Pharmacol Exp Ther,* 2011, 336, 30-7.

[10] Hendricks, WA; Pak, ES; Owensby, JP; Menta, KJ; Glazova, M; Moretto, J; Hollis, S; Brewer, KL; Murashov, AK. Predifferentiated embryonic stem cells prevent chronic pain behaviors and restore sensory function following spinal cord injury in mice. *Mol Med*, 2006, 12, 34-46.

[11] Castellanos, DA; Daniels, LA; Morales, MP; Hama, AT; Sagen, J. Expansion of formalin-evoked fos-immunoreactivity in rats with a spinal cord injury. *Neurosci Res,* 2007, 58, 386-93.

[12] Lee, JW; Furmanski, O; Castellanos, DA; Daniels, LA; Hama, AT; Sagen, J. Prolonged nociceptive responses to hind paw formalin injection in rats with a spinal cord injury. *Neurosci Lett,* 2008, 439, 212-5.

[13] Schwartz, GJ; Zeltser, LM. Functional organization of neuronal and humoral signals regulating feeding behavior. *Annu Rev Nutr,* 2013, 33, 1-21.

[14] Primeaux, SD; Tong, M; Holmes, GM. Effects of chronic spinal cord injury on body weight and body composition in rats fed a standard chow diet. *Am J Physiol Regul Integr Comp Physiol*, 2007, 293, 1102-9.

[15] Jung JI; Kim J; Hong SK; Yoon YW. Long term follow-up of cutaneous hypersensitivity in rats with a spinal cord contusion. *Korean J Physiol Pharmacol.* 2008;12: 299-306.

[16] Kriz, NA; Yamamotova, J; Tobias, RR. Tail flick latency and self-mutilation following unilateral differentiation in rats. *Physiol Res*, 2006, 55, 213-20.

[17] Kumar, S; Jain, S; Velpandian, T; Petrovich Gerasimenko, Y; D Avelev, V; Behari, J; Behari, M; Mathur, R. Exposure to extremely low-frequency magnetic field restores spinal cord injury-induced tonic pain and its related neurotransmitter concentration in the brain. *Electromagn Biol Med*, 2013, 32, 471-83.

[18] Alreja, M; Mutalik, P; Nayar, U; Manchanda, SK. The formalin test: a tonic pain model in the primate. *Pain,* 1984, 20, 97-105.

[19] Azizi, SA; Stokes, D; Augelli, BJ; DiGirolamo, C; Prockop, DJ. Engraftment and migration of human bone marrow stromal cells implanted in the brains of albino rats-similarities to astrocyte grafts. *Proc Natl Acad Sci USA,* 1998, 95, 3908-13.

[20] Nombela-Arrieta, C; Ritz, J; Silberstein, LE. The elusive nature and function of mesenchymal stem cells. *Nature Rev Mol Cell Biol,* 2011, 12, 126-31.

[21] Hofstetter, CP; Schwarz, EJ; Hess, D; Widenfalk, J; El Manira, A; Prockop, DJ; Olson, L. Marrow stromal cells form guiding strands in the injured spinal cord and promote recovery. *Proc Natl Acad Sci USA,* 2002, 99, 2199-2204.

[22] Ankeny, DP; Mctigue, DM; Jakeman, LB. Bone marrow transplants provide tissue protection and directional guidance for axons after contusive spinal cord injury in rats. *Exp Neurol,* 2004, 190, 17-31.

[23] Bakshi, A; Barshinger, AL; Swanger, SA; Madhavani, V; Shumsky, JS; Neuhuber, B; Fischer, I. Lumbar puncture delivery of bone marrow stromal cells in spinal cord contusion: a novel method for minimally invasive cell transplantation. *J Neurotrauma*, 2006, 23, 55-65.

[24] Wu, S; Suzuki, Y; Ejiri, Y; Bai, H; Kitada, M; Kataoka, K; Ohta, M; Chou, H; Ide, C. Bone marrow stromal cells enhance differentiation of cocultured neurosphere cells and promote regeneration of injured spinal cord. *J Neurosci Res,* 2003, 72, 343-51.

[25] Koda, M; Kamada, T; Hashimoto, M; Murakami, M; Shirasawa, H; Sakao, S; Ino, H; Yoshinaga, K; Koshizuka, S; Moriya, H; et al. Adenovirus vector mediated ex vivo gene transfer of brain-derived neurotrophic factor to bone marrow stromal cells promotes axonal regeneration after transplantation in completely transected adult rat spinal cord. *Eur Spine J,* 2007, 16, 2206-14.

[26] Taylor, L; Jones, L; Tuszynski, MH; Blesch, A. Neurotrophin-3 gradients established by lentiviral gene delivery promote short-distance axonal bridging beyond cellular grafts in the injured spinal cord. *J Neurosci,* 2006, 26, 9713-21.

[27] Kumar, S; Babiarz, J; Basak, S; Kim, JH; Barminko, J; Gray, A; Mendapara, P; Schloss, R; Yarmush, ML; Grumet, M. Sizes and sufficient quantities of MSC microspheres for intrathecal injection to modulate inflammation in spinal cord injury. *Nano Life*, 2015, 5, 1550004-14.

[28] Lee, J; Kuroda, S; Shichinohe, H; Ikeda, J; Seki, T; Hida, K; Tada, M; Sawada, K; Iwasaki, Y. Migration and differentiation of nuclear fluorescence-labeled bone marrow stromal cells after transplantation into cerebral infarct and spinal cord injury in mice. *Neuropathology,* 2003, 23, 169-80.

[29] Dasari, VR; Spomar, DG; Cady, C; Gujrati, M; Rao, JS; Dinh, DH. Mesenchymal stem cells from rat bone marrow downregulate caspase-3-mediated apoptotic pathway after spinal cord injury in rats. *Neurochem Res,* 2007, 32, 2080-93.

[30] Ness, TJ; San Pedro, EC; Richards, JS; Kezar, L; Liu, HG; Mountz, JM. A case of spinal cord injury-related pain with baseline rcbf brain SPECT imaging and beneficial response to gabapentin. *Pain,* 1998, 78, 139-43.

[31] Lee, BH; Lee, KH; Kim, UJ; Yoon, DH; Sohn, JH; Choi, SS; Yi, IG; Park, YG. Injury in the spinal cord may produce cell death in the brain. *Brain Res*, 2004, 1020, 37-44.

[32] Hains, BC; Saab, CY; Waxman, SG. Alterations in burst firing of thalamic vpl neurons and reversal by Na(V)1.3 antisense after spinal cord injury. *J Neurophysiol.* 2006, 95, 3343-52.

[33] Morrow, TJ; Paulson, PE; Danneman, PJ; Casey, KL. Regional changes in forebrain activation during the early and late phase of formalin nociception: Analysis using cerebral blood flow in the rat. *Pain,* 1998, 75, 355-65.

[34] Mena, NB; Mathur, R; Nayar, U. Amygdalar involvement in pain. *Indian J Physiol Pharmacol*, 1995, 39, 339-46.

[35] Mukherjee, K; Mathur, R; Nayar, U. Effect of VMH lesion on sucrose-fed nociceptive responses. *Jpn J Physiol,* 2000, 50, 395-404.

[36] Matthies, BK; Franklin, KB. Formalin pain is expressed in decerebrate rats but not attenuated by morphine. *Pain,* 1992, 51, 199-206.

[37] Sasaki, M; Radtke, C; Tan, AM; Zhao, P; Hamada, H; Houkin, K; Honmou, O; Kocsis, JD. BDNF-hyper-secreting human mesenchymal stem cells promote functional recovery; axonal sprouting; and protection of corticospinal neurons after spinal cord injury. *J Neurosci,* 2009, 29, 4932-41.

[38] Anand, BK; Brobeck, JR. Localization of a "feeding center" in the hypothalamus of the rat. *Proc Soc Exp Biol Med,* 1951, 77, 323-24.

[39] Soleimannejad, E; Naghdi, N; Khatami, Sh; Semnanian, S; Fathollahi, Y. Formalin pain increases the concentration of serotonin and its 5-hydroxyindoleacetic acid metabolite in the ca1 region of hippocampus. *DARU,* 2010, 18, 29-32.

[40] Magnusson, JE; Martin, RV. Additional evidence for the involvement of the basal ganglia in formalin-induced nociception: the role of the nucleus accumbens. *Brain Res*, 2002, 942, 128-32.

[41] Munro, G. Dopamine D1 and D2 Receptor agonism enhances antinociception mediated by the serotonin and nor-adrenaline reuptake inhibitor duloxetine in the rat formalin test. *European J Pharmacol,* 2007, 575, 66-74.

[42] Silva, E; Hernandez, L. Extracellular aminoacids in the amygdala and nucleus accumbens in the rat during acute pain. *Invest Clin*, 2007, 48, 213-24.

[43] Morgan, MM; Clayton, CC; Lane DA. Behavioral evidence linking opioid-sensitive gabaergic neurons in the ventrolateral periaqueductal gray to morphine tolerance. *Neuroscience,* 2003, 118, 227-32.

[44] Maione, S; Marabese, I; Oliva, P; de Novellis, V; Stella, L; Rossi, F; Filippelli, A; Rossi, F. Periaqueductal gray matter glutamate and gaba decrease following sub-cutaneous formalin injection in rat. *Neuroreport,* 1999, 10,1403-07.

[45] Sajedianfard, J; Khatami, S; Semnanian, S; Naghdi, N; Jorjani, M. In vivo measurement of noradrenaline in the locus coeruleus of rats during the formalin test: a microdialysis study. *Eur J Pharmacol,* 2005, 512, 153-56.

[46] King, BM. The rise; fall and resurrection of the ventromedial hypothalamus in the regulation of feeding behavior and body weight. *Physiol Behav,* 2006, 87, 221-44.

[47] Stanley, BG; Willett, VL; Donias, HW; Ha, LH; Spears, LC. The lateral hypothalamus: a primary site mediating excitatory amino acid-elicited eating. *Brain Res*, 1993, 630, 41-9.

[48] Giannakopoulos, G; Galanopoulou, P; Daifotis, Z; Couvaris, C. Effects of mesulergine treatment on diet selection; brain serotonin (5-ht) and dopamine (da) turnover in free feeding rats. *Prog Neuropsychopharmacol Biol Psychiatry*, 1998, 22, 803-13.

[49] Kelly, J; Grossman, SP. GABA and hypothalamic feeding systems. II. A comparison of GABA; glycine and acetylcholine agonists and their antagonists. *Pharmacol Biochem Behav,* 1979, 11, 647-52.

In: Manipulation of Stem Cells for Disease Benefits
Editor: Prasad Koka
ISBN: 978-1-53615-468-9

Chapter 13

PERIPHERAL BLOOD MONONUCLEOCYTES: AN EFFICIENT AND RELIABLE SOURCE OF INDUCED PLURIPOTENT STEM CELLS

***Riham M. Aly*[1,2,*] *and Marwa M. Ellithy*[1]**

[1]Basic Dental Science Department, Oral and Dental Research Division, National Research Centre Cairo, Egypt

[2]Stem Cell Laboratories, Centre of Excellence for Advanced Sciences, National Research Centre, Cairo, Egypt

ABSTRACT

Induced pluripotent stem cells (iPSCs) indeed hold great potential as a basis for cell-based therapies for multiple degenerative diseases. It involves the administration of transcription factors in order to transduce multiple terminally differentiated cell types into pluripotent embryonic-like stem cells. These cells can overcome the issues of immune rejection, as the cells are autologous, and also eliminate any ethical issues regarding the use of human embryos. Objective: Here we present a onetime transfection reprogramming protocol for peripheral blood mononucleocytes (PBMNCs) Methods: PBMNCs were cultured in conditions favoring hematopoietic progenitor population. Three plasmids encoding five reprogramming factors (Oct3/4, Sox2, Klf4, L-Myc and Lin28) in addition to EBNA1, an enhancer of transfection efficiency and episomal plasmids expression were applied to reprogram the isolated cells. Results: A single transfection of this plasmid combination was sufficient to generate pluripotent markers positive iPSC colonies. Colonies resembling human ES-like cells were observed as early as 20 days after episomal plasmid neucleofection. These colonies stained positively for alkaline phosphatase. Moreover, the generated iPSCs expressed stem cell markers TRA-

* Corresponding Author's E-mail: riham.aly@hotmail.com.

1-60, SSEA4, NANOG and OCT3/4 as determined by immunocytochemistry. These results demonstrated that iPSC could be effectively generated from PBMNCs using episomal plasmid vectors encoding OCT3/4, shRNA against p53, SOX2, KLF4, L-MYC and LIN28. Conclusion: Finally, it could be concluded that the method described in this research provides a promising approach for generating clinical grade induced pluripotent stem cells from highly accessible source of adult somatic cells.

Keywords: induced pluripotent stem cells, peripheral blood mononucleocytes, reprogramming, neucleofection

1. INTRODUCTION

Since its discovery in 2007, induced pluripotent stem cells (iPSCs) research has evolved exponentially offering promising insights to the future of regenerative medicine. Fibroblast derived from skin biopsy, was the first source of somatic cells described for generating iPSCs via reprograming [1]. Human iPSCs have since been reported to be generated from a broad array of cell types, including blood cells [1–5]. Peripheral blood mononucleocytes (PMNCs) offer a more convenient and abundant cell source than many other somatic sources. PBMNCs are generally comprised of a mixture of cells that include; T cells, B cells and myeloid cells in addition to a fraction of hematopoietic progenitor cells. However, blood mononucleocytes, are considered closer to embryonic stem cells (ESCs) than fibroblasts especially when cultured in conditions favoring the expansion of hematopoietic progenitor population [6]. A strong advantage of PBMNCs over fibroblasts is their decreased liability to mutation, which is attributed to their short life span. These cells were shown to possess favorable epigenetic profiles and gene patterns [7]. Originally, reprogramming was described using retroviruses that express Oct3/4, Sox2, Klf4 and c-Myc [1]. Though successful, this protocol needed consideration in terms of safety and reliability for applications in regenerative medicine and drug modeling. The most important of which was the derivation of IPS cells that do not integrate exogenous DNA in the hosts' genome. Plasmid vectors on the other hand pose as an efficient alternative for reprogramming cells. iPSCs lines were reported to be generated by single transfection of fibroblasts using a few plasmids encoding potent reprogramming factors [8, 9]. Thus, the use of episomal vectors represents an ideal approach for generating integration free iPSCs. Here we present a onetime transfection reprogramming protocol for PBMNCs that are cultured in conditions favoring hematopoietic pro-genitor population, using only three plasmids that encode (Oct3/4, Sox2, Klf4, L-Myc and Lin28) in addition to EBNA1, an enhancer of transfection efficiency and episomal plasmids expression.

2. Materials and Methods

2.1. Isolation and Culture of Blood MNCs of PBMNCs

All experimental protocols were reviewed and approved by the ethical committee of the National Research Centre. MNCs were isolated from fresh peripheral blood with Lymphoprep TM (Cosmo Bio Co., Tokyo, Japan). Isolated MNCs were cultured & expanded for 3 days in hematopoietic culture medium (HC media) serum free X-VIVO 10 (Lonza, Basel Switzerland) containing a cocktail of cytokines comprised of; 50 ng/mL IL-6 (Peprotech), 50 ng/mL SCF (Peprotech), and 20 ng/mL Flt3-ligand (R&D system, MN) according to previously published protocol with slight modifications Collectively these cytokines either act alone or synergistically in order to promote hematopoiesis and proliferation of pluripotent hematopoietic progenitor cells. SCF alone is a modest colony stimulating factor that exerts a pivotal role in the regulation of embryonic and adult hematopoiesis. Together with other cytokines such as Flt3-L, SCF promotes expansion of primitive hematopoietic stem cells and multi-potent progenitor cells in culture [10, 11]. IL 6 in combination with SCF has shown to promote survival and proliferation of pluripotent hematopoietic progenitor cell proliferation and differentiation in vitro [12–14]. Flt3-Ligand promotes the expansion of primitive hematopoietic cells in culture [15]. This cocktail of cytokines was applied in order to increase the reprogramming efficiency through creating an epigenetic state.

2.2. Generation of iPSCs from PMNCs with Episomal Vectors

In this study, cells were nucleofected with Epi5™ Episomal iPSC Reprogramming Kit (Life Technologies, cat.No.A15960) to reprogram PBMNCs. This kit consisted of a mixture of oriP/EBNA1-based expression constructs described earlier by Okita et al. [8]. Nucleofector 4D device (Lonza, Basel, Switzerland) was used to electroporate the plasmid mixture into 2.5 x 10^6 PMNCs supplemented with P3 Primary Cell 4D Nucleofector X kit L (Lonza, V4XP-3012) using EO-115 program following manufacturer's instructions. The gene transfer reagents were prepared by mixing; 164 µL P3 solutions, 36-µL Supplement solution and 2 µL of the above mentioned epi5 reprogramming kit. After reprogramming, cells were seeded onto six-well plates coated with recombinant human Vitronectin-N (VN) (Thermo Fisher Scientific). On days 3 & 5 after the transfection, 1 ml of Essential 8 medium (Life Technologies) was added into each well. On day 9 the culture medium was completely switched to iPSC medium supplemented with 1mM Y27632 (Wako, 253-00511). Medium change continued every other day. Subculturing and passaging were performed by detaching iPSC colonies using 0.5 X TrypLE Select (Life Technologies, A12859-01) at a ratio of 1:3 when colonies sizes increased. Approximately, after twenty days colonies that were 2mm were manually picked and transferred into a 6 well plate. A diagrammatic scheme describing the reprogramming steps is illustrated in Figure 1.

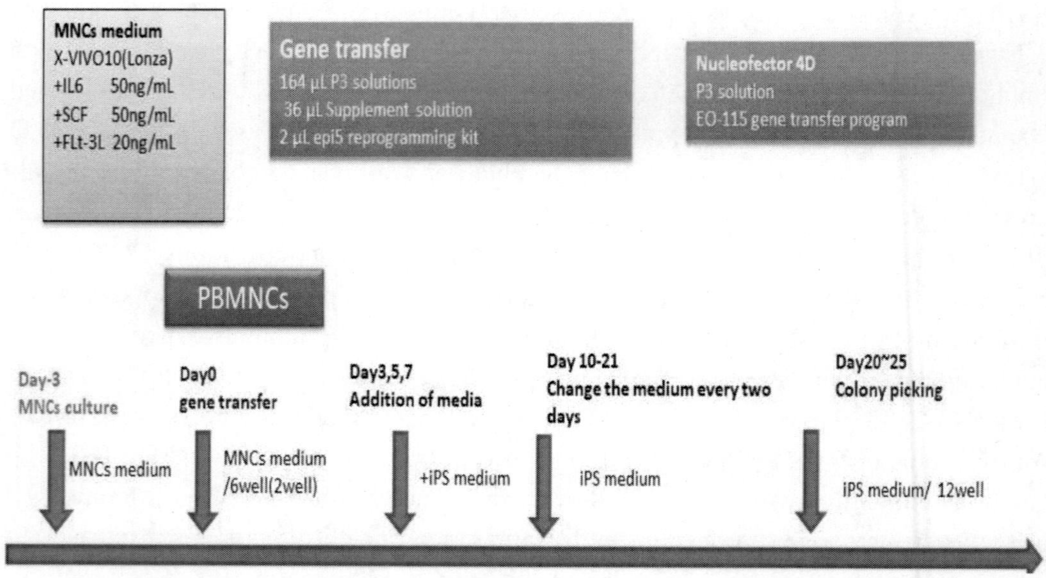

Figure 1. Schematic diagram illustrating steps required for generating iPS cell from PBMNC by Neucleofection. PBNCs were cultured with cytokines for 3 days, and then were subjected to single nucleofection by plasmids at day 0. Transfected cells were cultured into 6 wells coated with Vitronectin (VN). At day 3, 5, 7 iPSC medium was added. After 10 days, the medium was completely changed to iPSCs and media change was performed every two days. iPSCs were cultured for 20 to 25 days. Colonies were then manually picked.

2.3. Confirmation of Pluripotency of Reprogrammed PMNCs

2.3.1. Early Identification of iPSC by Alkaline Phosphatase Staining

iPSCs colonies were stained with leukocyte alkaline phosphatase kit (VECTOR, Burlingame, CA) following instructions of the manufacturer. Alkaline Phosphatase Stain permits identification of reprogrammed colonies and enables counting them. The number of stained iPSC colonies were manually counted under an inverted light microscope (Leica, 6000B-4) using Suite V3 (Leica) and enumerated at 20 days after nucleofection.

2.4. Quantitative RT-PCR

Total RNA was extracted using an RNeasy micro kit (QIAGEN), according to the manufacturer's instructions. Five hundred ng of total RNA were used to synthesize cDNA with QuantiTect Reverse Transcription Kit (QIAGEN). Then, quantitative PCR (qPCR) was performed with SYBR green PCR Master Mix (Life Technologies) and analyzed with a Step-One-PlusTM Real-Time PCR System (Life Technologies). The sequences of all primers used are listed in Table 1. Gene expression was normalized to that of GAPDH as the internal control and quantified by the 2-ΔΔCt method.

Table 1. List of primers used for q RT-PCR

OCT3/4	Forward GAAACCCACACTGCAGCAGA	Reverse TCGCTTGCCCTTCTGGCG
NANOG	Forward CTCAGCTACAAACAGGTGAAGAC	Reverse TCCCTGGTGGTAGGAAGAGTAAA
SOX2	Forward GGGAAATGGGAGGGGTGCAAAAGAGG	Reverse TTGCGTGAGTGTGGATGGGATTGGTG

2.5. Immunohistochemistry

Induced cells from PMNCs were fixed on dishes with 4% PFA overnight at 4°C, and then subjected to triple PBS washing. Anti-Oct3/4 [1:200; Santa Cruz, sc-5279], Anti-NANOG [1:200; ReproCell, RCAB 0003P], Anti-SSEA-4 [1:200; Chemicon, MAB4304] and Anti-TRA-1-60 [1:200; Chemicon, MAB4360] expression were investigated. Secondary antibodies labeled with Alexa Fluor 488 (1:500; A11008, Life Technologies) and Alexa Fluor 594 (1:500; A11062, Life Technologies) were used for visualization. Counterstaining with DAPI (D1306, Life Technologies) was performed and observed using Olympus IX71 fluorescence microscope.

3. Results

3.1. Successful Generation of iPSCs from PBMNCs

In this study, freshly isolated PBMNCs were cultured for 6 days prior to reprogramming to expand hematopoietic progenitors. After transfection with episomal plasmid vectors expressing human OCT3/4, shRNA against p53, SOX2, KLF4, L-MYC, LIN28, cells were cultured in X-VIVO10 serum-free hematopoietic medium, which was gradually changed to iPSC induction medium. At the time of seeding, cells were rounded with clear cell-to-cell boundaries. By the second week, cells adhered to each other. Colonies with flat human ESC-like morphology that is distinctive of human pluripotent stem cells started to appear at around day 20 after neucleofection. These colonies exhibited definite borders and contained tightly packed cells demonstrating increased nucleus/ cytoplasm ratios and prominent nucleoli (Figure 2).

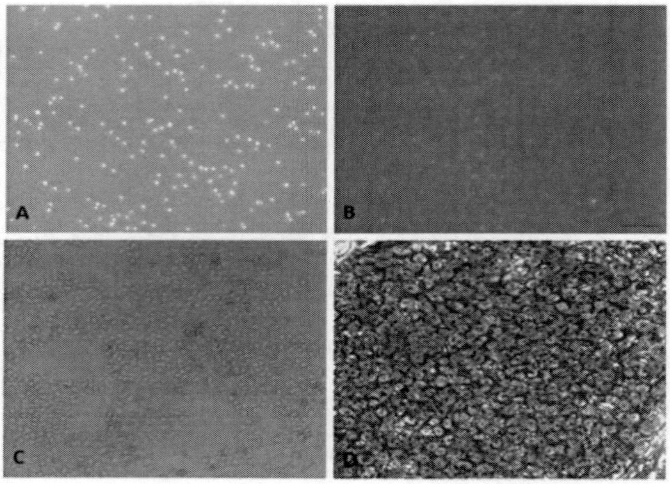

Figure 2. Photomicrograph illustrating (A) PBMNCs after 3 days of culture in X-VIVO10 serum-free hematopoietic medium. (B) PBMNCs at the time of seeding after reprograming, cells are rounded with clear cell-to-cell boundaries (C) Cells adhered to each other by the second week. (D) Colonies with flat human ESC-like morphology that is distinctive of human pluripotent stem cells started to appear at around day 20 after neucleofection. Scale bar (200 μm).

3.2. iPSCs Derived from PBMNCs Demonstrate Positive Alkaline Phosphatase Staining

The generated iPSCs were analyzed for alkaline phosphatase activity. Positive alkaline phosphatase staining denotes an undifferentiated pluripotent state. The average number of iPSCs colonies demonstrating positive alkaline phosphatase (ALP) staining was 30 ± 15. iPSCs generated as described above, proliferated successfully and were maintained and cultured for several passages under human iPSC culture conditions. Morphological appearance of the generated iPSCs colonies and positive alkaline phosphatase staining is illustrated in Figure 3.

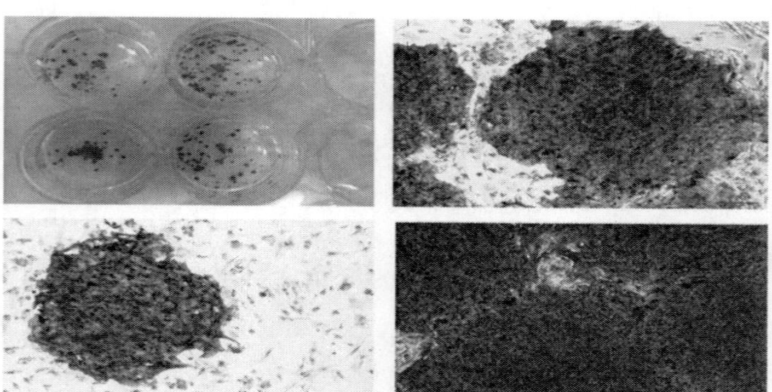

Figure 3. Photomicrograph illustrating positive alkaline phosphatase staining indicating an undifferentiated pluri-potent state of the derived colonies (Scale bar = 200 μm).

3.3. iPSCs Derived from PBMNCs Demonstrate Characteristics of Pluripotent Stem Cells

iPSCs generated illustrated positive staining for anti-NANOG and anti-OCT3/4 antibodies confirming pluripotency. We also analyzed cell membrane specific pluripotency markers using antibodies for SSEA-4 and TRA-1-60. Positive immunofluorescence staining of these markers by our generated cells further con-firmed that a pluripotent identity was assumed (Figure 4). Moreover, the expression of three endogenous pluri-potency-specific genes; OCT3/4, NANOG and SOX2 was analyzed using qRT-PCR (Figure 5). hESCs was used as control to compare the generated iPSCs to. Cells expressed OCT3/4, SOX2 and NANOG in comparison to hESCs. Together, the results demonstrate that iPSCs generated from PBMNCs are functionally comparable to pluripotent stem cells.

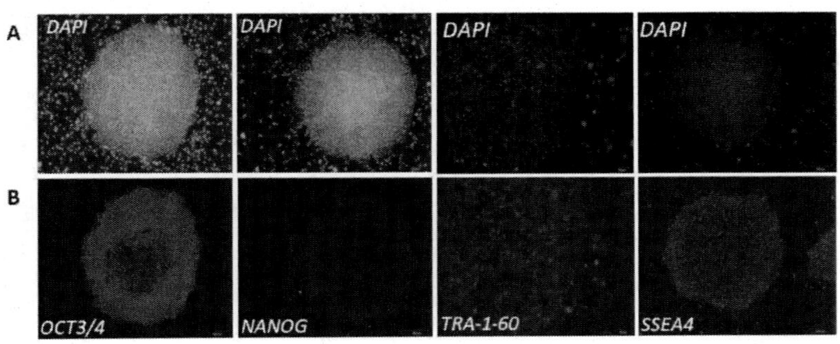

Figure 4. Immunostaining of pluripotency-related markers; OCT3/4, NANOG, SSEA-4 and TRA-1-60 of a representative iPSCs colonies. These markers were detected by specific antibodies and Alexa 594 (red) and Alexa 488 (green) conjugated secondary antibodies were used to visualize the expression Cells were counterstained with DAPI (blue) (Scale bar = 200 μm.).

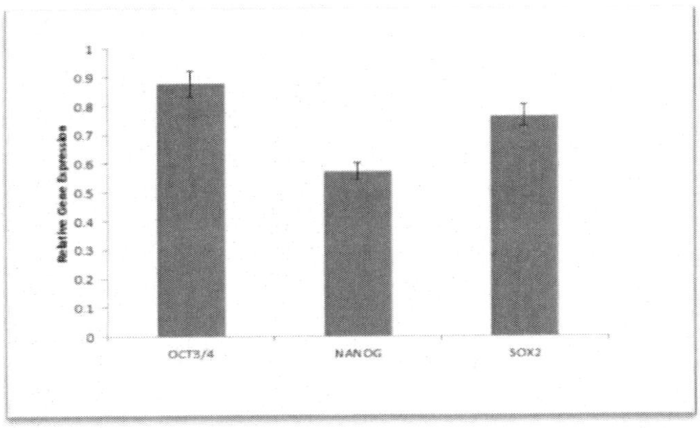

Figure 5. Expression of pluripotency-related genes OCT3/4, NANOG and SOX2 for reprogrammed PBMNCs. The data were analyzed by qRT–PCR and compared to HES1. Results are presented as mean ± SEM of three independent experiments (n = 3).

4. Discussion

In this report, we describe a simple method for transfection of PBMNCs using plasmid vectors. Blood MNCs are currently considered the cells of choice for the generation of iPSCs [9]. These cells are easily accessible and are somewhat protected from environmental mutagens [16]. In addition, blood cells demonstrate mutations that are found only in acquired blood disorders thus enabling researchers to investigate their pathogenesis thorough generation of disease specific iPSCs [16]. Unlike patient derived fibroblasts that require weeks of culturing prior to reprogramming, isolated PBMNCs can be cultured for as few as 4 days before reprogramming by standard protocols. In the present study, PBMNCs were briefly cultured in a mixture of cytokines that favored the growth of hematopoietic progenitor population. The cytokines (IL-6, SCf, Flt-3l) were used to mediate this culture condition prior to reprogramming. This culture condition allowed us to obtain a progenitor cell population from un-fractioned human blood MNC, prior to reprogramming. Previous studies have shown that the success of reprogramming human blood MNCs relies mainly on providing culture condition, that promotes the proliferation of a cell population that are not T or B cells before reprogramming is initiated. These studies have also shown that cells generated from human blood MNCs demonstrate a resemblance to human ESCs/ iPSCs in regards to their gene expression more than to fibroblasts and endothelial cells [9]. The success of iPSCs generation from hematopoietic cells after single DNA transfection was attributed to this unique gene expression signature. After culture of PBMNCs with the above mentioned cytokines for 3 days, PBMNCs were then transfected once and transferred to MEF feeder layered culture plates, following previously published transfection protocols for human blood cells with slight modifications [8,16,17]. Loh et al. was the first to report the use of human peripheral blood cells to generate iPSCs using retroviruses as vectors for delivering genes into CD34 blood cells [3]. This method was effective in generating iPSC, however it presented the donor with the inconvenience of receiving injections of granulocyte colony stimulating factor for three days prior to collection of the blood sample. To overcome the issues of virus integration, Seki et al. used Sendai virus as a non-integrating virus vector to induce iPSCs [18]. The cells used for iPSC induction were stimulated T cells derived from peripheral blood. However, safety concerns arose due to the use of infectious virus especially when encoding an oncogene like CMYC. In order to generate non-integrating iPSCs, episomal plasmids encoding Yamanaka factors were used [4, 8, 9, 19]. Plasmid based episomal vectors have been reported to efficiently reprogram different cell types generating integration free iPSCs depending on the incorporation of the EBNA1 gene and the OriP from the Epstein-Barr virus which permits a plasmid to divide extra chromosomally after single transfection as a circular chromosome [19–21]. In order to increase reprogramming efficiency especially for postnatal cells, a single improved EBNA1/OriP episomal vector was used to transfect peripheral or cord blood MNCS [9].

Okita et al. reported successful generation of iPSCs from a population of CD341 cord blood cells as well as peripheral blood using plasmid vectors with the addition of EBNA1 which enhanced the efficiency of iPSC generation [8]. It was previously reported that reprogramming efficiency was increased by transient inhibition of p53 by shRNA expressed by episomal and viral vectors [9, 22]. In accordance to Okita et al, we applied three plasmids expressing; OCT3/4, Sox2, Klf4, L-Myc, Lin28 and shRNA for TP53 in addition to an EBNA1 based plasmid that were transfected into the isolated PBMNCs. A single transfection of this plasmid combination was sufficient to generate pluripotent markers positive iPSC colonies. We observed colonies resembling human ES-like cells as early as 20 days after episomal plasmid neucleofection. These colonies stained positively for alkaline phosphatase. Moreover, the generated iPSCs expressed embryonic stem cell markers TRA-1-60, SSEA4, NANOG and OCT3/4 as determined by immunocytochemistry. The detection of these proteins on the reprogrammed cells is a sign of shifting of the transfected somatic cells into pluripotent cells [23]. Endogenous pluripotency markers NANOG, OCT3/4, and SOX2 expression by RT-PCR further confirmed the successful derivation of iPSCs. The expression of transcription factors OCT3/4 and NANOG is considered critical since they are key regulators of embryonic development. OCT4 is mainly responsible for maintenance of the pluripotent state [24,25] while, NANOG has been reported to be important for the derivation of both embryonic stem cells from blastocysts and iPSC from somatic cells together with OCT4 and SOX2 [23, 26, 27]. Collectively, our results demonstrated that iPSCs could be effectively and simply generated from PBMNCs utilizing the described episomal plasmids. Chou et al. attributed the increased efficiency of iPSCs generated from peripheral blood cells to the unique DNA methylation and gene expression signature of these cells [9]. Their findings together with our results support the hypothesis that the reprogramming efficiency of adult human cells as well as the quality of the derived iPSCs is strongly affected by epigenetic profiles of these cells [28]. In addition, PBMNCs required a short priming interval prior to reprogramming as opposed to dermal fibroblasts and other suggested sources. Finally, it could be concluded that the method described in this research provides an efficient approach for generating induced pluripotent stem cells from peripheral blood, which is a highly accessible source of adult somatic cells. However, we recommend further investigations on iPSCs generated from multiple donors in order for these cells to be effectively applicable for cell based therapies and disease modeling.

ACKNOWLEDGMENTS

This work was supported by the National Research Centre [In house project number; 11010 207].

Ethical Compliance

The authors have stated all possible conflicts of interest within this work. The authors have stated all sources of funding for this work. If this work involved human participants, informed consent was received from each individual. If this work involved human participants, it was conducted in accordance with the 1964 Declaration of Helsinki. If this work involved experiments with humans or animals, it was conducted in accordance with the related institutions' research ethics guidelines.

References

[1] Takahashi K, Tanabe K, Ohnuki M, Narita M, Ichisaka T, Tomoda K, et al. Induction of Pluripotent Stem Cells from Adult Human Fibroblasts by Defined Factors. *Cell*. 2007 Nov 30;131(5):861–72.

[2] Aasen, Trond Raya, Angel Barrero, Maria J Garreta, Elena Consiglio, Antonella Gonzalez, Federico Vassena, Rita Bilić, Josipa Pekarik, Vladimir Tiscornia G, Edel, Michael Boué S, Izpisúa Belmonte JC. Efficient and rapid generation of induced pluripotent stem cells from human keratinocytes. *Nat Biotechnol.* 2008;26(11):1276–84.

[3] Miller JD, Ng K, Daley GQ. Generation of induced pluripotent stem cells from human blood. *Blood.* 2009; 113(22):1–3.

[4] Mali P, Ye Z, Chou B-K, Yen J, Cheng L. An improved method for generating and identifying human induced pluripotent stem cells. *Methods Mol Biol*. 2010;636: 191–205.

[5] Choi KK, Yu J, Smuga-Otto K, Salvagiotto G, Rehrauer W, Vodyanik M, et al. Hematopoietic and endothelial differentiation of human induced pluripotent stem cells. *Stem Cells*. 2009 Mar;27(3):559–67.

[6] Dowey S, Huang X, Chou B, Ye Z, Cheng L. Generation of integration-free human induced pluri-potent stem cells from postnatal blood mononuclear cells by plasmid vector expression. *Nat Protoc*. 2012; 7((11)):2013–202.

[7] Su RJ, Baylink DJ, Neises A, Kiroyan JB, Meng X, Payne KJ, et al. Efficient Generation of Integration-Free iPS Cells from Human Adult Peripheral Blood Using BCL-XL Together with Yamanaka Factors. *PLoS One*. 2013;8(5).

[8] Okita K, Yamakawa T, Matsumura Y, Sato Y, Amano N, Watanabe A, et al. An efficient nonviral method to generate integration-free human-induced pluripotent stem cells from cord blood and peripheral blood cells. *Stem Cells*. 2013 Mar;31(3):458–66.

[9] Chou B-K, Mali P, Huang X, Ye Z, Dowey SN, Resar LM, et al. Efficient human iPS cell derivation by a non-integrating plasmid from blood cells with unique epigenetic and gene expression signatures. *Cell Res.* 2011 Mar 18;21(3):518–29.

[10] Martin FH, Suggs S V, Langley KE, Lu HS, Ting J, Okino KH, et al. Primary structure and functional expression of rat and human stem cell factor DNAs. *Cell.* 1990 Oct 5;63(1):203–11.

[11] Kent D, Copley M, Benz C, Dykstra B, Bowie M, Eaves C. Regulation of Hematopoietic Stem Cells by the Steel Factor/KIT Signaling Pathway. *Clin Cancer Res.* 2008 Apr 1;14(7):1926–30.

[12] Yang YC, Ciarletta AB, Temple PA, Chung MP, Kovacic S, Witek-Giannotti JS, et al. Human IL-3 (multi-CSF): identification by expression cloning of a novel hematopoietic growth factor related to murine IL-3. *Cell.* 1986 Oct 10;47(1):3–10.

[13] Dorssers L, Burger H, Bot F, Delwel R, Geurts van Kessel AH, Löwenberg B, et al. Characterization of a human multilineage-colony-stimulating factor cDNA clone identified by a conserved noncoding sequence in mouse interleukin-3. *Gene.* 1987;55(1):115–24.

[14] Broughton SE, Dhagat U, Hercus TR, Nero TL, Grimbaldeston MA, Bonder CS, et al. The GM-CSF/IL-3/IL-5 cytokine receptor family: from ligand recognition to initiation of signaling. *Immunol Rev.* 2012 Nov; 250(1):277–302.

[15] Hitchcock IS, Kaushansky K. Thrombopoietin from beginning to end. *Br J Haematol.* 2014 Apr;165(2): 259–68

[16] Ye Z, Zhan H, Mali P, Dowey S, Williams DMD, Jang YY-Y, et al. Human-induced pluripotent stem cells from blood cells of healthy donors and patients with acquired blood disorders. *Blood.* 2009 Dec 24;114(27):5473–80.

[17] Mali P, Ye Z, Hommond HH, Yu X, Lin J, Chen G, et al. Improved Efficiency and Pace of Generating Induced Pluripotent Stem Cells from Human Adult and Fetal Fibroblasts. *Stem Cells.* 2008 Aug;26(8):1998–2005.

[18] Seki T, Yuasa S, Oda M, Egashira T, Yae K, Kusumoto D, et al. Generation of Induced Pluripotent Stem Cells from Human Terminally Differentiated Circulating T Cells. *Cell Stem Cell.* 2010 Jul 2;7(1):11–4.

[19] Yu J, Hu K, Smuga-Otto K, Tian S, Stewart R, Slukvin II, et al. Human induced pluripotent stem cells free of vector and transgene sequences. *Science.* 2009 May 8;324(5928):797–801.

[20] Lindner SE, Sugden B. The plasmid replicon of Epstein-Barr virus: mechanistic insights into efficient, licensed, extrachromosomal replication in human cells. *Plasmid.* 2007 Jul;58(1):1–12.

[21] Marchetto MCN, Yeo GW, Kainohana O, Marsala M, Gage FH, Muotri AR. Transcriptional Signature and Memory Retention of Human-Induced Pluripotent Stem Cells. Reh TA, editor. *PLoS One.* 2009 Sep 18;4(9): e7076.

[22] Zhao Y, Yin X, Qin H, Zhu F, Liu H, Yang W, et al. Two Supporting Factors Greatly Improve the Efficiency of Human iPSC Generation. *Cell Stem Cell.* 2008 Nov 6;3(5):475–9.

[23] Stoyanova E, Mourdjeva M, Kyurkchiev S. Early selection of human fibroblast-derived induced pluri-potent stem cells. *Biotechnol Biotechnol Equip.* 2015; 29(5):942–8.

[24] Yeom YI, Ha HS, Balling R, Schöler HR, Artzt K. Structure, expression and chromosomal location of the Oct-4 gene. *Mech Dev.* 1991 Nov;35(3):171–9.

[25] Schöler HR, Ruppert S, Suzuki N, Chowdhury K, Gruss P. New type of POU domain in germ line-specific protein Oct-4. *Nature.* 1990 Mar 29;344(6265):435–9.

[26] Mitsui K, Tokuzawa Y, Itoh H, Segawa K, Murakami M, Takahashi K, et al. The homeoprotein Nanog is required for maintenance of pluripotency in mouse epiblast and ES cells. *Cell.* 2003 May 30;113(5):631–42.

[27] Schwarz BA, Bar-Nur O, Silva JCR, Hochedlinger K. Nanog Is Dispensable for the Generation of Induced Pluripotent Stem Cells. *Curr Biol.* 2014 Feb 3;24(3): 347–50.

[28] Kim K, Doi A, Wen B, Ng K, Zhao R, Cahan P, et al. Epigenetic memory in induced pluripotent stem cells. *Nature.* 2010 Sep 16;467(7313):285–90.

In: Manipulation of Stem Cells for Disease Benefits
Editor: Prasad Koka
ISBN: 978-1-53615-468-9

Chapter 14

IMPACT OF YOGA ON BLOOD GLUCOSE LEVEL AMONG PATIENTS WITH TYPE 2 DIABETES MELLITUS: A MULTICENTRE CONTROLLED TRIAL

***Amit Singh*[1,*], *Padmini Tekur*[1], *R. Nagaratna*[1,2] *and H. R. Nagendra*[1]**
[1]Division of Yoga and Life Sciences
[2]Holistic Health Center, SVYASA University, Bengaluru, India

ABSTRACT

Background: Type 2 Diabetes Mellitus (T2DM) is a metabolic condition characterized by chronic hyperglycemia. It is a highly prevalent medical problem across the globe and a leading cause of morbidity and mortality. Optimal blood glucose control is the primary goal of T2DM management. Yoga is a mind-body intervention found to be effective in various kinds of metabolic disorders including T2DM.

Aim: This study intended to assess the impact of 3 months Integrated Yoga (IY) intervention on fasting and post-prandial blood glucose level among patients with T2DM.

Methods: Total 251 patients with T2DM within the age range of 30-60 years (with average age; 46.04 ± 14.02 years) were enrolled in the study. Participants were divided into a yoga group (n = 137) and a control group (n = 114). Subjects in the yoga group received IY intervention consisted of Asanas, Surynamaskara, Pranayama and meditation every day for one hour/day, 6 days in a week for three months. Control group subjects followed their daily routines. Subjects on insulin therapy, with diabetic complications, uncontrolled hypertension, under steroid medication, or previous exposure to any form of yoga were excluded from the study. Fasting and post-prandial blood glucose level were assessed before and after 3 months for both the groups.

* Corresponding Author's E-mail: dramits90@gmail.com.

The results: Significant decrease in both fasting and postprandial blood glucose levels was observed in IY group after 3 months compared to baseline. No improvement was seen in the control group.

Conclusion: IY intervention helps in controlling blood glucose levels among patients with T2DM.

Keywords: yoga, T2DM, blood glucose

INTRODUCTION

Type 2 Diabetes Mellitus (T2DM) is a highly prevalent metabolic disorder characterized by chronic hyperglycemia [1]. It is one among the major public health problems and a leading cause of morbidity and mortality worldwide

The global prevalence of T2DM in 2010 was found to be 6.4%, which was estimated to increase by 7.7% by the year 2030. In Asia, 1 in 7 (15%) adults reported to have either elevated fasting glucose or impaired glucose tolerance. For every year 5 to 12% of these persons develop Type 2 diabetes. At present India is at second rank in having maximum number of T2DM patients in the world, this is expected to increase by 50% by the year 2030 [2].

Uncontrolled diabetes mellitus leads severe complications such as diabetic retinopathy, diabetic nephropathy, diabetic neuropathy and diabetic foot [3]. T2DM also cause micro-vascular and micro-vascular complications leading to cardiovascular disease, stroke, and cognitive impairment [3].

Optimal blood glucose control is the primary goal of diabetes management. Further, optimal blood glucose control in T2DM is associated with decreased risk of diabetic complications [4].

Conventional management of T2DM includes oral hypoglycaemic agents (OHA), insulin and lifestyle modification [5]. Despite taking regular OHA, the majority of T2DM patients showed poor blood glucose control, and a significant number of patients did not respond to OHA [6].

Stem cell therapy is also one of the most advanced approaches to treat T2DM [7]. It includes transplant of beta cell producing stem cells like embryonic stem cells. These are found to form functional pancreatic cells after transplant in rodents. Similar finding was observed in case of bone marrow harbours cells transplant in subjects with T2DM [8]. These observations suggest the promising role of stem cell therapy in the cure of T2DM.

Yoga is one among complementary and integrative medicines [9]. The practice of yoga has beneficial effects on several health domains. Yoga improves physical and mental health [10]. Earlier studies on yoga showed its potential role in improving blood glucose control, cardiac risk factors, nerve conduction among T2D patients [11]. Several RCTs have assessed the impact of yoga on blood glucose control and found yoga an effective intervention to improve blood glucose [12]. But literature showed lack of evidence from multi-centric trials on impact of yoga on blood glucose control in T2DM.

We conducted a multi-centric trial to assess the impact of 3 months IY intervention on fasting and post-prandial blood glucose level among patients with T2DM.

METHODOLOGY

Study Participants

Total 800 subjects' from 6 districts of South India were screened for the study criteria. From all districts total 320 subjects fulfilled the study criteria. 6 districts were randomly divided for either integrated yoga intervention or for control (3 for each IY and the control). Finally, there were 162 participants in IY group and 150 participants in the control group completed pre-assessments. 5 patients from the yoga group and 4 patients from the control group did not come from PPBS assessments hence, they were excluded from the study. 150 participants in the yoga group and 145 in the control group had a pre assessment and were followed up for 3 months. Anti-diabetic medication was kept constant through the entire study.

Inclusion Criteria

Subjects with T2DM, within the age range 30-60 years

Willing to participate in the study, both male and female participants were considered for the study.

Exclusion Criteria

- Subjects with uncontrolled diabetes or hypertension
- Subjects who had any kind of major surgery in the past one year
- Subjects on any type of anti-psychotic or steroid medication
- Subjects taking insulin
- Subjects who had previous exposure to any form of yoga in the past one year

Ethical Consideration

The study was approved by the Institutional Ethical Committee of Swami Vivekanand Yoga Anusandhan Samsthan (SVYASA-A deemed to be a University), Bengaluru, India.

A written Informed Consent Form was duly signed by all of the participants before the intervention.

Assessments

Subjects in both groups were assessed for fasting and post-prandial blood glucose level.

Fasting Blood Sugar (FBS) Level

Fasting blood glucose was measured from a blood sample collected early in the morning (between 6-7am) on empty stomach for all the subjects.

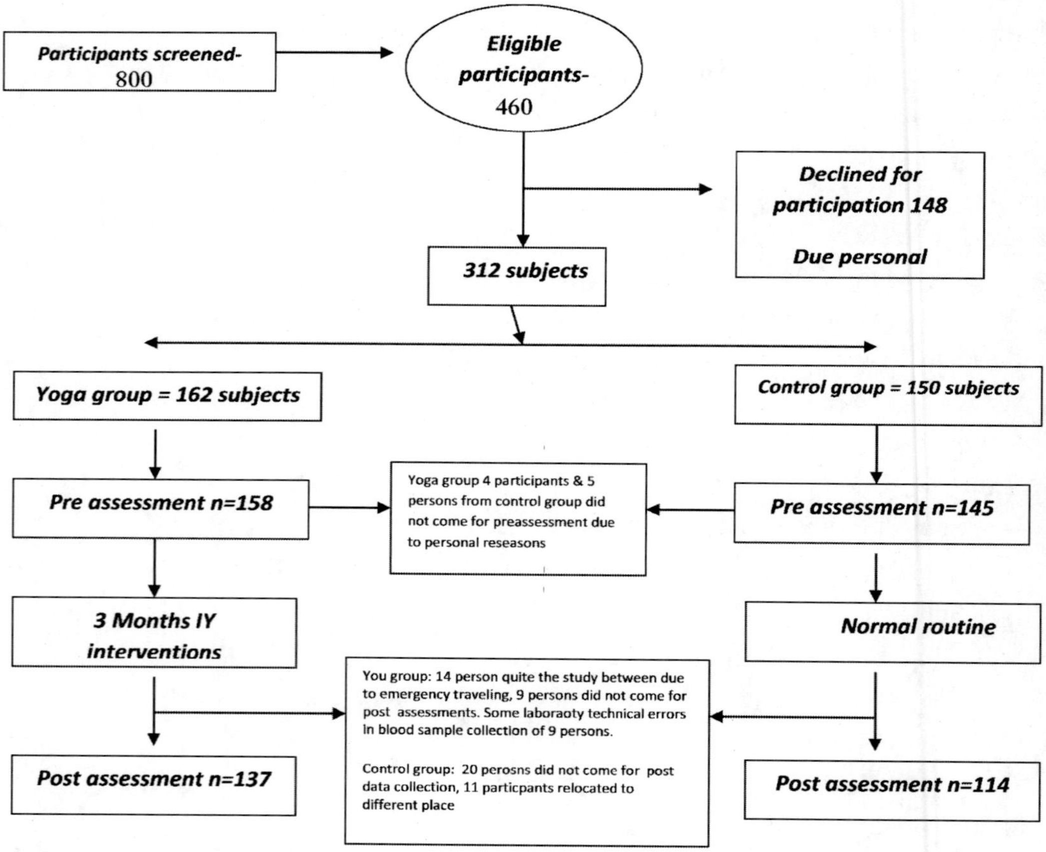

CONSORT Diagram: Recruitment of the participants.

Postprandial Blood Sugar (PPBS) Level

Participants were asked to have breakfast and after 2 hrs of breakfast once again blood sample was collected for PPBS assessment. All the subjects were asked to take their regular anti-diabetic medication as usual.

The blood test was done in an authenticated laboratory using the hexokinase method [13].

Intervention

Participants in the IY group received one hour of IY intervention (See Table 1) every day, 6 days a week for the period of 3 months. All the practices mentioned in the yoga module were used in the previous research studies and found useful in T2DM [14, 15].

Table 1. Details of special yoga technique for T2DM

Number	Name	Posture	Practices
1.	Breathing practices (5 minutes)	Standing	Hands Stretch Breathing
		Sitting	Rabit breathing Tiger Stretch Breathing
2.	Loosening practices Shitihilikarana vyayamah (5 minutes)	Standing	Padahastasana-Ardhachakrasana vyayama
			Trikonasana vyayama
			Kati parivartana vyayama (Spinal Twist)
		Sitting	Chakkichalana
			Bhunamanasana
		Supine	Pawanmuktasana Kriya
		Prone	Dhanurasana Swing
3.	Relaxation(5 minutes)		Instant Relaxation Technique
4.	Surya Namaskara (5 minutes)		12 steps
5.	Asanas (10 minutes each)	Standing	Ardhakatichakrasana
			ParivrittaTrikonasana
		Sitting	Vakrasana
			Ardhamatsyendrasana
		Prone	Bhujangasana Dhanurasana
		Supine	Pawanmuktasana Matsyasana
	Relaxation(10 minutes)		Deep Relaxation Technique
6.	Kriyas		Kapalabhati, Vaman Dhouti (Once a week)
7.	Pranayama (10 minutes)		Nadishuddhi
			Bhramari pranayama
			Om chanting
8.	Meditation (20 minutes)		Cyclic Meditation

Data Analysis

Data was presented as mean and standard deviation. The data were analysed using SPSS version 20 (IBM, Chicago, 2016). The paired sample t test was used for within group comparison and between group comparison was performed using an independent sample t test. *P* value more than 0.05 was considered as statistically significant change.

Blinding

Statistician and data collector were blinded as for groups and data scoring person was blinded as for groups

Results

Total 137 in yoga group and 114 in the control group completed the study.

Within Group Changes

In the yoga group, a significant decrease in FBS ($p > 0.001$, -32.68%) & PPBS ($p > 0.001$, -34.77%) was observed after 3 months of IY compared to the baseline. The Control group showed no significant improvement in FBS and PPBS after 3 months.

Between Group

Postintervention FBS & PPBS comparison between the groups showed significant difference suggestive of significantly lower FBS and PPBS in Yoga group compared to the control group.

Table 2. Prepost changes in mean & SD across the groups

Variables	**Yoga group (n = 137)**			**Control group (n = 114)**			**Between group Comparison**
	Baseline	Post	% change	Baseline	Post	% change	
FBS	142.99 ± 32.20	96.26 ± 11.92**[a]	-32.68	137.62 ± 34.33	133.59 ± 50.86	-2.98	>0.001[b]
PPBS	203.65 ± 45.92	132.83 ± 22.24** [a]	-34.77	190.97 ± 53.83	189.29 ± 78.11	-0.87	>0.001[b]

FBS-Fasting blood glucose level; PPBS-Post-prandial blood glucose level. **-Statistical significance at 0.001 level; [a] - Paired sample t test, [b] - Independent t test.

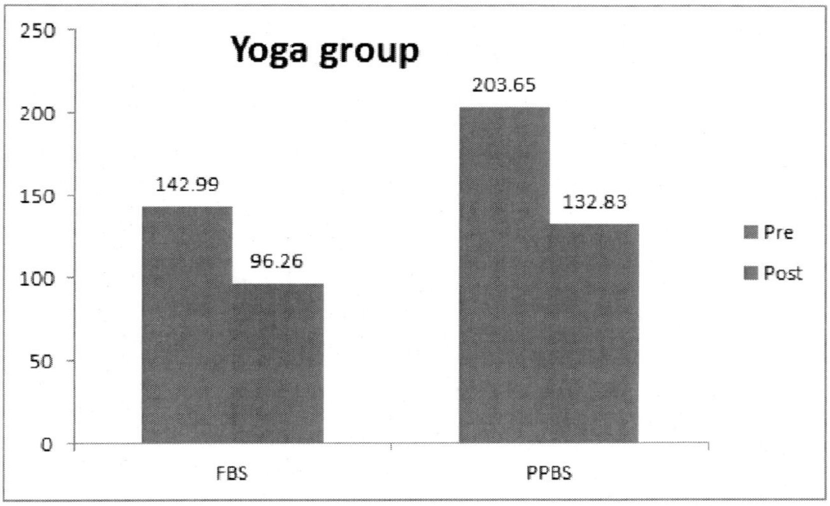

Figure 1. Prepost changes in FBS and PPBS the Yoga group.

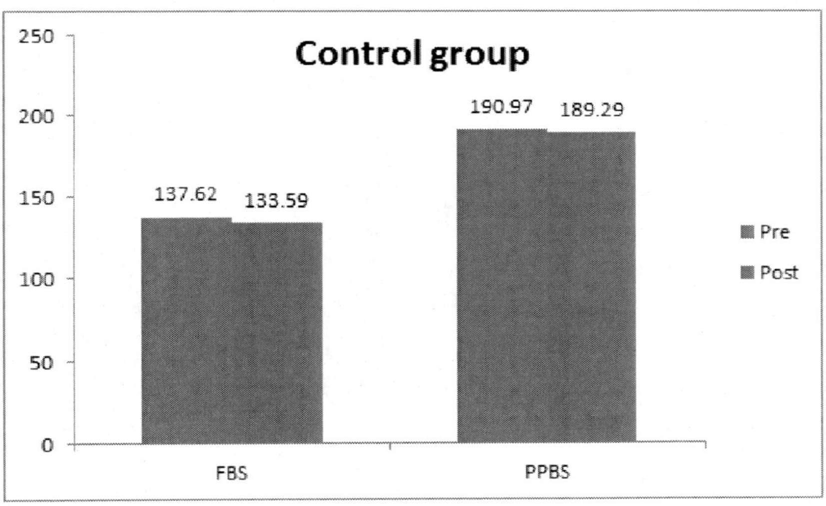

Figure 2. Prepost changes in FBS and PPBS the Control group.

DISCUSSION

The present study was intended to assess the impact of yoga on fasting and postprandial blood glucose level among T2DM patients. After three months of IY intervention significant decrease in fasting and postprandial blood glucose was observed. The control group did not show any changes. Group comparisons of post FBS & PPBS showed significant difference suggestive of superiority of yoga intervention.

Blood sugar control is a primary goal of treatment and in the present we found yoga intervention as an effective intervention to control the blood glucose level among T2DM patients. Thus, yoga can also be a potential preventive measure for T2DM complication.

The findings of the present study are supported by previous studies. A study by Lorenzo et al. 2008 reported significant decrease in blood glucose concentration following three months of Hath yoga intervention [16]. A similar study by Robi et al. 1992 found a significant decrease in fasting blood glucose level following three months of the yoga intervention in T2DM patients [17].

Similarly, we also reported a significant decrease in FBS and PPBS values after three months of IY intervention compared to baseline. This study reconfirms the usefulness of the yoga intervention in management of T2DM by showing its efficacy in reducing FBS and PPBS. However the present study differs from the previous study in term of sample size, frequency of yoga session in a week and type of yoga module used.

Several other treatment methods have been tested for their efficacy in the cure of the disease, stem cell therapy is one of these. Some studies have reported the promising role of stem cell therapy in the cure of T1DM and T2DM [18, 19]. The addition of the yoga intervention to such therapies may enhance the treatment outcome.

Changes in FBS and PPBS found in this study may attributed increased physical activity during asanas, suryanamaskar, and loosening practices, which is connected with increased insulin sensitivity and glucose uptake; slow breathing practice during pranayama is associated with reduced HPA axis activation which is related to increased insulin sensitivity.

Excess production of large sized of adipocytes is thought to be one of the important causes of insulin resistance in T2DM [20]. Large sized of adipocytes are involved in insulin resistance in T2DM. Impaired Production of large sized adepcytes, which may be via correcting the impairment in proliferation of differential capacity of mesenchymal cells [22, 23] in the present study IY module include lot of practice which increase the physical activity, which might have enhanced the mesanchymal cell proliferation and thus coto decrease insulin resistance.

Despite several RCTs available suggesting the significant impact of yoga in T2DM, the present study is unique in its type by being a multicentre trial with large sample size and 3 months intervention. The present study suggests the yoga as an adjunct intervention in management of T2DM.

This study has got a few limitations such as lack of monitoring diet control, other physical activities, and non-randomized study.

CONFLICT OF INTEREST

The authors declare no conflict of interest.

Ethical Compliance

The authors have stated all possible conflicts of interest within this work. The authors have stated all sources of funding for this work. If this work involved human participants, informed consent was received from each individual. If this work involved human participants, it was conducted in accordance with the 1964 Declaration of Helsinki. If this work involved experiments with humans or animals, it was conducted in accordance with the related institutions' research ethics guidelines.

References

[1] Inzucchi, S. E., & Sherwin, R. S. (2011). Type 2 diabetes mellitus. *Cecil Medicine.* 24th ed. Philadelphia, Pa: Saunders Elsevier.

[2] IDF, G. (2011). ISPAD guideline for diabetes in childhood and adolescence. *International Diabetes Federation, 131.*

[3] MacKnight, C., Rockwood, K., Awalt, E., & McDowell, I. (2002). Diabetes mellitus and the risk of dementia, Alzheimer's disease and vascular cognitive impairment in the Canadian Study of Health and Aging. *Dementia and Geriatric Cognitive Disorders, 14*(2), 77-83.

[4] American Diabetes Association. (2015). Standards of medical care in diabetes—2015 abridged for primary care providers. *Clinical diabetes: A Publication of the American Diabetes Association, 33*(2), 97.

[5] Gray A., Raikou M., McGuire A., Fenn P., Stevens R., Cull C, Stratton I, Adler A, Holman R, Turner R. Cost effectiveness of an intensive blood glucose control policy in patients with type 2 diabetes: economic analysis alongside randomised controlled trial (UKPDS 41). *BMJ.* 2000 May 20;320(7246):1373-8.

[6] Khattab M, Khader YS, Al-Khawaldeh A, Ajlouni K. Factors associated with poor glycemic control among patients with type 2 diabetes. *Journal of Diabetes and its Complications*. 2010 Mar 1;24(2):84-9.

[7] Lumelsky N., Blondel O., Laeng P., Vlesco I., Ravion R., McKay R. Differentiation of embryonic stem cells to insulin-secreting structures similar to pancreatic islets. *Science* 2001; 292: 1398–94.

[8] Zorina T. D., Subbotin V. M., Bertera S., et al. Recovery of endogenous cells function in the NOD model of autoimmune diabetes. *Stem Cells* 2003; 21: 377–88.

[9] Barnes, P. M., Bloom, B., & Nahin, R. L. (2008). Com-11. Plementary and alternative medicine use among adults and children: United States, 2007. *Natl Health Stat Rep, 12*, 1-23.

[10] US RAY, S. M., Purkayastha, S., Asnani, V., Tomer, O., Prashad, R., Thakur, L., & Selvamurthy, W. (2001). Effect of yogic exercises on physical and mental health of young fellowship course trainees. *Indian J Physiol Pharmacol*, *45*(1), 37-53.

[11] Siu, P. M., et al. (2015). "Effects of 1-year yoga on cardiovascular risk factors in middle-aged and older adults with metabolic syndrome: a randomized trial." *Diabetol Metab Syndr* **7**: 40.

[12] Aljasir, B., Bryson, M., & Al-shehri, B. (2010). Yoga practice for the management of type II diabetes mellitus in adults: A systematic review. *Evidence-Based Complementary and Alternative Medicine*, *7*(4), 399-408.

[13] Bondar, R. J., & Mead, D. C. (1974). Evaluation of glucose-6-phosphate dehydrogenase from Leuconostoc mesenteroides in the hexokinase method for determ-ining glucose in serum. *Clinical Chemistry*, *20*(5), 586-590.

[14] Hegde, S. V., Adhikari, P., Kotian, S., Pinto, V. J., D'Souza, S., & D'Souza, V. (2011). Effect of 3-month yoga on oxidative stress in type 2 diabetes with or without complications: a controlled clinical trial. *Diabetes care*, *34*(10), 2208-2210.

[15] Venugopal, V., Rathi, A., & Raghuram, N. (2017). Effect of short-term yoga-based lifestyle intervention on plasma glucose levels in individuals with diabetes and pre-diabetes in the community. *Diabetes & Metabolic Syndrome: Clinical Research & Reviews*, *11*, S597-S599.

[16] Gordon, L., Morrison, E. Y., McGrowder, D. A., Young, R., Garwood, D., Zamora, E., & Sanz, E. C. P. (2008). Changes in clinical and metabolic parameters after exercise therapy in patients with type 2 diabetes. *Archives of Medical Science*, *4*(4), 427-437.

[17] Monroe, R., Power, J., Kumar, A., & Nagarathna, R. (1992). *Yoga Therapy for NIDDM: A Controlled Trial.*

[18] Soria, B., Skoudy, A., & Martin, F. (2001). From stem cells to beta cells: new strategies in cell therapy of diabetes mellitus. *Diabetologia*, *44*(4), 407-415.

[19] Aguayo-Mazzucato, C., & Bonner-Weir, S. (2010). Stem cell therapy for type 1 diabetes mellitus. *Nature Reviews Endocrinology*, *6*(3), 139.

[20] Weyer C., Foley J. E., Bogardus C, Tataranni P. A., Pratley RE. Enlarged subcutaneous abdominal adipocyte size, but not obesity itself, predicts Type II diabetes independent of insulin resistance. *Diabetologia* 2000; 43: 1498–1506.

[21] Rangwala S. M., Lazar M. A. Transcriptional control of adipogenesis [In Process Citation]. *Annu Rev Nutr* 2000; 20: 535–559.

[22] Valero, M. C., Huntsman, H. D., Liu, J., Zou, K., & Boppart, M. D. (2012). Eccentric exercise facilitates mesenchymal stem cell appearance in skeletal muscle. *PloS One*, *7*(1), e29760.

[23] Ravussin, E., & Smith, S. R. (2002). Increased fat intake, impaired fat oxidation, and failure of fat cell proliferation result in ectopic fat storage, insulin resistance, and type 2 diabetes mellitus. *Annals of the New York Academy of Sciences*, *967*(1), 363-378.

In: Manipulation of Stem Cells for Disease Benefits
Editor: Prasad Koka
ISBN: 978-1-53615-468-9

Chapter 15

YOGA IN TYPE 2 DIABETES MELLITUS

Amit Singh*, Padmini Tekur, Kashinath Metri, Nagarathna Raghuram and H. R. Nagendra
Division of Yoga and Life Sciences, S-VYASA Yoga University, Bangalore, India

ABSTRACT

Type 2 Diabetes Mellitus (T2DM) is a chronic metabolic disorder and a leading cause of morbidity and mortality worldwide. Blood glucose control, prevention of DM complication and reducing the cardiovascular risk factors are the important goals of T2DM management. Having potential health benefiting effects, Yoga has become a popular alternative and complementary medicine in most of the countries around the world. There is large data evidence from RCTs for the efficacy of in various chronic problems including T2DM.

In this article, various benefits of yoga practice in T2DM patients are discussed. We did a review of recent scientific studies on beneficial effects of yoga in blood glucose control, CVD risk factors and complications in T2DM.

Our review found yoga as an effective intervention in reducing fasting blood sugar (FBS), postprandial blood sugar (PPBS), HbA1C and insulin resistance in T2DM. Yoga reduces cardiovascular complications in T2DM. Further, yoga improves nerve conduction velocity, cognitive function and it also improves mental health by reducing depression and stress in T2DM.

This review concludes that yoga is a cost effective, feasible and potent intervention for optimal blood glucose control, reducing CVD risk factors, to improve cognition and mental health among patients with T2DM.

Keywords: yoga, type 2 Diabetes Mellitus (T2DM), cardiovascular risk, blood glucose, cognition, mental health

* Corresponding Author's E-mail: dramits90@gmail.com.

Introduction

Type 2 Diabetes Mellitus (T2DM) is a metabolic disorder characterized by chronic hyperglycemia. It is one among the most prevalent metabolic disorders and a leading cause of death and disability all over the globe [1]. T2DM is the number one leading cause of chronic kidney disease, heart disease and blindness [2, 3]. It increases the risk of myocardial infarction and stroke by 4 folds [4]. T2DM is considered to be an important cause of cardiovascular disease, chronic kidney disease stroke and blindness [5, 6].

The global prevalence of T2DM varies from 5% to 20% [7]. Sedentary lifestyle, psychological stress, obesity, depression, unhealthy diet and addictions such as smoking and alcohol are considered to be the most common risk factors for T2DM [8, 9].

Progressive beta cell dysfunction is the hallmark of T2DM. By the time T2DM is diagnosed almost 50% of beta cell mass is lost this progresses further with the course of the disease [10]. Conventional management of T2DM targets on insulin resistance and insulin production, leaving the basic defects as it is [11]. The large number of patients with T2DM on anti-diabetic medication eventually shifts to insulin therapy. However, despite rigorous insulin therapy 24hrs glucose control keeps fluctuating contributing to T2DM complications. Hence, in order to correct the T2DM pathology beta cell mass enhancement is crucial. Stem cell therapy is an emerging field in the management of various kinds of disorders including T2DM. In a study 10 patients with T2DM received a stem cell transplant showed significant decrease in insulin requirement and a significant reduction in blood glucose level following stem cell therapy [12]. Stem cell transplant increase the beta cell mass and eventually insulin production. However, the research in the stem cell therapy has a long way to go.

Yoga is a form of mind body practice [13]. It is also a lifestyle which involves the practice moderation in diet, behavior and sleep pattern along with the practice of physical postures, a set of breathing techniques, relaxation techniques and meditation [14, 15]. Numerous scientific investigations have found significant role of yoga in the prevention and the management of several chronic health conditions including T2DM [16]. Yoga helps in T2DM with various aspects which are discussed below.

Objective of this review is review the different aspect of yoga health benefits in T2DM.

Yoga and Blood Glucose Control

Blood glucose control is the primary objective of the T2DM management. Optimal blood glucose control is associated with decreased risk of diabetic complications [17] and better quality of life in T2DM [18, 19]. Several RCTs have shown that yoga improves the blood glucose control among T2DM patients [20]. Yoga reduces the fasting blood glucose; post-prandial blood glucose and it also reduce HbA1C [21, 22, 23]. In a multicentric study, three months of intense yoga intervention reduced fasting and postprandial blood glucose by 32.6% & 34.7% respectively in subjects with T2DM [24]. Studies have also shown a decrease in anti-diabetic medication requirement following yoga practice [25]. Further, Yoga practice improves insulin resistance in T2DM [26, 27]. A meta-analysis has concluded that yoga can be a potential intervention to reduce blood glucose in T2DM [28].

Yoga and Cardiovascular Disease (CVD) in T2DM

Uncontrolled blood glucose level eventually leads to damage to the endothelial layer of micro and macro blood vessels leading to atherosclerosis. T2DM has been an independent risk factor for coronary artery disease and stroke. Prevalence of CAD and its severity are higher among T2DM subjects compared to the controls. Subjects with T2DM have 2 times higher risk of cardiac disease compared to non-diabetic population [29]. CAD has been a most important cause of mortality in T2DM. It is well documented that, yoga is helpful in improving various cardiac risk factors among subjects with high risk of CAD [30]. Yoga improves dyslipidemia, blood pressure, BMI and waist circumference which are considered to be an independent risk factor for CAD [31, 32, 33].

Hypertension is a frequently observed comorbid condition in T2DM [34] it is associated with increased risk of CVD in T2DM. 40% of T2DM patients found to have hypertension [35, 36]. Presence of hypertension as a co-morbid condition increases the risk of CAD by 4 folds. Each 10mmHg increase in the blood pressure increases the CAD risk by 1.5 fold. Control of blood pressure > 140/90 mmHg among T2DM is associated with decreased risk of CVD and End Stage renal disease in T2DM [37, 38].

Yoga reduces blood pressure in hypertensive individuals. Several RCTs has documented the decrease in the systolic, diastolic and mean arterial blood pressure following yoga in hypertension [39, 40, 41]. Studies have also reported the decrease in anti-hypertension medication requirement following yoga practices [42]. Their RCT studies documented the improvement in blood pressure after Yoga intervention among T2DM patient suggestive of yoga as potential intervention to reduce cardiac risk factor in T2DM [43].

Dyslipedemia

Dyslipedemia has been an independent risk for CVD. Dyslipidenia is associated with higher incidences of stroke and myocardial infarction among T2DM subjects.

Yoga practice reduces low density lipoprotein, cholesterol and triglycerides; it also improves high density lipoprotein among patients with dyslipidemia [44, 45]. The practice of yoga shown to help in improving dyslipidemia among T2DM which is shown in RCT study [46] Yoga practice reduces try glycerides, LDL and VLDL and it also improve HDL (good cholesterol) in T2DM subjects.

Yoga and Atherosclerosis

Endothelial dysfunction in T2DM leads to atherosclerosis. There are studies which have show a regression in atherosclerosis following yoga practice in patients with coronary artery disease [47]. A study found improvement in carotid artery lumen diameter following yoga intervention among patients with carotid artery stenosis, [48] which suggests the potential benefits of yoga in reducing risk of stroke [49].

T2DM increase the risk of T2DM by 4 folds. Yoga improves various cardiac risk factors such as dyslipidemia, blood pressure.

Improves Nerve Conduction

Diabetic neuropathy is a most commonly reported T2DM complication. Diabetic neuropathy eventually leads to diabetic foot, gangrene and amputation. Diabetic neuropathy is considered the number one leading cause for amputation. Studies on yoga have shown improvement in nerve conduction velocity following yoga practice [50] suggesting the potential role of yoga in the management and prevention of diabetic neuropathy.

Improves Cognitive Functions

Microvascular complications of T2DM lead to cognitive decline and eventually put the subjects at high risk of dementia and Alzheimer's disease [51]. Many longitudinal studies have reported the increased risk of cognitive decline among T2DM than the normal population [52].

Yoga is known to have cognition enhancing capacity [53].

In several studies yoga practice leads to improvement in various cognitive domains such as attention, processing speed memory, selective attention, concentration, etc. [54,

55]. A study found improvement in memory and attention following three months of yoga practice in subjects with T2DM [56].

Yoga and Mental Health in T2DM

Chronic stress and depression are the two important contributing factors to the cause of T2DM and they also accelerated the involved in the cause of TDM increased risk of T2DM and its complications. They are also associated with increased medication score and CVD risk in T2DM subjects. It is well evident that yoga practice reduces stress and depression and enhances mood [57, 58]. Yoga practice in T2DM reduces perceived stress and depression and helps in improving blood glucose control [59].

Chronic Stress and depression are considered to be an important risk factor for T2DM. Yoga found to be an effective intervention in reducing stress and its effects [60]. Yoga reduces depression and improves mood, helping to adopt good stress coping strategies [61, 62].

Autonomic Dysfunction

T2DM is characterized by autonomic dysfunction with increased sympathetic activity and reduced parasympathetic tone [63]. Increased sympathetic activity in T2DM is associated with increased risk of CVD and incident MI [64].

Yoga practice helps in reducing sympathetic activity and improves parasympathetic tone in T2DM patients shown by reducing low frequency and increased high frequency power [65, 66].

Mechanism: The exact of mechanism of yoga how it helps in improving various health parameters in T2DM is not fully understood; however, these changes can be attributed to decreased HPA (hypo-thalamo-pituitary adrenal axis) which is associated with decreased sympathetic arousal and increase cardiac autonomic function [67]. Various yogic postures and sukshmavyamas increase the glucose uptake and reduce insulin resistance [68, 69].

CONCLUSION

Thus, this review concludes that yoga is a cost effective, feasible and effective intervention which may help in blood glucose control, reducing cardiac risk factors and it may also help in prevention of cognitive decline and diabetic neuropathy.

Ethical Compliance

The authors have stated all possible conflicts of interest within this work. The authors have stated all sources of funding for this work. If this work involved human participants, informed consent was received from each individual. If this work involved human participants, it was conducted in accordance with the 1964 Declaration of Helsinki. If this work involved experiments with humans or animals, it was conducted in accordance with the related institutions' research ethics guidelines.

References

[1] UK Prospective Diabetes Study Group, 1998. Tight blood pressure control and risk of macrovascular and microvascular complications in type 2 diabetes: UKPDS 38. *BMJ: British Medical Journal*, 317(7160), p. 703.

[2] Cosentino, F; Assenza, GE. Diabetes and inflammation. *Herz*, 2004, 29, 749–59.

[3] American Diabetes Association. American Diabetes Association: Clinical Practice Recommendations. *Diabetes Care*, 2004, 27, S1–9.

[4] National Center for Chronic Disease Prevention and Health Promotion. *National Diabetes Fact Sheet,* (2002). Centers for Disease Control. Available at: http://www.cdc.gov/diabetes/pubs/estimates.htm.

[5] Esteves, J; Laranjeira, AF; Roggia, MF; Dalpizol, M; Scocco, C; Kramer, CK; et al. Diabetic retinopathy risk factors. *Arquivos brasileiros de endocrinologia e metabologia*., 2008, 52(3), 431–441.

[6] Garofalo, C; Iazzetta, N; Camocardi, A; Pacilio, M; Iodice, C; Minutolo, R; et al. Anti-diabetics and chronic kidney disease. *Giornale italiano di nefrologia: organo ufficiale della Societa italiana di nefrologia.*, 2015, 32(5), 1112–1114.

[7] Amos, AF; McCarty, DJ; Zimmet, P. The rising global burden of diabetes and its complications: estimates and projections to the year 2010. *Diabetic medicine*, 1997, 14(S5), pp. S7-S85.

[8] Turner, RC; Millns, H; Neil, HAW; Stratton, IM; Manley, SE; Matthews, DR; Holman, RR. Risk factors for coronary artery disease in non-insulin dependent diabetes mellitus: United Kingdom Prospective Diabetes Study (UKPDS: 23). *BMJ*, 1998, 316(7134), pp. 823-828.

[9] Eriksson, KF; Lindgärde, F. Prevention of Type 2 (non-insulin-dependent) diabetes mellitus by diet and physical exercise The 6-year Malmö feasibility study. *Diabetologia*, 1991, 34(12), pp. 891-898.

[10] American Diabetes Association. Diagnosis and classification of diabetes mellitus. *Diabetes Care*, 2008, 31, (Suppl. 1), S55–S60.

[11] Inzucchi, SE. Oral antihyperglycemic therapy for type 2 diabetes. *JAMA*, (2002), 287, 360–372.

[12] Bhansali, A; Upreti, V; Khandelwal, N; Marwaha, N; Gupta, V; Sachdeva, N; Sharma, RR; Saluja, K; Dutta, P; Walia, R; Minz, R. Efficacy of Autologous Bone Marrow–Derived Stem Cell Transplantation in Patients With Type 2 Diabetes Mellitus. *Stem Cells and Development*, 2009, Dec 1, 18(10), 1407-16.

[13] Schure, MB; Christopher, J; Christopher, S. Mind–body medicine and the art of self-care: teaching mindfulness to counseling students through yoga, meditation, and qigong. *Journal of Counseling & Development*, 2008, 86(1), pp. 47-56.

[14] Rao, M; Metri, KG; Raghuram, N; Hongasandra, NR. Effects of Mind Sound Resonance Technique (Yogic Relaxation) on Psychological States, Sleep Quality, and Cognitive Functions in Female Teachers: A Randomized, Controlled Trial. *Advances in Mind-Body Medicine*, 2017.

[15] Naoroibam, R; Metri, KG; Bhargav, H; Nagaratn, R. Effect of Integrated Yoga (IY) on psychological states and CD4 counts of HIV-1 infected Patients: A Randomized controlled pilot study. *International Journal of Yoga*, 2016.

[16] Singh, A; Tekur, P; Metri, K; Bhargav, H; Raghuram, N. Effect of a Residential Integrated Yoga Program on Blood Glucose Levels, Physiological Variables, and Anti-Diabetic Medication Score of Patients with Type 2 Diabetes Mellitus: A Retrospective Study. *Integrative Medicine International*, 2017.

[17] The Diabetes Control and Complications Trial Research Group The effect of intensive treatment of diabetes on the development and progression of long-term complications in insulin-dependent diabetes mellitus. *N Engl J Med*, 1993, 329, 977-986.

[18] American Diabetes Association, 1999. Quality of life in type 2 diabetic patients is affected by complications but not by intensive policies to improve blood glucose or blood pressure control (UKPDS 37). UK Prospective Diabetes Study Group. *Diabetes Care*, *22*(7), pp. 1125-1136.

[19] Nathan, DM; Singer, DE; Godine, JE; Harrington, CH; Perlmuter, LC. Retinopathy in older type II diabetics association with glucose control. *Diabetes*, 1986, 35(7), pp. 797-801.

[20] Innes, KE; Vincent, HK. The influence of yoga-based programs on risk profiles in adults with type 2 diabetes mellitus: a systematic review. *Evidence-Based Complementary and Alternative Medicine*, 2007, 4(4), pp. 469-486.

[21] Pardasany, A; Shenoy, S; Sandhu, JS. "Comparing the efficacy of tai chi chuan and hatha yoga in type 2 diabetes mellitus patients on parameters of blood glucose control and lipid metabolism," *Indian Journal of Physiotherapy and Occupational Therapy*, vol. 4, no. 3, pp. 11–16, 2010.

[22] Amita, S; Prabhakar, S; Manoj, I; Harminder, S; Pavan, T. "Effect of Yoga-Nidra on blood glucose level in diabetic patients," *Indian Journal of Physiology and Pharmacology*, vol. 53, no. 1, pp. 97–101, 2009.

[23] Subramaniyan, TG; Subramaniyan, N; Chidambaram, M. "Brisk walking and yoga as adjuvant therapy in management of type 2 diabetes mellitus," *International Journal of Students Research*, vol. 2, no. 1, pp. 43–46, 2012.

[24] Amit, Singh; Padmini, Tekur; Nagaratna, R; et al. Impact of Yoga on Blood Glucose Level among Patients with Type 2 Diabetes Mellitus: A Multicentre Controlled Trial. *Journal of Stem Cells*, Volume 13, Number 1.

[25] Nagarathna, R; Usharani, MR; Rao, AR; Chaku, R; Kulkarni, R; Nagendra, HR. "Efficacy of yoga based life style modification program on medication score and lipid profile in type 2 diabetes-a randomized control study," *International Journal of Diabetes in Developing Countries*, vol. 32, no. 3, pp. 122–130, 2012.

[26] Singh, S; Kyizom, T; Singh, KP; Tandon, OP; Madhu, SV. Influence of pranayamas and yoga-asanas on serum insulin, blood glucose and lipid profile in type 2 diabetes. *Indian Journal of Clinical Biochemistry*, 2008, *23*(4), pp. 365-368.

[27] Jyotsna, VP; Ambekar, S; Joshi, A; et al., "Prospective randomized controlled intervention trial: comprehensive yogic 20 Journal of Diabetes Research breathing program improves cardiac autonomic functions and quality of life in diabetes," *Indian Journal of Endocrinology and Metabolism*, vol. 16, supplement 2, pp. S489–S491, 2012.

[28] Innes, KE; Vincent, HK. The influence of yoga-based programs on risk profiles in adults with type 2 diabetes mellitus: A systematic review. *Evidence-Based Complementary and Alternative Medicine*, 2007, 4(4), pp. 469-486.

[29] Turner, RC; Millns, H; Neil, HAW; Stratton, IM; Manley, SE; Matthews, DR; Holman, RR. Risk factors for coronary artery disease in non-insulin dependent diabetes mellitus: United Kingdom Prospective Diabetes Study (UKPDS: 23). *BMJ*, 1998, 316(7134), pp. 823-828.

[30] Manchanda, SC; Narang, R; Reddy, KS; Sachdeva, U; Prabhakaran, D; Dharmanand, S; Rajani, M; Bijlani, R. Retardation of coronary atherosclerosis with yoga lifestyle intervention. *The Journal of the Association of Physicians of India*, 2000, 48(7), pp. 687-694.

[31] Jain, SC; Uppal, A; Bhatnagar, SOD; Talukdar, B. A study of response pattern of non-insulin dependent diabetics to yoga therapy. *Diabetes Research and clinical practice*, 1993, 19(1), pp. 69-74.

[32] Shantakumari, N; Sequeira, S. Effects of a yoga intervention on lipid profiles of diabetes patients with dyslipidemia. *Indian heart journal*, 2013, 65(2), pp. 127-131.

[33] Khatri, D; Mathur, KC; Gahlot, S; Jain, S; Agrawal, RP. Effects of yoga and meditation on clinical and biochemical parameters of metabolic syndrome. *Diabetes Research and Clinical Practice*, 2007, 78(3), pp. e9-e10.

[34] Sowers, JR. Epstein M Diabetes mellitus and associated hypertension, vascular disease, and nephropathy: an update. *Hypertension.*, 1995, 26(pt 1), 869–879.

[35] Harris, MI; Cowie, CC; Stern, MP; Boyko, EJ; Reiber, GE; Bennett, PH. editors. *Diabetes in America.* 2nd ed. Washington, DC: National Institutes of Health, National Institute of Diabetes and Digestive and Kidney Diseases, 1995.

[36] Hypertension in Diabetes Study (HDS): I. Prevalence of hypertension in newly presenting type 2 diabetic patients and the association with risk factors for cardiovascular and diabetic complications. *J Hypertens.*, 1993 Mar, 11(3), 309-17.

[37] UKPDS Group. Efficacy of atenolol and captopril in reducing risk of macrovascular and microvascular complications in type 2 diabetes: UKPDS 39. *BMJ.*, 1998, 317, 713–720.

[38] Tuomilehto, J; Rastenyte, D; Birkenhager, WH; Thijs, L; Antikainen, R; Bulpitt, CJ; Fletcher, AE; Forette, F; Goldhaber, A; Palatini, P; et al, for the Systolic Hypertension in Europe Trial Investigators. Effects of calcium channel blockers in older patients with diabetes and systolic hypertension. *N Engl J Med.*, 1999, 340, 677–684.

[39] Singh, S; Malhotra, V; Singh, KP; Madhu, SV; Tandon, OP. Role of yoga in modifying certain cardiovascular functions in type 2 diabetic patients. *JAPI*, 2004, 52, pp. 203-206.

[40] Innes, KE; Vincent, HK. The influence of yoga-based programs on risk profiles in adults with type 2 diabetes mellitus: a systematic review. *Evidence-Based Complementary and Alternative Medicine*, 2007, 4(4), pp. 469-486.

[41] Kumar, K; Sivasankaran, S; Pollard-Quintner, S; Sachdeva, R; Pugeda, J; Hoq, SM; Zarich, SW. Reversing Hypertension through Yogic Intervention. The effect of a six-week program of yoga and meditation on brachial artery reactivity: Do psycho-social interventions affect vascular tone? *Clinical Cardiology*, 2006, 29(9), pp. 393-398.

[42] Bijlani, RL; Vempati, RP; Yadav, RK; Ray, RB; Gupta, V; Sharma, R; Mehta, N; Mahapatra, SC. A brief but comprehensive lifestyle education program based on yoga reduces risk factors for cardiovascular disease and diabetes mellitus. *Journal of Alternative & Complementary Medicine*, 2005, 11(2), pp. 267-274.

[43] Wiwanitkit, V. Yoga and lipid profile. *International Journal of Yoga*, 2011, 4(1), p. 39.

[44] Vyas, R; Dikshit, N. Effect of meditation on respiratory system, cardiovascular system and lipid profile. *Indian Journal of Physiology and Pharmacology*, 2002, 46(4), pp. 487-491.

[45] Kerr, D; Gillam, E; Ryder, J; Trowbridge, S; Cavan, D; Thomas, P. An Eastern art form for a Western disease: randomised controlled trial of yoga in patients with poorly controlled insulin-treated diabetes. *Pract Diabetes Intern*, 2002, 19, 164–6.

[46] Manchanda, SC; Narang, R; Reddy, KS; Sachdeva, U; Prabhakaran, D; Dharmanand, S; Rajani, M; Bijlani, R. Retardation of coronary atherosclerosis with yoga lifestyle intervention. *The Journal of the Association of Physicians of India*, 2000, 48(7), pp. 687-694.

[47] Manchanda, SC; Mehrotra, UC; Makhija, A; Mohanty, A; Dhawan, S; Sawhney, JPS. Reversal of Early Atherosclerosis in Metabolic Syndrome by Yoga-A Randomized Controlled Trial. *Journal of Yoga & Physical Therapy*, 2013, 3(1), p. 1.

[48] Manchanda, SC; Narang, R; Reddy, KS; Sachdeva, U; Prabhakaran, D; Dharmanand, S; Rajani, M; Bijlani, R. Retardation of coronary atherosclerosis with yoga lifestyle intervention. *The Journal of the Association of Physicians of India.*, 2000 Jul, 48(7), 687-94.

[49] Malhotra, V; Singh, S; Tandon, OP; Madhu, SV; Prasad, A; Sharma, SB. Effect of Yoga asanas on nerve conduction in type 2 diabetes. *Indian journal of physiology and pharmacology*, 2002, 46(3), pp. 298-306.

[50] Roberts, RO; Geda, YE; Knopman, DS; Christianson, TJ; Pankratz, VS; Boeve, BF; Vella, A; Rocca, WA; Petersen, RC. Association of duration and severity of diabetes mellitus with mild cognitive impairment. *Archives of Neurology*, 2008, 65(8), pp. 1066-1073.

[51] Cukierman, T; Gerstein, HC; Williamson, JD. Cognitive decline and dementia in diabetes—systematic overview of prospective observational studies. *Diabetologia*, 2005, 48(12), pp. 2460-2469.

[52] Froeliger, B; Garland, EL; Modlin, LA; McClernon, FJ. (2012). Neurocognitive correlates of the effects of yoga meditation practice on emotion and cognition: a pilot study. *Frontiers in Integrative Neuroscience*, 6, p. 48.

[53] Ross, A; Thomas, S. The health benefits of yoga and exercise: a review of comparison studies. *The Journal of Alternative and Complementary Medicine*, 2010, 16(1), pp. 3-12.

[54] Oken, BS; Zajdel, D; Kishiyama, S; Flegal, K; Dehen, C; Haas, M; Kraemer, DF; Lawrence, J; Leyva, J. Randomized, controlled, six-month trial of yoga in healthy seniors: effects on cognition and quality of life. *Alternative Therapies in Health and Medicine*, 2006, 12(1), p. 40.

[55] Rajani, SN; Indla, YR; Archana, R; Rajesh, P. Role of yoga on cardic autonomic function tests and cognition in type 2 diabetes. *International Journal of Research in Ayurveda and Pharmacy*, 2015, 6(6), p. 764.

[56] Khalsa, SB; Hickey-Schultz, L; Cohen, D; Steiner, N; Cope, S. Evaluation of the mental health benefits of yoga in a secondary school: a preliminary randomized controlled trial. *The Journal of Behavioral Health Services & Research.*, 2012, Jan 1, 39(1), 80-90.

[57] Büssing, A; Michalsen, A; Khalsa, SB; Telles, S; Sherman, KJ. Effects of yoga on mental and physical health: A short summary of reviews. *Evidence-Based Complementary and Alternative Medicine*., 2012, 2012.

[58] Agte, VV; Tarwadi, K. Sudarshan kriya yoga for treating type 2 diabetes: a preliminary study. *Alternative & Complementary Therapies*., 2004, Aug 1, 10(4), 220-2.

[59] West, J; Otte, C; Geher, K; Johnson, J; Mohr, DC. Effects of Hatha yoga and African dance on perceived stress, affect, and salivary cortisol. *Annals of Behavioral Medicine*, 2004, 28(2), pp. 114-118.

[60] Kozasa, EH; Santos, RF; Rueda, AD; Benedito-Silva, AA; De Moraes Ornellas, FL; Leite, JR. Evaluation of Siddha Samadhi Yoga for anxiety and depression symptoms: A preliminary study. *Psychological Reports*, 2008, 103(1), pp. 271-274.

[61] Woolery, A; Myers, H; Sternlieb, B; Zeltzer, L. A yoga intervention for young adults with elevated symptoms of depression. *Alternative Therapies in Health and Medicine*, 2004, 10(2), p. 60.

[62] Vinik, AI; Ziegler, D. Diabetic cardio-vascular autonomic neuropathy. *Circulation*, 2007, 115(3), pp. 387-397.

[63] Pop-Busui, R; Evans, GW; Gerstein, HC; Fonseca, V; Fleg, JL; Hoogwerf, BJ; Genuth, S; Grimm, RH; Corson, MA; Prineas, R. and ACCORD Study Group, 2010. Effects of cardiac autonomic dysfunction on mortality risk in the Action to Control Cardio-vascular Risk in Diabetes (ACCORD) trial. *Diabetes Care*, 33(7), pp. 1578-1584.

[64] Tyagi, A; Cohen, M. Yoga and heart rate variability: a comprehensive review of the literature. *International Journal of Yoga*, 2016 Jul, 9(2), 97.

[65] Vempati, RP; Telles, S. Yoga-based guided relaxation reduces sympathetic activity judged from baseline levels. *Psychological Reports*, 2002 Apr, 90(2), 487-94.

[66] Manchanda, SC; Narang, R; Reddy, KS; Sachdeva, U; Prabhakaran, D; Dharmanand, S; Rajani, M; Bijlani, R. Retardation of coronary atherosclerosis with yoga lifestyle intervention. *The Journal of the Association of Physicians of India*, 2000, 48(7), pp. 687-694.

[67] Kim, SD. Effects of yogic exercises on life stress and blood glucose levels in nursing students. *Journal of Physical Therapy Science*., 2014, 26(12), 2003-6.

[68] Innes, KE; Bourguignon, C; Taylor, AG. Risk indices associated with the insulin resistance syndrome, cardio-vascular disease, and possible protection with yoga: a systematic review. *The Journal of the American Board of Family Practice*., 2005, Nov 1, 18(6), 491-519.

In: Manipulation of Stem Cells for Disease Benefits
Editor: Prasad Koka
ISBN: 978-1-53615-468-9

Chapter 16

IMPROVEMENT IN BIOCHEMICAL AND PSYCHOPATHOLOGIES IN WOMEN HAVING PCOS THROUGH YOGA COMBINED WITH HERBAL DETOXIFICATION

Vibhuti Rao[1], Kashinath Metri[2,*], Shubhashankari Rao[1] and R. Nagaratna[2]
[1]Shubha Ayurveda Center, Basavangudi, Bengaluru, India
[2]Division of Yoga and Life Science, S-VYASA University, Bengaluru, India

ABSTRACT

Aim: To study the efficacy of Yoga as a supportive therapy modality to Ayurveda treatment in improving endocrine parameters and psychopathologies in PCOS.

Methods: We selected 64 women with PCOS within the age range 18 to 40 years (mean age = 29.24 years) who visited to *Ayurveda* center to seek *Ayurveda* treatment for PCOS. Subjects were randomly assigned to two groups of 32 each in *Ayurveda* group-AY and *Ayurveda* + *Yoga* group-AY + Y respectively. Women who had had; medical history of uterine fibroids, endometriosis, pelvic inflammatory disease, tubal blockage and or had exposure to yoga practices in the past 2 years were excluded from the study. All the women in AY group received cleansing therapy based on *Ayurveda* prescription which was followed by oral herbal medication intake for three months. Women in AY + Y group received 3 months of yoga intervention 1 hr daily, 5 day/week for 3 months along with *Ayurveda* treatment. The assessment of the study was for endocrine variables, ovary mass and psychological states using perceived stress scale and hospital anxiety depression invent-tory, at the baseline and after 3 months.

Results: In the AY + Y group a significant decrease was observed for 9 variables (1) prolactin ($p = 0.003$), 2) LH ($p = 0.006$), 3) testosterone ($p = 0.003$), 4) HbA1C ($p = 0.006$), 5) AMH ($p = 0.004$), 7) T4 ($p = 0.001$), 8) TSH ($p = 0.035$), 9) right ovary mass

* Corresponding Author's E-mail: kgmhetre@gmail.com. Dr. Kashinath G Metri. Associate Professor.

(p = 0.003). In AY Group significant reduction was found for 3 variables 1) AMH (p = 0.006), HbA1C (p = 0.003), T4 (p = 0.03). In the between group comparison A+Y group showed significantly greater reduction in HbA1C ($p < 0.001$) and TSH (p = 0.002), left (p = 0.04) and right (p = 0.006) ovary mass as compared to AY group. We noticed significant improvement in anxiety, depression, & perceived stress in Y+A group.

Conclusion: The present study suggests that addition of yoga intervention to the herbal medication for PCOS have additional benefits compared to only herbal treatment. This study also suggest that combination of complimentary therapies have synergetic effects in management of PCOS.

Keywords: ayurveda, yoga, PCOS, hormones, alternative medicine

INTRODUCTION

Poly Cystic Ovary Syndrome (PCOS) is a common endocrine disorder prevailing in women of reproductive age [1]. It is an independent risk factor for other reproductive problems such as infertility, endometrial cancer, and late menopause [2, 3] and metabolic disorder. PCOS significantly contributes to the risk of co-morbid metabolic conditions such as obesity, type 2 diabetes mellitus (T2DM) and hyper-tension [4, 5]. Nearly half of women with PCOS tend to develop obesity [6] and 2/3rd PCOS women developT2DM and cardiovascular disease [7].

Statistics show that PCOS affects more than 10% of women worldwide. A survey reported that prevalence of PCOS in Indian adolescent girls is about 9.13% [8] whereas in South Indian adolescent prevalence of PCOS is as high as 22%. [9]. Studies also show that 6.5% women in Spain [10] and 14% Iranian adolescent girls suffer from PCOS [11]. Conventional management and front-line treatment of PCOS includes oral insulin-sensitizing agents such as metformin, hormonal therapy, and surgery. The mentioned treatments are not only associated with some side effects but also have no definite cure [12].

In recent years there has been a shift in the treatment methods of chronic health problems including PCOS with the increase in trend of complementary and alternative medicine (CAM) use.

Ayurveda and Yoga, both are time proven therapeutic system and procedure since time immemorial. The development, study, and application of Ayurveda and Yoga has been dated more than 5000 years old with the aim of promotion of health of the healthy person and to cure the disease of the diseased individual. Ayurveda has proved its beneficial role in various health conditions such as diabetes, hyper-tension, arthritis, anxiety, depression, etc. [13, 14, 15, 16].

Several studies have shown a promising results of administration of Ayurveda herbs in the management of PCOS, it reduce menstrual irregularity, excess menstrual bleeding, dysmenorrhea, weight, the bulk mass of ovary, FHS/LH ratio and improved pregnancy rate in women having PCOS [17, 18, 19, 20].

Yoga includes proven practices to alleviate the discord and disorder of mind and body. The practices of limbs of yoga such asana, pranayama, meditation and cleansing practices aid to the normal functioning of both mind and body at various levels. Thus, the practice of yoga is known to have beneficial effects on the physical, physiological and psychological health of an individual and based on scientific evidence, the beneficial effect of Yoga has been known in various chronic health problems like diabetes, hypertension, Parkinson's disease and rheumatoid arthritis [21, 22, 23].

The practice of Yoga has shown to reduce AMH, LH, and testosterone, the mFG score for hirsutism and improvement in menstrual frequency in adolescent girls with PCOS [24]. It has proven to be more effective as compared to conventional physical exercises in improving blood glucose level, lipid profile and insulin resistance values in adolescent girls with PCOS [25] and also reduces anxiety and improves the quality of life of PCOS patients [26, 27].

However, there are lack of studies showing the combined effects of Yoga and ayurveda herbs in management of PCOS. The present study intended to study the efficacy of Yoga and ayurveda herb administration on biochemical variables and psycho-pathologies among women with PCOS.

METHODOLOGY

Study Participants

Women Participant who visited an Ayurveda center in Bangalore city of South India, between December 2015 and June 2017 to seek Ayurveda treatment for PCOS were enrolled in this study. All women were between the age ranges 18- 40 years.

Recruitments

We screened 94 women with PCOS for inclusion criteria. Of 94 screened, 64 satisfied study criteria, potential participants were randomly assigned to either yoga + Ayurveda (AY + Y) group (32 women) or Ayurveda (AY) group (32 subjects). 3 women dropped due to personal problem and 1 women didn't come for post assessment.

Among them, 30 women were randomly assigned to Ayurveda group and 30 women in Ayurveda & Yoga group using random number generator table. Both groups were comparable in terms of age, socio-economic status and PCOS history.

- *We included the subjects;* who fulfilled Rotterdam criterion of PCOS; within the age range 18 years to 40 years; willing to participate in the study; who can read, write and understand English.
- *We excluded the subjects if they;* were adolescence girls and women aged more than 40 years; did not fall under Rotterdam criteria of PCOS; were under any kind of medication; were suffering from uterine Fibroids, Endometriosis, Pelvic Inflammatory Disease and Tubal blockage; they had previous exposure to any form of Yoga in last 2 years.

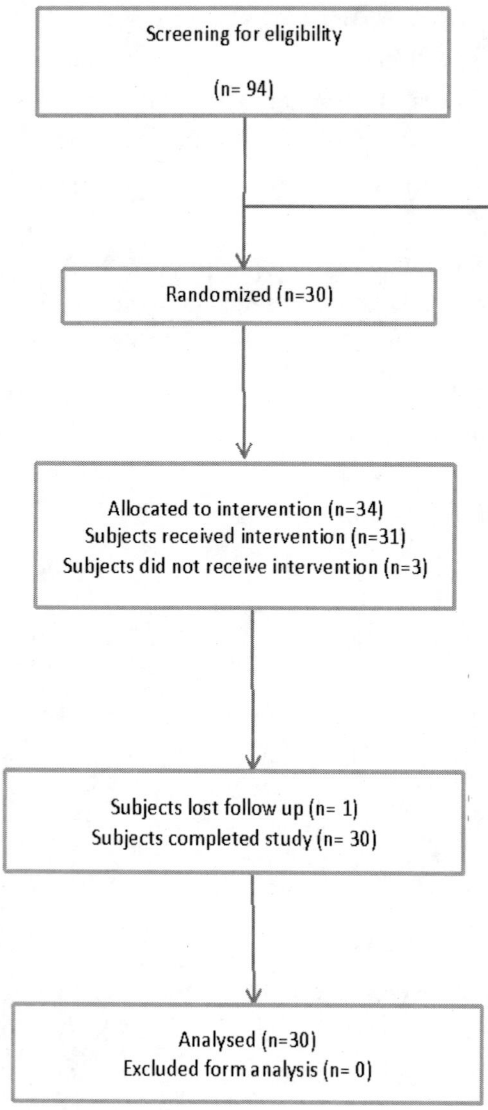

Figure 1. Flow chart.

Ethics and Informed Consent

The study was approved by the Departmental Project Evaluation Committee of DDE, Swāmi Vivekānanda Yoga Anus and hāna Samsthāna (SVYASA), University. Written informed consent was obtained from the women who agreed to participate in the study.

Outcome Measures

- Endocrine Measures
  - Antimullerian Hormone (AMH).
  - Prolactin hormone (Prolactin).
  - Testosterone (Testosterone).
  - Follicle stimulating hormone (FSH) and Luteinizing hormone (LH).
  - Thyroid profile (T3, T4, and TSH) were also assessed before and after the study.
- Ovary Mass
  - Right and left ovary mass (Length, Width & breadth) were measured by abdominal ultrasound sonography.
- HbA1C

Blinding and Masking

Double blinding was not possible as this was an interventional study. The medical officer, ultra-sinologist and the laboratory staff were blind to the groups. Also, the statistician who did the randomization and the final analysis was blind to the source of the data.

ASSESSMENTS

Endocrine Variables

Abdominal ultrasound scanning of the pelvis with special attention to the ovaries was carried out by an expert ultra-sinologist using a Philips HD 11XE ultrasound system. Fasting sample of venous blood (10mL) was drawn between 6:00 AM and 8:00 AM at the Ayurveda hospital. The samples were packed in ice and maintained at 3 degrees C to 4 degrees C and transported to the laboratory within 2 hours. Serum was separated by centrifugation and stored at – 20C until it was analyzed at certified laboratories. Hormone estimates including total testosterone, LH, FSH, and prolactin were done by fully automated bidirectional interfaced chemiluminescent immuno-assay.

Thyroid-stimulating hormone was measured by ultrasensitive sandwich chemiluminescent immuno-assay. Serum AMH levels were assessed by using a 2nd generation enzyme immunoassay (AMH-EIA kit; Immuno-tech, a Beckman Coulter Company, Marseilles, France). The intra and inter assay coefficients of variation were 5.1% and 6.6%, respectively for AMH, 3.8% and 4.3% for FSH, 4.9% and 6.5% for LH, and 4.0% and 5.6% for testosterone.

INTERVENTION

Ayurveda Herbal Treatment (Table 1)

Both the groups received Ayurveda herbal medication and cleansing therapies prescribed by Ayurveda expert. Treatment was carried out in following steps;

1. Therapeutic cleansing (*Panchakarma*) using ayurveda herbs- It consisted of Vamana Karma (therapeutic vomiting), Virechana Karma (Therapeutic cleansing), Two type of Basti Chikitsa and (medicated enema) followed by oral medications.
2. Internal medicines-Ayurvedic medicines and formulations which are specifically mentioned for female reproductive related problems such as Ashoka arishtam, Sukumar Ghrita, Dashamoola Kashaya, Nishamlaki tablets, Krishna-jeeraka, Sahachara and PhalaSarpis.

All the subjects in Ayurveda + Yoga group along with Ayurveda treatment mentioned above, received 3 months of yoga practices, consisting of Asanas (physical postures), Pranayama(breathing practices), relaxation techniques and meditation sessions which were followed in previous Yoga studies (See table) for 1 hour on a daily basis and for 5 days a week.

Statistical Analysis

All statistical analysis was performed using SPSS version 16.0. RM-ANOVA was applied to see pre-post changes in within group and between groups.

Table 1. Yoga module followed in Ayurveda + Yoga intervention group

Name of the Practice
• Starting prayer
• Loosening practices.
• Pawanamukthasana series ...1
• Full butterfly
• Twisting practices
• Cat pose 5
• Pawanamukthasana series
• Shavasana relaxation
• ASANAS.
• SITTING POSTURES
• Baddhakonasana
• Squat(pranamasana)
• Paschimitthanasana
• Churning mill pose
• STANDING POSTURES
• Triangle pose
• Intensive leg stretching pose
• PRONE POSTURES
• Bhujangasana
• Shalabhasana
• Dhanurasana
• SUPINE POSTURES
• Viparithakarani (aswini mudra)
• Sarvangasana
• Halasana
• Surya namaskar 3 ROUNDS
• OM meditation/Antarmouna
• PRANAYAMA
• Kapalbhati
• Cooling pranayama
• Naadishodana
• Bhramari 2min
• Full yogic breathing
• YOGA NIDRA

Table 2. Ayurveda intervention

- Administration of deepana and pachana drugs: Oral administration of drugs to improve digestive fire
- Administration of Ayurvedic therapeutic cleansing procedures
- Oral administration of herbal preparations

RESULTS

Demographics (Table 3) No between group differences were noticed in terms of age of subjects, marital years, number of working women and years of educational and socioeconomic status.

Marital Status

Most of the participants in both the groups were married (Table 4).

Education Level

In both the groups, participants were highly educated and most of them had a bachelor's degree (Table 5).

Table 3. Age of the participants: (n-number of participants)

Age Group (Years)	Yoga + Ayurveda Group (n)	Ayurveda Group (n)
18-25	7	5
26- 33	15	21
34-40	8	4
Mean (sd.) of Age	29.23 (5.34)	29.27 (5.06)

Table 4. Marital life (duration) of the participants

Marital Duration (Years)	Yoga + Ayurveda Group (n)	Ayurveda Group (n)
Unmarried	4	7
1-5 years	11	14
6-10 years	12	7
10 plus years	3	2

Table 5. Education level of the participants

Education Level	Yoga + Ayurveda Group (n- Number of Participants)	Ayurveda Group (n- Number of Participants)
Bachelor's Degree	24	21
Master's Degree	6	9

Occupation

Most of the participants in the Ayurveda group were in paid job and they were almost of equal numbers in Yoga + Ayurveda group (Table 6).

History of PCOS

More than 50% of the participants in Yoga + Ayurveda and Ayurveda group were diagnosed with PCOS since past five years (Table 7).

Outcome Variables (Table 8)

Maximum number of subjects (26) was between age ranges 26 to 33 years.

Tables below show the demographic data of both the groups. The age group for the study was restricted to 18 to 40 years. Most of the women fall between 26 and 33 years in both the groups. The Mean Age (M) of participants was 29.23 years.

In both the groups, participants were highly educated and most of them had a bachelor degree (Table 4).

Most of the participants in both the groups were married (Table 5).

Most of the participants in the Ayurveda group were in paid job and they were almost of equal numbers in Yoga + Ayurveda group (Table 6).

More than 50% of the participants in Yoga + Ayurveda and Ayurveda group were diagnosed with PCOS since past five years (Table 7).

Table 6. Occupation of the participants

Occupation	Yoga + Ayurveda Group (n)	Ayurveda Group (n)
Housewife	14	11
Paid work-professional	13	14
Unpaid-student	3	5

Table 7. Duration of PCOS among participants

Duration of PCOS (Years)	Yoga + Ayurveda Group (n)	Ayurveda Group (n)
1-5	18	17
6-10	9	13
11 plus years	3	0
Mean (std.)	5.167 (3.82)	2.61)

Table 8. Pre-post comparison of all the variables within and between groups

Groups Variables	Yoga+ Ayurveda				Ayurveda				Between Group Comparison
	Pre Mean ± SD	Post Mean ± SD	Mean Difference	P value	Pre Mean ± SD	Post Mean ± SD	Mean Difference	P value	
Weight	65.04 ± 14.96	62.97 ± 18.00	- .514	0.607	66.65 ± 9.37	67.04 ± 9.78	- .849	.396	.286
Prolactin	13.67 ± 6.52	10.74 ± 5.52	- 2.958	0.003**	10.69 ± 6.64	9.62 ± 4.22	- 1.459	.145	.409
FSH	8.96 ± 17.69	8.09 ± 14.23	- .348	0.728	5.68 ± 3.29	6.31 ± 3.42	- 1.231	.218	.523
LH	10.44 ± 7.24	8.94 ± 5.07	- 2.770	0.006**	10.84 ± 5.25	10.23 ± 4.87	- 1.270	.204	.334
Testosterone	11.60 ± 8.17	7.68 ± 5.24	-2.937	0.003**	9.85 ± 7.05	8.59 ± 5.50	- 1.111	.266	.668
AMH	4.17 ± 3.14	3.84 ± 1.41	- 2.860	0.004**	5.87 ± 4.92	3.82 ± 1.82	- 2.757	.006**	.938
HBA1C	5.71 ± 0.63	5.35 ± 0.42	- 1.134	0.017*	5.72 ± 0.55	5.85 ± 0.47	- 2.111	.035*	< 001**
T3	2.09 ± 1.32	1.97 ± 0.92	- .081	0.936	2.13 ± 1.52	2.36 ± 1.20	- .762	.446	.122
T4	6.45 ± 2.97	4.96 ± 2.89	- 3.967	0.001	6.13 ± 3.11	4.96 ± 2.20	- 2.213	.027*	.882
TSH	5.05 ± 5.60	2.98 ± 2.14	- 2.11	0.035**	5.21 ± 4.22	4.81 ± 2.61	- .229	.819	.002**
PSS	33.80 ± 3.66	15.97 ± 4.84	- 6.371	< 001**	29.23 ± 7.00	23.90 ± 6.45	- 3.996	< 001**	< 001**
Anxiety	17.10 ± 3.69	9.70 ± 3.39	- 6.302	< 001**	15.40 ± 2.63	11.20 ± 3.54	- 4.636	< 001**	< 001**
Depression	13.67 ± 3.86	7.70 ± 3.83	- 6.078	< 001**	12.53 ± 3.01	9.60 ± 3.89	- 3.793	< 001**	< 001**
Right ovary mass	11.11 ± 5.40	9.06 ± 3.03	- 1.703	.003	13.62 ± 5.61	11.82 ± 3.24	- .994	.376	.006
Left ovary mass	12.36 ± 4.51	9.38 ± 3.07	- 2.757	.089	13.31 ± 7.10	11.69 ± 3.47	- 1.250	.167	.045

Within Group Comparison

In AY + Y group a significant decrease was observed for 9 variables (1) prolactin ($p = 0.003$), 2) LH ($p = 0.006$), 3) testosterone ($p = 0.003$), 4) HbA1C ($p = 0.006$), 5) AMH ($p = 0.004$), 7) T4 ($p = 0.001$), 8) TSH ($p = 0.035$), 9) right ovary mass ($p = 0.003$). In AY Group significant reduction was found for 3 variables 1) AMH ($p = 0.006$), HbA1C ($p = 0.003$), T4 ($p = 0.03$).

Between Group Comparison

A + Y group showed significantly more reduction in HbA1C ($p < 0.001$) and TSH ($p = 0.002$), left ($p = 0.04$) and right ($p = 0.006$) ovary mass as compared to AY group.

DISCUSSION

The present study was intended to study the effect of Yoga as a support therapy modality to Ayurveda treatment of PCOS. It was observed that there was a significant improvement in various endocrine parameters, psychological aspects, perceived stress and ovary mass in both the groups. The results for all the assessed parameters for Yoga + Ayurveda group showed much better results as compared to Ayurveda group.

To the best of our knowledge, based on literature review, there was no study conducted to analyze the effect of both Ayurveda and Yoga as a synthesized module in the management of PCOS prior to the present study.

Previous studies on Yoga and Ayurveda used as a separate tool for maintenance and treatment have shown a beneficial effect on endocrine parameters, symptoms and psychological variables in subjects with PCOS. This study suggests that combining Yoga and Ayurveda in the management of PCOS have better results as compared to just Ayurveda intervention.

In a study, Nidhi et al. demonstrated a significant decrease in fasting insulin and lipid profile, AMH, testosterone PCOS symptoms and anxiety following three months of Yoga practice in adolescent girls having PCOS [28, 29, 30]. Similarly in the present study, it was found that there is a significant improvement in AMH, testosterone, and anxiety. In this study, there was no assessment done on lipid profile and fasting insulin. Instead of insulin, the assessment was done on HbA1C and results showed that there was a significant improvement in Yoga + Ayurveda group.

A study conducted by Dayani et al. showed a significant improvement in 6 months of Ayurveda intervention consisting of Panchakarma and oral administration of Ayurveda medicine in PCOS symptoms like menstrual irregularity, hirsutism, follicle maturity and LH/FSH ratio. It was also reported that 75% of women conceived after 6 months of intervention. Ayurveda intervention implemented in the present study is similar to the previous study but the duration of intervention is comparatively less (3 month). The previous study reported significant improvement in FSH and LH ratio but in the present study, there was no significant improvement in FSH and LH. The possible reason could be because of 6 months of Ayurveda intervention in the previous study and 3 months of intervention could be a lesser time duration for the effect to be positive in assessing in FHS/LH [31].

Similarly, another study by Bhagyashree et al. 3 months administration of 5gms Ayurvedic herbal preparation twice a day for a period of 3 months showed significant improvement in PCOS symptoms such as menstrual irregularities and duration of menstrual bleeding. In this study, they had not assessed any hormonal change but reported symptomatic improvement in PCOS symptoms which may be due to improvement in hormonal level. The present study did not assess the symptoms methodologically but it was noticed that there is a significant improvement in menstrual problems and hirsutism.

Metformin is most widely used medicine in the conventional management of PCOS. In a review role of Metformin in PCOS, it was concluded that metformin is effective in inducing the ovulation and there are marginal benefits in metabolic parameters in PCOS along but it has a significant number of side effects as well. Metformin is recommended along with lifestyle modification but it is not an alternative for diet and exercise [32].

In another study by Deo, 6-month administration of Metformin 1700mg/day in 18 adolescent girls (2 drop outs due to side effects) with PCOS showed improvement in PCOS symptoms, serum progesterone levels, and testosterone. There is no side effect reported in the present study in both the groups, patients comply was 100% for both the treatment groups and results showed significant improvement in testosterone. Also, it was observed that there was a significant improvement in AMH value even with the shorter intervention of 3 months. This indicated that combination of Ayurveda and Yoga can be used as an alternative for Metformin in PCOS treatment. The comparisons discussed indicate alternative therapies such as Ayurveda and Yoga has upper hand and edge over conventional treatment methods in improving endocrine parameters and symptoms in PCOS without any kind of side effects. However, further studies should be confirmed with randomized control trial.

MECHANISM

The exact mechanism and elements of Ayurveda and Yoga in improving endocrine and psychological variables in this study is not known. Some possible reasons could be:

(a) Usage of different herbal drugs in Ayurveda treatment such as saraca asoka (the major component in Ashokaristha), tinas poracardifolia (guduchi) and aloe vera. The mentioned drugs are known to have a positive influence one estrogen and progesterone hormone and have tonic activity on female reproductive organs [33, 34]. The formulations used in ashokaristha has proved to be effective in correcting various female reproductive related problems such as manorrhagia, dysmenorrhea [35].

The practice of Yoga is known to help in reducing sympathetic activity and improve vagal tone by reducing hypothalamo-pituitary-adrenal axis, [36, 37] this might have supported in reducing activity of hypothalamo-ovarian axis which led to improvement in endocrine functions. Further, Yoga practices have proved to be effective in reducing anxiety and depression by reducing cortico-limbic activity.

Studies have shown that women with PCOS frequently suffer from anxiety and depression, also it is well documented that yoga reduces and corrects anxiety and depression. As increased serum cortisol is associated with anxiety and depression and practice of yoga has shown to reduce serum cortisol [38, 39, 40].

Strengths of the Study

First study in records, using both Ayurveda herbs and Yoga as a treatment method for PCOS, No adverse effects was observed in any of the group during the intervention, the adherence rate was excellent due to high participation rate influenced by weekly follow-up and use of social media.

Limitations of the Study

No control group, small sample size, lack of follow-up after the intervention, dietary elements were not strictly followed, only interested participants could take the benefit of weekly meetings and social gathering.

(b) No side effect and low cost associated with the Yoga intervention makes it more acceptable among PCOS women than conventional medicines.
(c) Yogic intervention works at both body and mind level to enhance the quality of life and a sense of wellbeing among PCOS women.

Suggestions for future work-

- Future studies should include the randomized control trials with larger sample size.
- Long term follow-up should be done.

- Longer duration of follow-up with continued home practice for about six months.
- Studies should be focused on the mechanism of action.

Conclusion

The present study suggests that addition of yoga intervention to the herbal medication for PCOS have additional benefits compared to only herbal treatment. This study also suggest that combination of complimentary therapies have synergetic effects in management of PCOS.

References

[1] Azziz, R; Woods, KS; Reyna, R; Key, TJ; Knochenhauer, ES; Yildiz, BO. The prevalence and features of the polycystic ovary syndrome in an unselected population. *J Clin Endocrinol Metab.*, 2004, 89, 2745-2749. 10.1210/jc.2003-032046.

[2] Tehrani, FR; Solaymani-Dodaran, M; Hedayati, M; Azizi, F. Is polycystic ovary syndrome an exception for reproductive aging? *Hum Reprod.*, 2010, 25, 1775-1781, 10, 1093/humrep/deq088.

[3] Balen, AH; Conway, GS; Kaltsas, G; Techatrasak, K; Manning, PJ; West, C; Jacobs, HS. Polycystic ovary syndrome: The spectrum of the disorder in 1741 patients. *Hum Reprod.*, 1995, 10, 2107-2111.

[4] Christakou, CD; Diamanti-Kandarakis, E. Role of androgen excess on metabolic aberrations and cardiovascular risk in women with polycystic ovary syndrome. *Womens Health* (LondEngl)., 2008, 4, 583-594. 10.2217/17455057.4.6.583.

[5] El-Mazny, A; Abou-Salem, N; El-Sherbiny, W. Insulin resistance, dyslipidemia, and metabolic syndrome in women with polycystic ovary syndrome. *Int J Gynaecol Obstet.*, 2010, 109, 239-241. 10.1016/j.ijgo.2010.01.014.

[6] Messinis, IE; Messini, CI; Anifandis, G; Dafopoulos, K. Polycystic ovaries and obesity. *Best Practice & Research Clinical Obstetrics & Gynaecology.*, 2015, May 31, 29(4), 479-88.

[7] Goodarzi, MO; Dumesic, DA; Chazenbalk, G; Azziz, R. Polycystic ovary syndrome: etiology, pathogenesis and diagnosis. *Nature Reviews Endocrinology.*, 2011, Apr 1, 7(4), 219-31.

[8] Nidhi, R; Padmalatha, V; Nagarathna, R; Amritanshu, R. Prevalence of polycystic ovarian syndrome in Indian adolescents. *Journal of Pediatric and Adolescent Gynecology.*, 2011, Aug 31, 24(4), 223-7.

[9] Joshi, B; Mukherjee, S; Patil, A; Purandare, A; Chauhan, S; Vaidya, R. A cross-sectional study of polycystic ovarian syndrome among adolescent and young girls in Mumbai, India. *Indian Journal of Endocrinology and Metabolism*, (2014), 18(3), 317-324. doi:10. 4103/2230-8210.131162.

[10] Asuncion, M; Calvo, RM; San Millan, JL; Sancho, J; Avila, S. Escobar-Morreale HF2000 A prospective study of the prevalence of the polycystic ovary syndrome in unselected Caucasian women from Spain. *J Clin Endocrinol Metab*, 85, 2434–2438.

[11] Tehrani, FR; Simbar, M; Tohidi, M; Hosseinpanah, F; Azizi, F. The prevalence of polycystic ovary syndrome in a community sample of Iranian population: Iranian PCOS prevalence study. *Reproductive Biology and Endocrinology.*, 2011, Mar 25, 9(1), 1.

[12] Norman, RJ; Noakes, M; Wu, R; et al. Improving reproductive performance in overweight/obese women with effective weight management. *Hum Reprod Update*, 2004, 10, 267–280.

[13] Hardy, ML; Coulter, I; Venuturupalli, S; Roth, EA; Favreau, J; Morton, SC; Shekelle, P. Ayurvedic *Interventions for Diabetes Mellitus: A Systematic Review: Summary.*

[14] Bhogayata, K; Sharma, PP; Patel, BR. A clinical evaluation of Saptaparna (Alstoniascholaris L., R. Br.) on essential hypertension. *AYU (An International Quarterly Journal of Research in Ayurveda).*, 2009, Jul 1, 30(3), 318.

[15] Chopra, A. Ayurvedic medicine and arthritis. *Rheumatic Disease Clinics of North America.*, 2000, Feb 1, 26(1), 133-44.

[16] Sairam, K; Dorababu, M; Goel, RK; Bhattacharya, SK. Antidepressant activity of standardized extract of Baco-pamonniera in experimental models of depression in rats. *Phytomedicine.*, 2002, Dec 31, 9(3), 207-11.

[17] Khot, BM; Lad, MD; Jagannath, A. Clinical Efficacy of Ayurveda Treatment on Polycystic Ovarian Syndrome. *IOSR Journal of Pharmacy*, www.Iosrphr.org Volume. 2013, 3, 21-5.

[18] Siriwardene, SD; Karunathilaka, LP; Kodituwakku, ND; Karunarathne, YA. Clinical efficacy of Ayurveda treatment regimen on Subfertility with poly cystic ovarian syndrome (PCOS). *AYU (An International Quarterly Journal of Research in Ayurveda).*, 2010, Jan 1, 31(1), 24.

[19] Raman, S; Palep, HS. Alternative therapies in polycystic ovarian syndrome. *Insulin.*, 2010, 1(2), 3.

[20] Kadam, K; Allahbadia, G; Arora, S; Gandhi, G; Allahbadia, S; Kaur, K. Hyponiddan Indian with poly-cystic ovarian syndrome. Abstracts of the 22nd Annual Meeting of the ESHRE, Prague, Czech Republic, 1821 June 2006. K. Kadam, G. Allahbadia, S. Arora, G. Gandhi, S. Allahbadia, K. Kaur. *Hyponiddan Indian Herbomineral Preparation is Equally*, P-468.

[21] Schure, MB; Christopher, J; Christopher, S. Mind-body medicine and the art of self-care: Teaching mindfulness to counseling students through yoga, meditation, and qigong. *Journal of Counseling and Development*: *JCD.*, 2008, Jan 1, 86(1), 47.

[22] Mohanty, S; Metri, K; Nagaratna, R; Nagendra, HR. Immediate Effect Of Mind Sound Resonance Technique (Msrt-A Yogic Relaxation Technique) On Cognitive Function In Type 2 Diabetes. *Voice of Research.*, 2015 Jun, 44.

[23] Yoga for rheumatoid arthritis. K Metri. *Alternative and Complementary Therapies*, 22 (4), 175-179.

[24] Nidhi, R; Padmalatha, V; Nagarathna, R; Amritanshu, R. Effects of a holistic yoga program on endocrine parameters in adolescents with polycystic ovarian syndrome: a randomized controlled trial. *The Journal of Alternative and Complementary Medicine.*, 2013, Feb 1, 19(2), 153-60.

[25] Nidhi, R; Padmalatha, V; Nagarathna, R; Ram, A. Effect of a yoga program on glucose metabolism and blood lipid levels in adolescent girls with polycystic ovary syndrome. International *Journal of Gynecology & Obstetrics.*, 2012 Jul, 31, 118(1), 37-41.

[26] Nidhi, R; Padmalatha, V; Nagarathna, R; Amritanshu, R. Effect of holistic yoga program on anxiety symptoms in adolescent girls with polycystic ovarian syndrome: A randomized control trial. *International Journal of Yoga.*, 2012, Jul 1, 5(2), 112.

[27] Nidhi, R; Padmalatha, V; Nagarathna, R; Amritanshu, R. Effect of yoga program on quality of life in adolescent polycystic ovarian syndrome: a randomized control trial. *Applied Research in Quality of Life.*, 2013, Sep 1, 8(3), 373-83.

[28] Nidhi, R; Padmalatha, V; Nagarathna, R; Ram, A. Effect of a yoga program on glucose metabolism and blood lipid levels in adolescent girls with polycystic ovary syndrome. International *Journal of Gynecology & Obstetrics.*, 2012 Jul, 31, 118(1), 37-41.

[29] Nidhi, R; Padmalatha, V; Nagarathna, R; Amritanshu, R. Effects of a holistic yoga program on endocrine parameters in adolescents with polycystic ovarian syndrome: A randomized controlled trial. *The Journal of Alternative and Complementary Medicine.*, 2013, Feb 1, 19(2), 153-60.

[30] Nidhi, R; Padmalatha, V; Nagarathna, R; Amritanshu, R. Effect of holistic yoga program on anxiety symptoms in adolescent girls with polycystic ovarian syndrome: A randomized control trial. *International Journal of Yoga.*, 2012, Jul 1, 5(2), 112.

[31] Siriwardene, SD; Karunathilaka, LP; Kodituwakku, ND; Karunarathne, YA. Clinical efficacy of Ayurveda treatment regimen on Subfertility with poly cystic ovarian syndrome (PCOS). *AYU* (*An International Quarterly Journal of Research in Ayurveda*)., 2010, Jan 1, 31(1), 24.

[32] Diamanti-Kandarakis, E; Economou, F; Palimeri, S; Christakou, C. Metformin in polycystic ovary syndrome. *Annals of the New York Academy of Sciences*., 2010, Sep 1, 1205(1), 192-8.

[33] Mitra, SK; Gopumadhavan, S; Venkataranganna, MV; Sarma, DN; Anturlikar, SD. Uterine tonic activity of U-3107 (EveCare), A herbal preparation in rats. *Indian Journal of Pharmacology*., 1999, 31, 200-3.

[34] Satyavathi, GV; Raina, MK; Sharma, M. *Indian Medicinal Plants*, New Delhi, ICMR Publications, 1976, 45.

[35] Akhtar, Y; Alamgir, M; Khan, MT; Hannan, JM; Choudhuri, M. A single blind randomised placebo controlled clinical trial of a classical Ayurvedic formulation Ashokarista in the treatment of menorrhagia and dysmenorrhoea. *Oriental Pharmacy and Experimental Medicine*., 2007, 7(4), 372-8.

[36] Telles, S; Nagarathna, R; Nagendra, HR. Breathing through a particular nostril can alter metabolism and autonomic activities. *Indian Journal of Physiology and Pharmacology*., 1994, Apr 1, 38, 133.

[37] Ross, A; Thomas, S. The health benefits of yoga and exercise: a review of comparison studies. *The Journal of Alternative and Complementary Medicine*., 2010, Jan 1, 16(1), 3-12.

[38] Benson, S; Hahn, S; Tan, S; et al. Prevalence and implications of anxiety in polycystic ovary syndrome: Results of an Internet-based survey in Germany. *Hum Reprod*, 2009, 24, 1446–1451.

[39] Kerchner, A; Lester, W; Stuart, SP; Dokras, A. Risk of depression and other mental health disorders in women with polycystic ovary syndrome: A longitudinal study. *Fertil Steril*, 2009, 91, 207–212.

[40] Telles, S; Gaur, V; Balkrishna, A. Effect of a yoga practice session and a yoga theory session on state anxiety. *Percept Mot Skills*, 2009, 109, 924–930.

In: Manipulation of Stem Cells for Disease Benefits
Editor: Prasad Koka
ISBN: 978-1-53615-468-9

Chapter 17

Effect of Integrated Yoga as an Add-On to Physiotherapy on Walking Index, ESR, Pain, and Spasticity among Subjects with Traumatic Spinal Cord Injury: A Randomized Control Study

Monali Madhusmita[1,*], T. M. Srinivasan[1], John Ebnezar[1], H. R. Nagendra[1] and Patita Pabana Mohanty[2]
[1]SVYASA University, Bangalore, India
[2]Department of Physiotherapy, SVNIRTAR, Odisha, India

Abstract

Introduction: Traumatic Spinal Cord Injury (TSCI) is an injury to the spinal cord that results in temporary or permanent motor, sensory, and cognitive deficits.

The current conventional approach of TSCI management includes surgery, pharmacology, and physical therapy, which have some limitations and are associated with side effects. Yoga is a form of mind-body medicine found to be effective in several neurological disorders as an add-on to other therapies.

Aim: The present study intended to see the effect of Integrated Yoga (IY) intervention as an add-on to the physiotherapy on walking index, ESR, pain and spasticity among subjects with TSCI.

Methods: The study was conducted in a Rehabilitation Centre at Swami Vivekananda National Institute of Rehabilitation, Training and research (SVNIRTAR), Odisha. A total of 125 paraplegics within age range 18-60 years were randomly assigned to either integrated Yoga therapy + physiotherapy group (IY + PT) group (n = 62, age = 33.97 ± 10.00) or Physiotherapy (PT) group (n = 63, age = 32.84 ± 9.47). The participants in PT + IY group received one month of integrated yoga intervention consisting of yogic

* Corresponding Author's E-mail: monaliyoga@gmail.com.

postures, yogic breathing techniques & chanting, and yogic relaxation practices along with physical therapy. Yoga session lasted for 75 mins per day and 6 days per week. PT group participants received only physiotherapy intervention for one month. All the participants were assessed for Erythrocyte Sedimentation Rate (ESR), Walking Index for Spinal Cord Injury II (WISCI II), Multidimensional Pain Inventory (MPI), and Modified-Modified Ashworth Scale (MMAS) at the baseline and after one month.

Results: We found statically significant changes in 4 variables for IY + PT group 1) Erythrocyte Sedimentation Rate ($P < 0.001$), 2) WISCI II ($P < 0.001$) MPI-S1 ($P < 0.001$), MPI-S2 ($P = 0.003$), & MPI-S3 ($P = 0.003$), and 4) MMAS ($P < 0.001$) after one month of intervention compared to baseline.

Compared to PT group, IY + PT group showed significantly better improvement in WISCI II ($P < 0.001$), MPI-S3 ($P = 0.003$), and MMAS ($P < 0.001$).

Conclusion: The resent study suggests the usefulness of an IY intervention add on to physiotherapy in the management of patients with paraplegia.

INTRODUCTION

Traumatic Spinal cord injury (TSCI) is a medically complex and life-disrupting condition. It is an insult to the spinal cord which leads to temporary or permanent, sensory, motor and autonomic deficits resulting in severe disability (Alexander, Biering-Sorensen, Bodner, et al., 2009). Paraplegia is most commonly observed condition after TSCI. Paraplegia affects the activities of daily living and puts socioeconomic burden on family of an individual (Wyndaele & Wyndaele, 2006). Spasticity is the most common complication which affects gait and activities of daily living to a higher degree. It is also involved in pain aggravation, deformities and contractures (Burchiel, Kim, et al., 2001). Evidences from several studies suggest that paraplegia characterized by increased systematic inflammation shown by increased ESR (Hausmann, 2003). Systematic inflammation in individual with paraplegia is associated with increased respiratory and bladder infection, further it affects the prognosis of TSCI (Diana, Cardenas, Thomas, Hooton, 1995; Gris, Hamilton, Weaver, 2008).

Available treatment for paraplegia in convention medicine is surgery, pharmacological intervention and physical therapies. Despite, large portion of paraplegics report persistent functional disability, spasticity and pain. Further, conventional therapies have limited efficacy in improving systematic inflammation (Bethea, John; Dietrich, Dalton, 2002).

In order to enhance the present management of paraplegia and to get better treatment outcome addition of other supportive therapies has become mandatory.

Yoga is a form of mind body interventions. Yoga is a lifestyle meant for physical, mental, social and spiritual growth of an individual. In present days Yoga is perceived as practice of asanas, pranayama, and meditation and various kinds of yogic relaxation methods (Manas, Kashinath, Nagaratna, Nagendra, 2017).

Several evidences from scientific studies suggest the variety of health benefiting effects of yoga. Yoga has been found useful in many chronic health conditions including various neurological disorders such as multiple sclerosis, stroke, Parkinson's disease etc. Studies on Yoga shows to improve gait, spasticity, pain, inflammation and QoL among neurologically impaired patients (Mishra, Singh, Bunch, Zhang, 2012).

For individuals with SCI, the injury permanently transforms their lives. Indeed, SCI can result in diverse motor, sensory and autonomic problems (Hou, Rabchevsky, 2014). Mobility impairment (e.g., paraplegia and tetraplegia), bowel and bladder incontinence, loss of sensation and sexual dysfunction are common following SCI (Guilcher, Craven, Lemieux-Charles, et al, 2013). As a result, individuals with SCI have complex health needs as their condition includes chronic multi-morbidity, mainly associated with the development of several secondary health conditions (e.g., pain and pressure ulcers) (Guilcher, Craven, Lemieux, Charles, et al., 2013). In addition, compared with community estimates, higher rates of psychological disorders can be present in 17%–25% of individuals with SCI (Khazaeipour, Taheri-Otaghsara, Naghdi, 2015). Particularly, between 18% and 37% of individual with SCI experience depression (Williams, Murray, 2015).

From a clinical perspective, understanding the needs of individuals with SCI, knowing the person and working with the family can be beneficial to guide their healthcare and improve outcomes (Stiens, Fawber, Yuhas, 2013). As unmet needs have a direct relationship with diminished quality of life (Sweet, Noreau, Leblond, et al., 2014), it is mandatory to understand them and to find ways to meet them. In consequence, obtaining a comprehensive picture of needs by integrating the different perspectives of professionals, family caregivers and individuals with SCI is paramount. The challenge is in understanding the evolution of these needs as they change over time. The literature on SCI needs indicates that in the first-year post discharge, the fulfilment of critical needs (e.g., housing and transportation) is below 60% (Beauregard, Guindon, Noreau, et al., 2012),while the long-term care needed is higher than the care received for information and psychosocial care needs (van Loo, Post, Bloemen, et al, 2010).Rehabilitation plays a central role in maximizing function and facilitating community reintegration following SCI (Anthony, Ralph, Sukhvinder, et al., 2017).

Strategies that seek out the complementary effects of combination treatments and that efficiently integrate relevant technical advances in biomechanics represent an untapped potential and are likely to have an immediate impact. There are no published randomized control trials till date available to explore the efficacy of combination of complementary alternative therapies with conventional main stream rehabilitation treatments, in the management of SCI.

Hence, in present study we assessed the impact of one month of yoga intervention as an add-on to physiotherapy on ESR, walking Index, pain and spasticity among participants with paraplegia.

METHODOLOGY

Study Participants

Patient admitted to the Rehabilitation Centre at Swami Vivekanand National Institute of Rehabili-tation, Training and research (SVNIRTAR), Odisha.

Participants in this study were patients with post traumatic paraplegia within age range 18-60 years after 6 months of primary rehabilitation. Both male and female individuals were considered for the study.

Sample Size

The sample size was calculated using G-power software from the previous study (Sander et al., 2013), with the effect size: 0.546 of the Spinal Cord Independence Measure (SCIM); Adjustment scale being: Alpha = 0.05, Beta = 0.85. Calculated sample size was 124.

Inclusion and Exclusion Criteria

Patients admitted to Swami Vivekananda National Institute Rehabilitation, Training and Research (SVNIRTAR), Odisha, of both genders and within age range of 18 – 60 years, those who have sustained a traumatic spinal cord injury for a minimum of 6 months prior to consent and have completed their primary rehabilitation, and are Incomplete SCI patient with American spinal injury Association impairment scale (AIS)C and (AIS)D with injury to the spinal cord from level anywhere between T1 to L5.

Participants with contraindications to FES such as cardiac pacemaker, epilepsy, lower limb fracture or pregnancy, who are likely to experience clinically significant autonomic dysreflexia and/or orthostatic hypotension in response to electrical stimulation or prolonged upright postures, having chronic systemic diseases, e.g., hepatitis C or HIV-AIDS, having an existing stage 3 or 4 pressure ulcer according to the National Pressure Ulcer Advisory Panel classification, have had recent major trauma or surgery within the last 6 months, having degenerative myelopathy, neoplasm, or congenital spinal cord anomalies and concomitant medical problems that might have influenced everyday function, such as malignancy, brain injury or mental diseases were excluded.

SCREENING TOOL

Standardized neurological examination protocol of the American Spinal Injury Association (ASIA).

International Standards for Neurological Classification of Spinal Cord Injury (ASIA Impairment Scale) classifies motor and sensory impairment as follows:

- ***ASIA A*** – No motor or sensory function is preserved below the level of injury (and in the sacral segments S4 – S5).
- ***ASIA B*** – Sensory but not motor function is preserved below the neurological level (includes the sacral segments S4 – S5).
- ***ASIA C*** – Motor function is preserved below the neurological level, but too little to represent a practically usable function (more than half of key muscles below the neurological level have a muscle grade less than 3).
- ***ASIA D*** – Motor function is preserved below the neurological level, to an extent that provides practically usable function (at least half of key muscles below the neurological level have a muscle grade of 3 or more on a scale from 0 to 5).
- ***ASIA E*** – Motor and sensory functions are normal.

ASIA A implies a complete injury, **ASIA B – D** describe incomplete injuries.

ETHICAL CONSIDERATIONS

The study protocol was passed by S-VYASA's Institutional Ethics Committee. All procedures were performed according to the Declaration of Helsinki research ethics. Signed informed consent of all subjects was obtained after explaining the nature of study in detail and the voluntary nature of participation. Confidentiality was assured as part of the research process.

DESIGN OF THE STUDY

Two group pre–post randomized wait-list control (WLC) design is adopted.

RANDOMISATION

To avoid selection biases Sequentially Numbered Opaque Sealed Envelops (SNOSE) is adopted. After screening, the patients are asked to select an opaque envelop from the bunch which is randomly arranged and the number it contains is not visible outside. The envelopes are sequentially numbered but the number it contains is not visible outside. The patients are then allocated to the experimental or WLC group according to the number they receive. Each number is separately assigned to either Experimental or WLC group randomly.

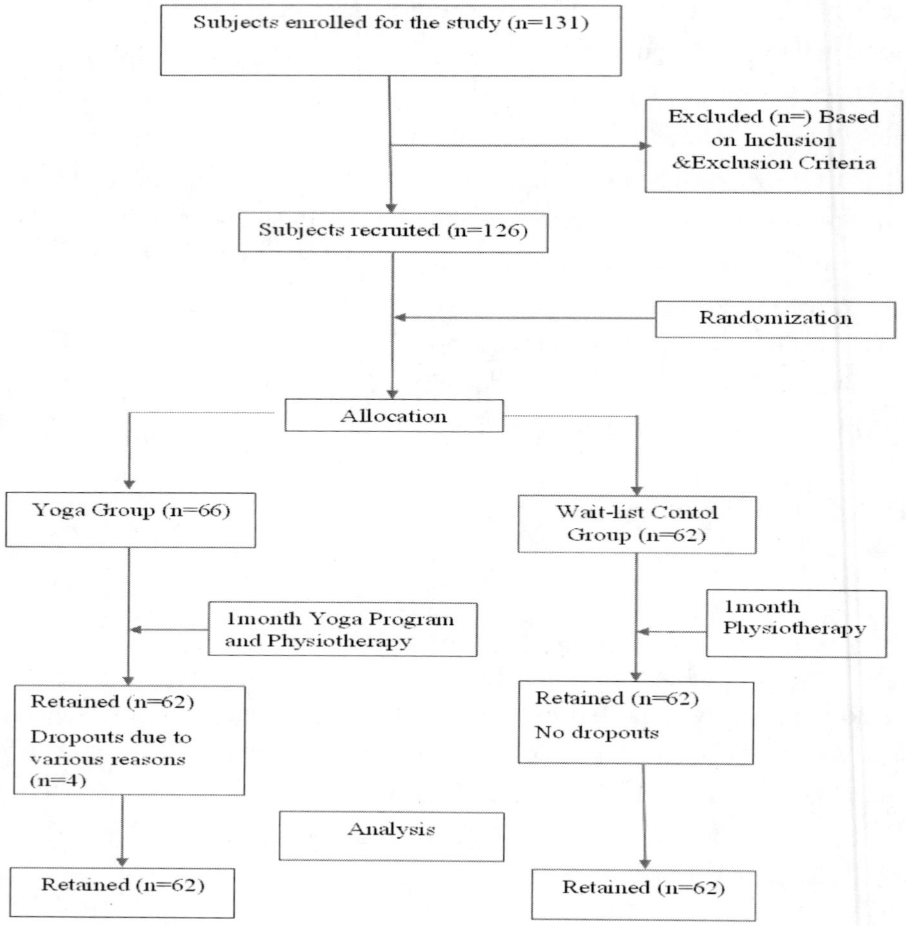

Figure 1. Trial Profile.

Objective Assessment Tools

Walking Index for SCIII (WISCIII)

Walking Index for Spinal Cord Injury (WISCI II) assesses the amount of physical assistance needed, as well as devices required, for walking following paralysis that results from Spinal Cord Injury (SCI). Designed to be a more precise measure of improvement in walking ability specific to SCI. It rank orders the ability of a person to walk 10m after a spinal cord injury from most to least severe impairment (Ditunno & Dittuno, 2001).

American Spinal Injury Assessment (ASIA) Motor and Sensory Scores

The ASIA Impairment Scale builds on the earlier Frankel scale, but includes a number of significant improvements. The International Standards for Neurological Classification of Spinal Cord Injury (ISNCSCI) were developed by the American Spinal Injury Association (ASIA) as a universal classification tool for spinal cord injury (SCI), depending upon motor and sensory impairment that results from a SCI. It assesses Functional Mobility, Strength and Upper Extremity Function. A tapered piece of cotton and a safety pin is required to administer the test, which usually takes 10-60 minutes (Furlan et al., 2008).

Modified Ashworth Scale to Measure Spasticity

Originally developed to assess the effects of antispasticity drugs on spasticity in Multiple Sclerosis. Modified Ashworth: measures spasticity in patients with lesions of the Central Nervous System. Original Ashworth Scale: Tests resistance to passive movement about a joint with varying degrees of velocity scores range from 0-4, with 5 choices. A score of 1 indicates no resistance and 5 indicates rigidity. Modified Ashworth Scale: Similar to Ashworth, but adds a 1+ scoring category to indicate resistance through less than half of the movement. Thus scores range from 0-4, with 6 choices (Bohannon & Smith, 1987).

Anthropometry: Body Mass Index (BMI)

The body mass index (BMI), or Quetelet index, is a measure of relative weight based on an individual's mass and height. It is defined as the individual's body mass divided by the square of their height – with the value universally being given in units of kg/m^2 (Eknoyan and Garabed, 2007).

Bio-Markers

Erythrocyte Sedimentation Rate (ESR)

An erythrocyte sedimentation rate (ESR) is a type of blood test that measures how quickly erythrocytes (red blood cells) settle at the bottom of a test tube that contains a blood sample. Normally, red blood cells settle relatively slowly. A faster-than-normal rate may indicate inflammation in the body. Inflammation is part of your immune response system. It can be a reaction to an infection or injury. ESR can be marker of altered immune response seen in people with SCI (Edsberg, Jennifer, Rajna, et al., 2015).

Assessments

The assessments were done on day1 and day30. Fasting blood was drawn from the study participants early in the morning and send to the Institute's Pathology Lab to test for ESR. The Physical Examination tests like MMAS and WISCI II were carried out by an Expert Physiotherapist who was blinded to the study design. MPI was filled by the participants with the guidance of trained staff.

Subjective Assessment Tools

Multidimensional Pain Inventory (Spinal Cord Injury Version) – MPI-SCI

A spinal cord injury version of the MPI that assesses the severity and impact of chronic pain, emotional and physical adaptation to persistent pain, and social support. The internal consistency of the MPI-SCI sub-scales ranged from fair (.60) for affective distress to substantial (.94) for pain interference with activities. With the exception of the support and life control sub-scales, all others showed adequate test-retest reliability. The MPI-SCI measures impact of pain on activities of daily living, which corresponds to achievements and activities of daily living, and subjective evaluations and reactions of Dijker's Model. Each item is scored on a 7-point scale. Scale scores are computed by summing over all items and then the mean is composed based on the number of scale items. It is not possible to obtain a total score (Turk et al., 1983).

INTERVENTION

This study is conducted in a residential rehabilitation centre at SVNIRTAR, Odisha and the intervention period is one month.

PT Intervention for Both Groups

Proprioceptive Neuro-muscular Facilitation, slow and sustained stretching, prolong icing, strengthening of anti-gravity muscles, functional electrical stimulation & gait training.

Add-On for Group YPT: For One Month, IAYT with Physiotherapy

The specific module of 'Integrated approach of Yoga therapy (IAYT)' for Spinal Cord injury management was developed by using the concepts from traditional yoga scriptures (Patanjali Yoga Sutras, Upanishads and Yoga Vasishtha) that highlights a holistic approach to health management at physical, mental, emotional and intellectual levels. The practices consisted of asana chosen specifically for Spina Cord Injury (yoga postures), pranayama, kriyas, relaxation techniques, Chanting of *OM* and *Mahamrytunjaya Mantra* and yogic counselling for stress management. The physical practices (spinal cord injury special techniques) progressed from safe yogic movements to yoga postures to provide traction like effect and channelize the vital energy flow all through the spine.

Table 1. Time-table for Yoga and Physiotherapy group

Therapy	Intervention	Time Period
Active Therapy	1. Yoga Special Technique for Spinal Cord Injury	45 minutes
	2. Mind Sound Resonance Technique (MSRT)	30 minutes
Passive Therapy	3. Proprioceptive Neuro-muscular Facilitation	20 minutes
	4. Slow and Sustained stretching	45 minutes
	5. Prolong icing	30–45 min
	6. Strengthening of Anti-spastic muscles	45-60 min
	7. Functional Electrical Stimulation	30 min
	8. Gait training	15 min
Counseling	Yogic Counseling	40 min. twice/week

Table 2. Time-table for Physiotherapy group

Therapy	Intervention	Time Period
Active Therapy	1. Active range formation exercise (AROM)	45 minutes
	2. Listening to soothing music	30 minutes
Passive Therapy	3. Proprioceptive Neuro-muscular Facilitation	20 minutes
	4. Slow and Sustained stretching	45 minutes
	5. Prolong icing	30–45 min
	6. Strengthening of Anti-spastic muscles	45-60 min
	7. Functional Electrical Stimulation	30 min
	8. Gait training	15 min
Counseling	Psychological Counseling	40 min. twice/week

Data Analysis

Data were analysed using the R-Studio. The research team applied the Shapiro-Wilk test to assess normality. The paired sample test and Wilcoxon's signed-rank test were used to find differences within a group, for normal and non-normal data, respectively. $P < .05$ was considered as statistically significant change for all the variables Gender and other categorical variables were analysed using $\chi2$ test. The independent sample t-test was used to check the difference between groups for demographic measures.

RESULTS

One-hundred-twenty-five paraplegic patients participated in the study. Both groups were comparable at the baseline in terms of age (p = 0.519, independent t-test) and gender distribution (p = 0.636, $\chi 2$ test).

Table 3. Comparison of the continuous variables of experimental and wait-list control group before intervention (baseline), at end of therapy

Experimental Group				Control Group			
Variables	Pre	Post	% Change	Pre	Post	P value	% Change
WISCI II	7.03 ± 3.87	11.79 ± 4.15***@@@	67.68	6.57 ± 2.16	7.87 ± 2.33***	<0.001	90.82
ESR	42.13 ± 26.14	27.63 ± 18.75***@@@	34.42	42.57 ± 26.58	41.52 ± 21.42	0.58	2.48
MPI-SCI_S1	4.36 ± 1.03	3.73 ± 1.22***	14.38	4.5 ± 1.87	4.13 ± 1.89***	<0.001	8.27
MPI-SCI_S2	3.45 ± 0.84	3.11 ± 0.81**	9.69	3.58 ± 0.99	3.55 ± 0.97	0.54	0.75
MPI-SCI_S3	2.53 ± 1.34	2.07 ± 1.1**@@	18.23	2.92 ± 1.2	2.74 ± 1.3	0.023	6.13

Legends: WISCI II (Walking index for SCIII), ESR (Erythrocyte Sedimentation Rate), MPI-SCI_S1 (Multidimensional Pain Inventory-Section1), MPI-SCI_S2 (Multidimensional Pain Inventory-Section2), MPI-SCI_S3 (Multidimensional Pain Inventory-Section3).

Table 4. Comparison of the categorical variables of experimental and WLC groups

Categorical Variables							
Variable		**PRE1(G1)**	**PRE2 (G2)**	χ^2	**POST1 (G1)**	**POST2(G2)**	χ^2
MMAS	Grade: 1	4 (6.45%)	9 (14.3%)	0.505	36 (58.06%)	16 (25.4%)	<0.001
	Grade: 2	30 (48.4%)	28 (44.44%)		26 (41.9%)	34 (53.97%)	
	Grade: 3	26 (41.9%)	25(39.68%)		0	13 (20.6%)	
	Grade: 4	2 (3.23%)	1(1.6%)		0	0	

* P<0.05, ** P<0.01, *** P<0.001; Within group: pre compared with post.

@@@P <0.001, @@P <0.01; Comparison between group: Pre compared with Pre, and Post compared with Post.

The tables show the number of participants with grade of spasticity before and after the study across the groups.

Within-Group Comparisons

Experimental group: At the completion of one-month practice of Integrated Yoga with Physio-therapy, the study found significant reductions in Variables: (1) 34.42% for Erythrocyte Sedimentation Rate (P < 0.001), 67.68% for Walking index for SCIII

(WISCI II) (P = 0.001), 14.38% for Multi-dimensional Pain Inventory (MPI-S1) (P < 0.001), 9.69% for MPI-S2 (P = 0.003), 18.23% for MPI-S3 (P = 0.003), and Modified-Modified Ashworth Scale (MMAS) (P < 0.001).

Control group: At the completion of one-month practice of Physiotherapy only, the study found significant reductions in Variables: 2.48% for Erythrocyte Sedimentation Rate (P = 0.58), 19.82% for Walking index for SCIII (WISCI II) (P < 0.001), 8.27% for Multidimensional Pain Inventory (MPI-S1), P < 0.001, 0.75% for MPI-S2, P = 0.54, 6.13% for MPI-S3, P = 0.023, and Modified-Modified Ashworth Scale (MMAS).

Between-Group Comparisons

When the groups were compared, the study found the Experimental group's results for five variables were significantly different than those of the control group: Erythrocyte Sedimentation Rate (ESR), P < 0.001, Walking index for SCIII (WISCI II), P < 0.000,Multidimensional Pain Inventory: MPI-S1, P = 0.43,MPI-S2, P = 0.07, MPI-S3, P = 0.003 and Modified-Modified Ashworth Scale (MMAS), P < 0.000. Baseline scores were matched for other variables except for MPI-S3.

Variable	**PRE(G1) Vs PRE(G2)**	**POST(G1) Vs POST(G2)**
WISCI II	0.411	<0.001
ESR	0.925	<0.001
MPI-S1	0.476	0.427
MPI-S2	0.097	0.067
MPI-S3	0.007	0.003

DISCUSSION

This study aimed to compare the effect of add-on of IY intervention to Physiotherapy, in the management of spinal cord injury (SCI) patients. At the end of one-month the study found significant reductions in Variables: Erythrocyte Sedimentation Rate, Walking index for SCIII (WISCI II), Multidimensional Pain Inventory: MPI-S1, (MPI-S2), MPI-S3 and Modified-Modified Ashworth Scale (MMAS).

The current study clearly shows that add-on of IAYT was effective make the performance of YG was better than WLC.

Mechanisms underlying the beneficial effects of Yoga practice on spinal cord injury patients are not yet well understood. Yoga represents a form of mind-body fitness. IAYT includes a combination of asanas, pranayama, meditation and relaxation, and internally directed mental focus on awareness of self, breathing, and energy (Rajashree, Hankey, Nagendra, Mohanty, 2016). However, Muscle conditioning during yoga's intense stretching postures helps by improving oxidative capacity and strength of skeletal muscles, flexibility, endurance, coordination, power, static and dynamic stability, decreasing glycogen utilization, in turn improving physical performance and increasing walking pace and stride length (Katiyar, Bihari, 2006). This possibly explains for the improvement in scores of Walking Index for SCIII (WISCI II), and shows significant difference between the groups post intervention.

MSRT technique leads to deep relaxation, which helps in downregulating the hypothalamus-pituitary-axis and reduces anxiety (Hewitt, 2009) and stress (Robins, Hendin, Trzesniewski, 2001). By reducing the activation and reactivity of the sympathoadrenal system and the hypothalamic pituitary adrenal (HPA) axis and promoting feelings of well-being, Yoga may alleviate the effects of stress and bring up multiple positive downstream effects on neuroendocrine status, metabolic function and related systemic inflammatory responses. These results may also explain the improvements in pain in YG more than WLC {Multidimensional Pain Inventory: MPI-S1, (MPI-S2), MPI-S3}, and reduction in Erythrocyte Sedimentation Rate (ESR) values which is highly significant in YG.

Deep relaxation technique, an important component of IAYT showed significant reductions in the yoga group's spasticity, possibly due to modulation of cardiac autonomic function and cardiorespiratory efficiency (Tomas, 2011). It may also synchronize neural elements in the brain, leading to ANS changes, resulting parasympathetic dominance and blunted sympathetic activity leading to reduced spasticity. Pranayama modifies various inflatory and deflatory lung reflexes and interacts with central neural elements to improve homeostatic control (Tandon, Tripathi, 2012).

Cerebrospinal Fluid (CSF) and Traumatic Spinal Cord Injury (TSCI)

The spinal cord injury may result in cellular alterations in cerebrospinal fluid (CSF) of the TSCI patients. These changes can be experimentally evaluated *ex vivo* by isolating the CD34+ progenitor stem cells from the CSF of the pre and post TSCI patients. Any severe damage to CSF of these TSCI patients may be reflected in the CD34+ stem cells differentiation. Since the colony formation is controlled by cytokines, these growth factor changes may also be measured using ELISA, on the CSF of the pre and post TSCI patients. Hence, whether cytokine therapy could be considered for the TSCI patients may be of relevance.

Scope and Limitations of the Study

This is the first randomized controlled study of yoga for spinal cord injured patients with ASIA score C and D (paraplegics). It used IAYT, and its reasonable sample size offers good evidence for the benefits of yoga-based rehabilitation. Having additional subgroups stratified as motor and sensory complete and incomplete would have made the study more vigorous. In addition, we did not investigate radiological findings, such as MRI, CT-scan or X-rays, which would have detailed clearly the clinical outcomes, providing a fuller picture of subject's anatomy and physiology. Similarly, assessments of neurological biomarkers (e.g., neuroproteomics) in body fluids would throw light on mechanisms. Objective measurement of bio-energy fields of patients with GDV or BIOWELL would also explore the positive changes in energy state and mood. We would recommend a multicentre RCT to confirm results of the study, with a longer follow-up of 6 months or more to evaluate long-term efficacy.

Conclusion

Present study indicated that addition of integrated yoga intervention to physiotherapy have beneficial effects in terms of improving pain, inflammation, gait and spasticity among patients with paraplegia. Further, this study also suggest the implementation of yoga intervention in the conventional rehabilitation program for traumatic spinal injury patients.

Conflict of Interest

Authors declare no conflict of interest.

Acknowledgments

We are thankful to all the participants of this study. We also thank you to all the staff members of rehabilitation center.

Ethical Compliance

The authors have stated all possible conflicts of interest within this work. The authors have stated all sources of funding for this work. If this work involved human participants, informed consent was received from each individual. If this work involved human participants, it was conducted in accordance with the 1964 Declaration of Helsinki. If this work involved experiments with humans or animals, it was conducted in accordance with the related institutions' research ethics guidelines.

REFERENCES

Botterell EH, Jousse AT, Kraus AS, Thompson MG, Wynne Jones M, Geisler WO. A model for the future care of acute spinal cord injuries. *Ann R Coll Phys Surg Can.* 1975;8:193-218.

De Vivo MJ. Epidemiology of traumatic spinal cord injury. In: Kirshblum S, Campagnolo DI, De Lisa JA, eds. *Spinal Cord Medicine.* Baltimore, Md: Lippincott Williams & Wilkins;2002:69-81.

Dean CM, Richards CL, Malouin F. Task-related circuit training improves performance of locomotor tasks in chronic stroke: A randomized, controlled pilot trial. *Arch Phys Med Rehabil.* 2000;81:409–17.

Ditunno PL, Patrick M, Stineman M, B Morganti, Townson AF and Ditunno JF, Cross-cultural differences in preference for recovery of mobility among spinal cord injury rehabilitation professionals, *Spinal Cord*. 2006;44, 567-575.

Garland SJ, Stevenson TJ, Ivanova T. Postural responses to unilateral arm perturbation in young, elderly, and hemiplegic subjects. *Arch Phys Med Rehabil*. 1997;78: 1072–7.

Gjone R, Nordlie L. Incidence of traumatic paraplegia and tetraplegia in Norway: a statistical survey of the years 1974 and1975. *Paraplegia* 1978;16:88-93.

Go BK, De Vivo MJ, Richards JS. The epidemiology of spinal cord injury. In: Stover SL, De Lisa JA, Whiteneck GG, eds. *Spinal Cord Injury*. Gaithersburg, Md: Aspen; 1995: 21-55.

Harvey, Lisa A, Adrian J Byak, Marsha Ostrovskaya, Joanne Glinsky, Lyndall Katte and Robert Herbert, Randomised trial of the effects of four weeks of daily stretch on extensibility of ham string muscles in people with spinal cord injuries, *Australian Journal of Physiotherapy*. 2003 Vol. 49, 176– 181.

Kahn NN, Feldman SP, Bauman WA. Lower extremity functional electrical stimulation decreases platelet aggregation and blood coagulation in persons with chronic spinal cord injury: a pilot study. *J Spinal Cord Med.* 2010; 33(2):150-8.

Katiyar SK, Bihari S. Role of pranayama in rehabilitation of COPD patients a randomized controlled study. *Indian J Allergy Asthma Immunol* 2006;20:98e104. (Katiyar, Bihari, 2006).

Kim E. Innes, Heather K. Vincent. The Influence of Yoga-Based Programs on Risk Profiles in Adults with Type 2 Diabetes Mellitus: A Systematic Review. *Evid Based Complement Alternat Med.* 2007 Dec;4(4):469-86. doi: 10.1093/ecam/nel103.

Kraus JF. Injury of the head and spinal cord: the epidemiology relevance of the medical literature published from 1960 to1978. *J Neurosurg* 1980;53:3-10.

Krause JS, Sternberg M, Lottes S, et al. Mortality after spinal cord injury: an 11 year prospective study. *Arch Phys Med Rehabil*. Aug1997;78(8):815-21.

Kurtzke JF. Epidemiology of spinal cord injury. *Exp Neurol* 1975;48:163-236.

Li M, Yang CW. Current situation and prospect in treatment of spine and spinal cord injuries. *Chin J Traumatol.* 2009Jun;12(3):131-2.

Lundgren T, Dahl J, Yardi N, Melin L. Acceptance and Commitment Therapy and yoga for drug-refractory epilepsy: A randomized controlled trial. *Epilepsy Behav.* 2008;13:102–8.

Lynskey James V., Adam Belanger, and Ranu Jung, Activity-dependent plasticity in spinal cord injury, *J Rehabil Res Dev.* 2008;45(2):229-240.

Minaire P, Castanier M, Girard R, Berard E, Deidier C, Bourret L. Epidemiology of spinal cord injury in the Rhône-Alpes region, France, 1970-1975. *Paraplegia* 1978;16:76-87.

Oken BS, Kishiyama S, Zajdel D, Bourdette D, Carlsen J, Haas M, et al. Randomized controlled trial of Yoga and exercise in multiple sclerosis. *Neurology.* 2004;62:2058–64.

Pearson KG, Topical Review: Could enhanced reflex function contribute to improving locomotion after spinal cord repair? *Journal of Physiology.* 2001, 533. 1, pp. 75-81.

Rajashree Ranjita, Alex Hankey, HR. Nagendra, Soubhagyalaxmi Mohanty. Yoga-based pulmonary rehabilitation for the management of dyspnea in coal miners with chronic obstructive pulmonary disease: A randomised controlled trial. *J Ayurveda Integr Med.* 2016 Jul - Sep;7(3):158-166. doi: 10.1016/j.jaim.2015.12.001. Epub 2016 Aug 18.

Rhee P, Kuncir EJ, Johnson L, et al. Cervical spine injury is highly dependent on the mechanism of injury following blunt and penetrating assault. *J Trauma.* Nov 2006;61(5): 1166-70.

Santo Tomas LH. Emphysema and chronic obstructive pulmonary disease in coal miners. *Curr Opin Pulm Med* 2011;17:123e5. (Tomas, 2011).

Schwab ME. Repairing the injured spinal cord. *Science.* 2002; 295:1029-1031 (review).

Tandon OP, Tripathi Y, editors. *Best and Taylor's physiological basis of medical practice.* 13th ed. Gurgaon: Wolters Kluwer Health/Lippincott Williams and Wilkins Publishers; 2012. (Tandon, Tripathi, 2012).

Velikonja O, Curic K, Ozura A, Jazbec SS. Influence of sports climbing and yoga on spasticity, cognitive function, mood and fatigue in patients with multiple sclerosis. *Clin Neurol Neurosurg.* 2010;112:597–601.

Water RL, Adkins RH, Yakura JS. *Definition of complete spinal cord injury.* Paraplegia. Nov. 1991;29(9):573-81.

Waters RL, Meyer PR, Adkins RH, Felton D. Emergency, acute, and surgical management of spinal trauma. *Arch Phys Med Rehabil* 1999;80:1383-1390.

Winterholler M, Erbguth F, Neundörfer B. The use of alternative medicine by multiple sclerosis patients--patient characteristics and patterns of use. *Fortschr Neurol Psychiatr.* 1997;65:555–61.

Zwick D. Integrated Iyengar Yogain to rehab for spinal cord injury. *Nursing*. 2006Oct;36. SupplPT:18– 22.

In: Manipulation of Stem Cells for Disease Benefits ISBN: 978-1-53615-468-9
Editor: Prasad Koka

Chapter 18

INTEGRATING YOGA IN REHABILITATION OF SPINAL CORD INJURY TO IMPROVE BENEFITS OF STEM CELL THERAPIES

Monali Madhusmita[1,*], John Ebnezar[2], Thaiyar Madabusi Srinivasan[3], Kashinath G Metri[4] and Patita Pabana Mohanty

[1]Division of Yoga and Life Sciences,
S-VYASA University, Bangalore, India
[2]Department of Orthopedics, Ebnezar Orthopaedic Centre,
Parimala Specialty Hospital, Bangalore, India
[3]Division of Yoga and Physical Sciences,
S-VYASA University, Bangalore, India
[4]Division of Yoga and Life Sciences,
S-VYASA University, Bangalore, India
[5]Department of Physiotherapy, SVNIRTAR, Odisha, India

ABSTRACT

Spinal cord injury (SCI) leads to severe disability contributing to poor quality of life. Cell-based or cell-related therapies have emerged as breakthrough therapies, both in regeneration of spinal cord and enhanced functional recovery. This review aims to discuss the therapeutic benefits of yoga in the rehabilitation of SCI in enhancing neural plasticity and emerging as an important add-on to support stem cell therapies. Conventional treatment for SCI does not bring out full recovery of loss of function. Chronic systemic inflammation prevailing years after injury is one of the obstacles in

* Corresponding Author's E-mail: monaliyoga@gmail.com.

sensory and motor function improvement. Recurrence of secondary infections, risk of neural tissue death and depression disorders leading to poor quality of life are some of the factors which are barriers to recovery of SCI. Cell replacement strategies provide cells that can replace the lost function. They provide a regenerative pathway for injured adult neurons, which would then promote the regeneration of adult neurons. Transplantation of cells mostly leads to the rejection of the donor material due to a combination of humoral and cellular immune responses. Evidences how that yoga modulates immune function which is otherwise compromised by stress. It can promote neurogenesis and angiogenesis resulting from increase production of neurotrophins. Yoga as an immune modulator can thus enhance the acceptance of implanted stem cells leading to the regeneration of the spinal cord circuitry and restore function after injury. It is thus hypothesized that yoga's therapeutic benefits may prove as an approach to alleviate the barriers of cellular therapies if necessary evidences are generated.

Keywords: spinal cord injury (SCI), stem cells, stem cell therapy, yoga, neuroplasticity, neurotrophins, neurogenesis, angiogenesis

INTRODUCTION

Spinal Cord Injury Pathophysiology

Spinal cord injury (SCI) is a disastrous condition, with sudden loss of sensory, motor and autonomic functions distal to the level of trauma. The primary effects of the trauma are necrosis, edema, hemorrhage, and vasospasm. An avalanche of secondary pathophysiology includes: i) ischemia, ii) apoptosis, iii) fluid and electrolyte disturbances, iv) excitotoxicity, v) lipid peroxidation, vi) production of free radicals, and vii) an inflammatory response, resulting in further catastrophe due to swelling and blood flow reduction. Finally, a large fluid filled cavity or cyst forms in the center of the cord, surrounded by a subpial rim containing some preserved axons, mostly demyelinated. Hypertrophic astrocytes, macrophages, and other cells secrete extracellular matrix and inhibitory molecules to form glial scar, culminating in a physical and chemical barrier to regeneration. Although there are major advances in the medical and surgical care of SCI patients, still no effective treatment exists for the neurological deficits resulting from SCI. These damages result in serious disability and multiple secondary health conditions (SHCs; multi-morbidity due to co-morbidities/complications) that require progressing management [19]. Further, it is said, "Persons with SCI have a specific constellation of ongoing health problems that are not being addressed by the mainstream health care system, and that demand the attention of the health services research community" [4].

Multimorbidity associated with SCI makes it a very costly condition and it costs around $21,450 per annum, to care for 1 person with chronic SCI in the United States [5]. Generally, men are at higher risk of SCI than women; the gender ratio ranged from 0.99:1 in Taipei, Taiwan to 13.5:1 in India [19]. Employment of emergency services includes treatment for urinary tract infections, pneumonia, and other SHCs such as pressure ulcers and depression [10]. But 17% of these health care service utilization could be categorized under "preventable" [7].

'Divergent' antipsychotic medications and drugs used in some neurological disorders such as SCI are associated with metabolic side effects such as weight gain, diabetes, and dyslipidemias [38]. First and second generation antidepressants are linked to cardiovascular and sexual dysfunction complications. The therapeutic use of these medications is also partial. Thus, there is a clear demand for complementary non-psycho-pharmacological intervention for psychiatric, neurological and various other dis-orders [18]. Many studies suggest that yoga acts as a preventive measure and helps in patient's psychological healing process [23].

Current Therapeutic Strategies for Spinal Cord Injury

Surgical Decompression

Urgent surgical decompression within 24 h after injury significantly increased post-operative motor and sensory functions according to American Spinal Injury Association (ASIA) score. Although early decompression reduces the risk of respiratory failure and sepsis, neurological surgery for the treatment of SCI is still associated with complications such as incidental durotomy or meningitis.

Therapeutic Hypothermia

Beneficial effects of modest (32–34_C) systemic hypothermia induced by intravascular cooling catheter and difference between the temperature at the spinal cord lesion and core body temperature have been successfully resolved by localized cooling of the injury site during surgical decompression. Systemic hypothermia as well as local cooling attenuate main pathophysiological processes during SCI including neuronal metabolism, neuro- inflammation, oxidative stress, excitotoxicity, and apoptosis. At the same time, decreased temperature protects the spinal cord from further injury by preserving the blood-spinal cord barrier (BSCB) and reducing edema, and induces neuro-repair by enhancing angiogenesis and neurogenesis.

Pharmacotherapy

Because of their anti-inflammatory effects and capacity to reduce oxidative stress and excitotoxicity, corticosteroids are used in many preclinical and clinical studies as therapeutic agents for the treatment of SCI. Use of methyl prednisolone in patients with SCI has become controversial, because of high rate of complications such as sepsis, pulmonary embolism, and gastrointestinal hemorrhage [47].

Barriers in Neuronal Regeneration/Functional Recovery in SCI

Inflammation

Inflammation leads to apoptosis of neurons and oligodendrocytes, scar formation and finally in the reduction of neuronal function. Managing inflammation will decrease secondary degeneration and the functional deficit after SCI [51].

Secondary Infections

Urinary tract infection, pressure ulcers, pulmonary and cardiovascular problems are some SCI complications which cause psychosocial distress for patients and delay of integration with society [49].

Chronic Pain Syndrome

Chronic pain in SCI is mostly referred to as 'central pain' and is very debilitating in nature and results in poor rehabilitation outcomes [54].

Respiratory Failure and Fatigue

Respiratory complications remain the most common cause of mortality following SCI [49].

Yoga as a Therapeutic Tool

Yoga is a promising mind-body intervention for improving health and well- being in a number of able-bodied and clinical populations.[40] It is an ancient Indian physical, mental and spiritual practice and the word "yoga" comes from Sanskrit, "yuj," meaning "yoke" or "union" [18]. Yoga has been observed to treat symptoms of some neurological and psychiatric disorders through an array of physiological mechanisms pertinent to either the aerobic factors of yoga (the changing sequel of asanas) or the breathing and meditative components of yoga (pranayama and dhyana). The aerobic components of yoga augment mental health through a variety of pathways such as stimulating the central nervous system for the release of endorphins monoamines, and brain-derived neuro-trophic factor (BDNF) in the hippocampus [33]. The meditative part consists of controlled breathing, relaxation, and meditation techniques and works with multiple possible mechanisms which lead to a decrement in sympathetic and increase in para-sympathetic tone, which further has been linked with emotional regulation and empathic response [18]. Secondly, there may be increase in heart-rate variability (HRV) and respiratory sinus arrhythmia (RSA). The reduction in these parameters has been associated with anxiety, panic disorder, depression, irritable bowel syndrome, early Alzheimer's, and obesity. Finally, meditative practices lead to increases in EEG synchrony and coherence, which are associated with improved integrated brain functioning and problem-solving.

Various studies show that meditation increases the levels of Brain-derived neurotrophic factor (BDNF) [41]. Other consequences include increase in vagal tone, down-regulation of the hypothalamic-pituitary-adrenal axis and decrease in serum cortisol, increase in gamma-aminobutyric acid (GABA) levels and serum prolactin. Upgrading of frontal electro-encephalogram (EEG) alpha wave activity improves relaxation [11, 12, 30].

Some studies have linked an increase in melatonin and a decrease in cortisol, to the meditative components of yoga [3]. Increases in melatonin impacts promotion of sleep, stimulates the immune system by acting as a powerful antioxidant, and decreases blood pressure. Further, Tooley et al. observed higher levels of plasma melatonin in patients immediately after yogic meditation sessions, as compared with control [36]. They hypothesized two possible mechanisms: First, meditation reduces blood flow to the liver, slowing the metabolism of melatonin. Secondly, these practices increase the levels of serotonin, which is converted to melatonin in the pineal gland. Harinath et al. also observed an increase in melatonin levels after a 3-month practice of asanas, pranayama, and meditation [8]. Meditation has also been associated with reduction in levels of cortisol. Studies have found a significant positive correlation between levels of cortisol, negative affect, and depression. Vagal or parasympathetic activity is responsible for calming the body's stress response systems, and is associated with decreased levels of cortisol. Thus, components of yoga apart from aerobic exercise, such as controlled breathing and meditation techniques, is known to decrease cortisol levels [13, 24].

More active practices followed by relaxing ones lead to deeper relaxation than relaxing practices alone, documented by research from Swami Vivekananda Yoga University, Bangalore, India and possibility of neural plasticity bringing changes in the hypo-pituitary–pancreatic axis [2].

Rehabilitation of SCI Patients: Potential of Yoga

Severed spinal cord due to SCI leads to disruption of communication in parts that are innervated at or below the lesion. Neuroprotective drugs such as methylprednisolone are being used for the treatment for spinal injuries and may prevent cell death. SCI is followed by several complications for which there is a need for rehabilitation [44]. Teams of nurses, physicians, physical and occupational therapists, psychologists, and social workers, avail inter-disciplinary health care services for rehabilitation of SCI patients. Yoga as a therapy is a holistic approach, which is believed to stimulate neural pathways and neurotransmitters. Thus, different yogic techniques may act as a valuable healing tool, with proper modification and supervised facilitation, leading to regeneration of nerve fibers in SCI patients [30].

Iyengar Yoga for SCI Patients

Evidences shows that special form of yoga known as Iyenger yoga using props and other innovative modalities is able to handle special challenges of SCI patients [45]. With guided assistance this form of yoga develops strength, flexibility, and physical balance through proper stretching of muscles and building up symmetric and asymmetric postures. Enhancement of body awareness through integration of pranayama into these postures and focus on time and weight management of muscle contraction and relaxation is the mainstay of this form of yoga. Literature review reveals that specific forms and different limbs of yoga helps in alleviating dysfunctions such as bowel, bladder, sexual, pain and depression in individuals with SCI [10].

Integrated Yoga for Traumatic SCI Patients

Another recent study conducted at a rehabilitation centre in Odisha, India, indicated that the addition of integrated yoga intervention to physiotherapy has beneficial effects in terms of improving pain, inflammation, gait, and spasticity among patients with paraplegia. Further, it also suggested the integration of yoga practices in conventional rehabilitation programs for traumatic spinal injury patients [46].

Effect of Yoga on Neurotrophins and Neurotransmitters

A review elaborates the effect of yoga on various neurotransmitters and neurotrophins.[36] Endogenous dopamine production was raised during Yoga Nidra meditation, as demonstrated by a PET study and increase in brain GABA levels following 60-min yoga session as compared to controls performing a 60-min reading, as demonstrated by another study [15, 32]. Furthermore, other evidences revealed that yogic practice daily for one hour for a period of 3 months helps in lowering ACTH and cortisol, while elevating serotonin, dopamine, and BDNF in healthy active men [23].

Stem Cell Therapy

Stem cells are defined as cells that have the capacity to recreate themselves perpetually and possess pluripotent ability to differentiate into many cell types. Mammalian pluripotent stem cells which have been identified are of two types:

embryonic stem cells (ESCs) derived from the inner cell mass of blastocysts and embryonic germ cells (EGCs) obtained from post implantation embryos. These stem cells give rise to various organs and tissues [5, 27, 36]. Currently, there is identification of generation of a new class of pluripotent stem cells known as induced pluripotent cells (iPS cells) from adult somatic cells such as skin fibroblasts by introduction of embryogenesis-related genes [22, 33, 43]. As an addendum to ESCs and iPS cells, tissue-specific stem cells have been isolated from various tissues such as hematopoietic stem cells, bone marrow mesenchymal stem cells, adipose tissue derived stem cells, amniotic fluid stem cells, and neural stem cells. Multipotent neural stem cells (NSCs) found in developing or adult mammalian brain which has attribute of indefinite growth and multipotent potential. They differentiate into three major Central Nervous System (CNS) cell types: neurons, astrocytes, and oligodendrocytes [8, 13, 17, 38]. Recently, it is evident that stem cells which were thought to be responsible for generation of mature differentiated cells of one organ may have the ability to also differentiate across lineages and contribute to generation of other types of tissues. For instance, hematopoietic stem cells can differentiate into neuronal tissue, suggesting that easily accessible stem cells sources may one day be useful in the therapy of ischemic (stroke) and other degenerative diseases of CNS [26.]

Stem cell therapy despite of its various challenges is a very promising treatment modality for treating the spinal cord injury and recovering functional ability. The ability of stem cells to differentiate into various other cell types and producing substances such as cytokine, growth factor, and trophic factor, in turn promote neuroprotection and regeneration. Schwann cells, embryonic stem cells, mesenchymal stem cells/bone marrow stem cells, olfactory ensheathing cells and neural stem cells are various types of stem cells used for implantation in SCI. Among various types of stem cells, bone marrow derived mesenchymal stem cells is highly used in SCI. Research showed that direct intra-medullary injection to the injured spinal cord site in sub-acute phase is most effective [45].

In a recent study, CD34C cells from human UCB (Umbilical Cord Blood) were ingrained into immune-compromised animals that had undergone a stroke 48 hours earlier. There were reports of neo-vascularization in the ischemic zone, leading to neuronal regeneration, mainly owing to endogenous neuro-genesis [32]. Similar results have been observed for animals that were treated with granulocyte colony stimulating factor (G-CSF), an agent that mobilizes hematopoietic progenitors from the bone marrow into the blood [28].

Many in vivo studies shows that non-neural stem cells also has significant functional impact in the clinical management of stroke and spinal cord injury, and other neurodegenerative disorders by inducing angiogenesis, recruiting endogenous stem cells, guiding axons or secreting neurotrophic factors. As already demonstrated in animal models and in clinical studies in ischemic heart disorders [1, 5, 39] these results have clinical significance, despite the fact that the injected cell population did not itself generate neural cells. A large number of studies in last 5–10 years have showed that non-neural stem cells are competent of generating neurons or glia in vitro and in vivo [25].

Spinal cord injury is a devastating condition in humans leading to significant disability with immense loss of quality of life and economic output. Till date there is no adequate clinical cure and overall prognosis is mostly poor. Research in the last two decades shows that cellular or cell-related therapies have unlatched exhilarating therapeutic possibilities.

For spinal cord regeneration, stem cell trans-plantation still holds the best future and amongst them, human embryonic stem cells (hESC) and olfactory ensheathing cells (OEC) are presently the leading prospects [14]. Inflammation after traumatic SCI is non-resolving and it will be present in chronic injury stages also. It plays a key role in the pathophysiology of SCI, and it has been associated with further neurodegeneration and development of neuropathic pain. Neuropathic pain is a huge challenge, and cellular or cell-related therapies are rapidly gathering momentum to combat it. These therapies aspires to attain analgesic effects from different perspectives such as preventing neuronal damage due to inflammation, cell cycling, or dysfunctional regeneration; inducting biological minipumps using adrenal medullary chromaffin tissues, engineered cell lines, or astrocytes; and lastly, regulating the internal milieu using trans-plant of bone marrow of bone marrow mesenchymal stem cells [15]. Neural precursor cells (NPCs) have been shown to reduce acute and sub-acute inflammatory responses after SCI [24]. The role of yoga practices in stem cell regeneration and regulation is under investigation, and as this study implies, it is possible that targeted exercises and pranayama could stimulate stem cell organization in SCI. More on this is presented later.

Barriers in Stem Cell Therapy for SCI

Immune Response

Transplantation of cells may leads to the rejection of the stem cells due to a combination of humoral and cellular immune responses [53].

Reduced Angiogenesis

Reduced angiogenesis leads to failure in neural plasticity [52].

Reduced Neurogenesis

Insignificant neurogenesis due to various reasons may lead to failure in neural regeneration and functional recovery in SCI [52].

Decreased Level of Growth Factors

Different types of growth factors helps in directing differentiation of neural stem cells and their deficiency acts as a barrier to stem cell therapy [50].

Neuroplasticity

Brain plasticity is seen to be influenced by several factors including neurotrophic factors, neurotransmitters, endocrines, cytoskeleton proteins and neuronal electrical activity to name a few. Practice of yoga produces brain plasticity leading to improvement in cognitive function and alleviation of symptoms such as depression, anxiety etc. [23]. It has great potentials in treating neurological diseases as well. Neurotrophic factors are key molecules which are involved in the development and differentiation of the nervous system and play a major role in neuronal plasticity. Synaptic neuroplasticity induced by neurotrophins like BDNF or VEGF may be responsible for the therapeutic benefit of yoga in various psychiatric and neuro-degenerative diseases. A study in patients with depression has shown reduction in cortisol level along with increased blood plasma BDNF content following yoga practice [22]. Figure 1 illustrates the possible mechanism of impact of integrating yoga therapy in rehabilitation SCI to improve benefits of stem cell therapies.

CONCLUSION

This study concludes that yoga is an immune-modulator and can be instrumental in overcoming barriers of conventional treatment and stem cell therapy to achieve functional recovery in SCI. Yoga is an emerging therapy having potential to enhance stem cell therapy by increasing production of neurotrophins and other neurotransmitters, decreasing systemic inflammation, enhancing neurogenesis and angiogenesis; thus, it may also help in minimizing the barriers of stem cell therapy. All these potential beneficial effects of yoga may help in improving the benefits of stem cell therapy out come in patients with SCI.

Management of SCI is challenging and also incurs huge economic burden on the individual, family and care- takers and the health care system of the state. Loss of man-power due to SCI is a serious issue to be addressed with the rise in road traffic accidents (RTA). Yoga has shown promising results to combat the deleterious aftereffects of SCI and in alleviating secondary complications. Quality of life enhancement resulting from adaptation of yogic lifestyle is a boon for individuals with SCI. Yoga therapy practice is also known to enhance neural plasticity by promoting expression of neuro-transmitters and neurotrophins in the CNS.

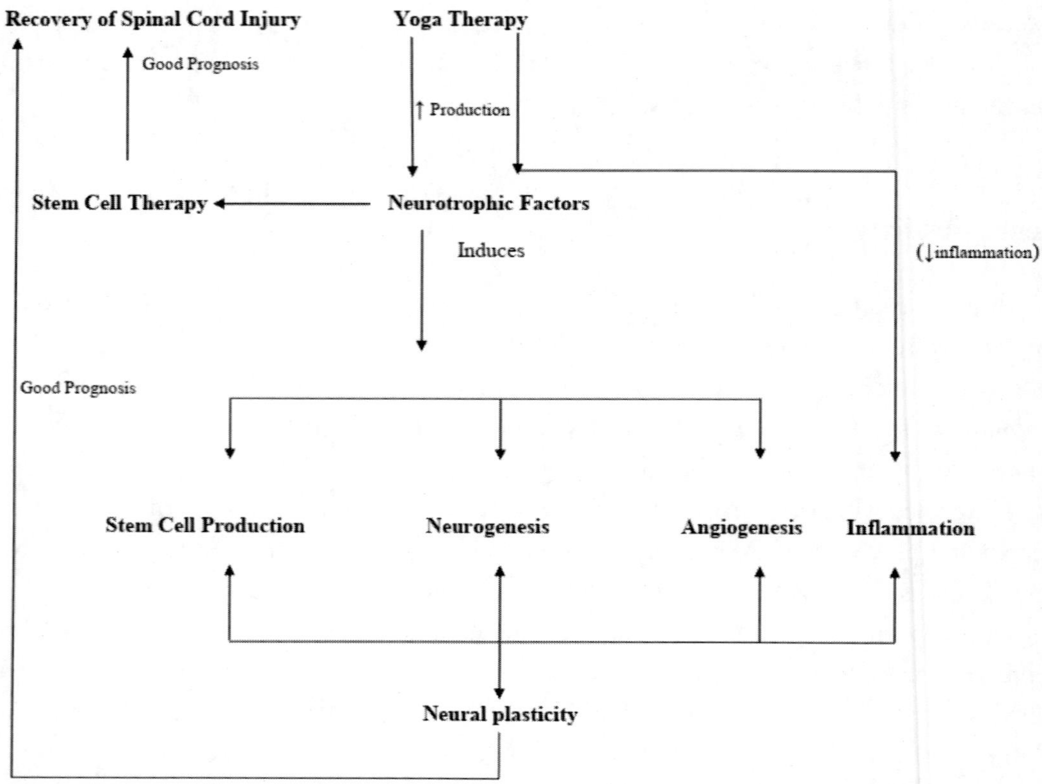

The above flow chart shows the impact of integrating yoga therapy in the rehabilitation of SCI to improve the outcome of cell -based strategies by enhancing neuro-glial plasticity with reduction of inflammation and increase production of neurotrophins leading to neurogenesis, angiogenesis and increase production of stem-cells.

Increase in levels of neurotrophins in blood plasma resulting from yogic practices induces neurogenesis and angiogenesis further enhancing synaptic plasticity. Cellular therapies such as stem cell therapies are emerging as promising therapeutic tools, leading SCI management towards a more satisfactory clinical cure. However till date, the success rate of such cell-based therapies is minimal and associated with many shortcomings. Success rate of stem cell therapy in acute or fresh spinal cord injuries of few weeks is very high with acceptance of grafted tissue and translation of its effect to neurological recovery. But in chronic phase following SCI, the problem of tissue rejection and administration of immunosuppressant drugs after stem cell therapy, makes prognosis poor. Incorporation of yoga therapy into rehabilitation programs of SCI patients can possibly enhance the likelihood of acceptance of induced stem cells by the body, lowering the possibility of tissue rejection and intake of immunosuppressant drugs leading to significant functional recovery. Stem cell therapy works by inducing angiogenesis, recruiting endogenous stem cells, guiding axons and secreting neurotrophic factors etc. Yoga therapy could contribute hugely for successful implementation of stem cell therapy as a breakthrough treatment for SCI patients' rehabilitation. Scientific literature also indicates that the state of brief intermittent hypoxia produced during practice of pranayama might stimulate migration of the stem cells from their milieu to the site of injury and facilitate neuronal regeneration [33]. Thus, integration of yoga therapy into rehabilitation of SCI may be one of the approaches to alleviate the limitations of cellular therapies.

References

[1] Noonan VK, Fallah N, Park SE, Dumont FS, Leblond J, Cobb J, et al. Health care utilization in persons with traumatic spinal cord injury: The importance of multi-morbidity and the impact on patient outcomes. *Top Spinal Cord Inj Rehabil* [Internet]. 2014 [cited 2018 Aug 10]; 20(4):289–301. Available from: http://www.ncbi.nlm.nih.gov/pubmed/25477742.

[2] Ning GZ, Wu Q, Li YL, Feng SQ. Epidemiology of traumatic spinal cord injury in Asia: a systematic review. *J Spinal Cord Med* [Internet]. 2012 Jul [cited 2018 Aug 10];35(4):229–39. Available from: http://www.ncbi.nlm.nih.gov/pubmed/22925749.

[3] Jaglal SB, Munce SEP, Guilcher SJ, Couris CM, Fung K, Craven BC, et al. Health system factors associated with rehospitalizations after traumatic spinal cord injury: A population-based study. *Spinal Cord* 2009 Aug 10 [cited 2018 Aug 10];47(8):604–9. Available from http://www.ncbi.nlm.nih.gov/pubmed/19274059.

[4] Guilcher SJT, Craven BC, Calzavara A, McColl MA, Jaglal SB. Is the emergency department an appropriate substitute for primary care for persons with traumatic spinal cord injury? *Spinal Cord* [Internet]. 2013 Mar 13 [cited 2018 Aug 10];51(3):202–8. Available from: http://www.ncbi.nlm .nih.gov/pubmed/23147131.

[5] Wirshing DA, Boyd JA, Meng LR, Ballon JS, Marder SR, Wirshing WC. The effects of novel antipsychotics on glucose and lipid levels. *J Clin Psychiatry* [Internet]. 2002 Oct [cited 2018 Aug 16];63(10):856–65. Available from: http://www.ncbi.nlm.nih.gov/pubmed/12416594.

[6] Meyer HB, Katsman A, Sones AC, Auerbach DE, Ames D, Rubin RT. Yoga as an Ancillary Treatment for Neurological and Psychiatric Disorders: A Review. *J Neuropsychiatry Clin Neurosci* [Internet]. 2012;24(2): 152–64. Available from: .http://psychiatryonline.org/doi /abs/10.1176/appi.neuropsych.11040090.

[7] Wren AA, Wright MA, Carson JW, Keefe FJ. Yoga for persistent pain: New findings and directions for an ancient practice. *Pain* [Internet]. 2011 Mar [cited 2018 Aug 16];152(3):477–80. Available from: http://www. ncbi.nlm.nih.gov/pubmed/21247696.

[8] Taylor CB, Sallis JF, Needle R. The relation of physical activity and exercise to mental health. *Public Health Rep* [Internet]. [cited 2018 Aug 16];100(2):195–202. Available from: http://www.ncbi.nlm.nih.gov/pubmed/ 3920718.

[9] 9. Xiong GL, Doraiswamy PM. Does Meditation Enhance Cognition and Brain Plasticity? *Ann N Y Acad Sci* [Internet]. 2009 Aug [cited 2018 Aug 16];1172(1): 63–9. Available from: http://www.ncbi.nlm.nih.gov/pub med/197 43551

[10] Kamei T, Toriumi Y, Kimura H, Kumano H, Ohno S, Kimura K. Decrease in Serum Cortisol during Yoga Exercise is Correlated with Alpha Wave Activation. *Percept Mot Skills* [Internet]. 2000 Jun [cited 2018 Aug 16];90(3):1027–32. Available from: http://www.ncbi. nlm.nih.gov/pubmed/10883793.

[11] Janakiramaiah N, Gangadhar BN, Naga Venkatesha Murthy PJ, Harish MG, Subbakrishna DK, Veda-murthachar A. Antidepressant efficacy of Sudarshan Kriya Yoga (SKY) in melancholia: A randomized comparison with electro-convulsive therapy (ECT) and imipramine. *J Affect Disord* [Internet]. [cited 2018 Aug 16];57(1–3):255–9. Available from: http://www.ncbi.nlm.nih.gov/pubmed/1070 8840.

[12] Streeter CC, Whitfield TH, Owen L, Rein T, Karri SK, Yakhkind A, et al. Effects of yoga versus walking on mood, anxiety, and brain GABA levels: a randomized controlled MRS study. *J Altern Complement Med* [Internet]. 2010 Nov [cited 2018 Aug 16];16(11):1145–52. Available from: http://www.ncbi.nlm.nih.gov/pub med/ 20722471.

[13] Balasubramaniam M, Telles S, Doraiswamy PM. Yoga on our minds: A systematic review of yoga for neuro-psychiatric disorders. *Front Psychiatry*. 2013;3 (JAN): 1–16.

[14] Tooley KM, Traxler MJ, Swaab TY. Electro-physiological and behavioral evidence of syntactic priming in sentence comprehension. *J Exp Psychol Learn Mem Cogn* [Internet]. 2009 [cited 2018 Aug 16];35(1):19–45. Available from: http:// doi.apa.org/get doi.cfm?doi=10.1037/a0013984.

[15] Rael Cahn B, Goodman MS, Peterson CT, Maturi R, Mills PJ, Thwing Emeny R, et al. Yoga, Meditation and Mind-Body Health: Increased BDNF, Cortisol Awakening Response, and Altered Inflammatory Marker Expression after a 3-Month Yoga and Meditation Retreat. *Frontiers* 2017 [cited 2018 Aug 14]; Available from: www.frontiersin.org.

[16] Balaji PA, Varne SR, Ali SS. Physiological effects of yogic practices and transcendental meditation in health and disease. *N Am J Med Sci*. 2012;4(10): 442–8.

[17] Zhang N, Yin Y, Xu SJ, Wu YP, Chen WS. Inflamm-ation & apoptosis in spinal cord injury. *Indian J Med Res* [Internet]. 2012 Mar [cited 2018 Aug 16]; 135:287–96. Available from: http://www.ncbi.nlm.nih .gov/pubmed/22561613.

[18] Smith EN, Boser A. Yoga, vertebral fractures, and osteoporosis: research and recommendations. *Int J Yoga Therap* [Internet]. 2013 [cited 2018 Aug 16];23(1):17–23. Available from: http://www.ncbi.nlm.nih.gov/pub med/240 16820.

[19] Zwick D. Integrating Iyengar yoga into rehab for spinal cord injury. *Nursing* (Lond) [Internet]. 2006 Oct [cited 2018 Aug 16];36 Suppl P T:18–22. Available from: http:// www.ncbi.nlm.nih.gov/pubmed/17038855.

[20] Iyengar B. *Light on Yoga: Yoga Daipikaa*, [Internet]. New York: Schocken Books; 1966 [cited 2018 Aug 16]. Available from: http://www.worldcat.org/title/light-on-yoga -yoga-daipikaa/oclc/908875553.

[21] Telles S, Sayal N, Nacht C, Chopra A, Patel K, Wnuk A, et al. Yoga: Can It Be Integrated with Treatment of Neuropathic Pain? *Integr Med Int* [Internet]. 2017 [cited 2018 Jul 24];4:69–84. Available from: www.karger.com /imi.

[22] Streeter CC, Whitfield TH, Owen L, Rein T, Karri SK, Yakhkind A, et al. Effects of Yoga Versus Walking on Mood, Anxiety, and Brain GABA Levels: A Randomized Controlled MRS Study. *J Altern Complement Med* [Internet]. 2010 Nov [cited 2018 Aug 15];16(11):1145–52. Available from: http://www.ncbi.nlm.nih.gov/pub med/207 22471.

[23] Kjaer TW, Bertelsen C, Piccini P, Brooks D, Alving J, Lou HC. Increased dopamine tone during meditation-induced change of consciousness [Internet]. Vol. 13, *Cognitive Brain Research.* 2002 [cited 2018 Aug 15]. Available from: www.elsevier.com/locate/bres.

[24] Pal R, Singh SN, Chatterjee A, Saha M. Age-related changes in cardiovascular system, autonomic functions, and levels of BDNF of healthy active males: role of yogic practice. *Age* (Omaha) [Internet]. 2014 Aug 11 [cited 2018 Aug 14];36(4):9683. Available from: http:// www.ncbi.nlm .nih.gov/pubmed/25012275.

[25] Thomson JA, Itskovitz-Eldor J, Shapiro SS, Waknitz MA, Swiergiel JJ, Marshall VS, et al. Embryonic stem cell lines derived from human blastocysts. *Science* [Internet]. 1998 Nov 6 [cited 2018 Aug 30];282(5391): 1145–7. Available from: http://www.ncbi.nlm.nih.gov/ pubmed/9804556.

[26] Shamblott MJ, Axelman J, Wang S, Bugg EM, Littlefield JW, Donovan PJ, et al. Derivation of pluri-potent stem cells from cultured human primordial germ cells. *Proc Natl Acad Sci USA* [Internet]. 1998 Nov 10 [cited 2018 Aug 30]; 95(23): 13726–31. Available from: http://www.ncbi.nlm .nih.gov/pubmed/9811868.

[27] Donovan PJ, Gearhart J. The end of the beginning for pluripotent stem cells. *Nature* [Internet]. 2001 Nov 1 [cited 2018 Aug 30];414(6859):92–7. Available from: http:// www.ncbi.nlm.nih.gov/pubmed/11689953.

[28] Takahashi K, Tanabe K, Ohnuki M, Narita M, Ichisaka T, Tomoda K, et al. Induction of Pluripotent m,Stem Cells from Adult Human Fibroblasts by Defined

Factors. *Cell* [Internet]. 2007 Nov 30 [cited 2018 Aug 30];131(5):861–72. Available from: http://www.ncbi. nlm.nih.gov/pubmed/ 18035408.

[29] Yu J, Vodyanik MA, Smuga-Otto K, Antosiewicz-Bourget J, Frane JL, Tian S, et al. Induced Pluripotent Stem Cell Lines Derived from Human Somatic Cells. *Science* (80) [Internet]. 2007 Dec 21 [cited 2018 Aug 30];318(5858): 1917–20. Available from: http://www. ncbi.nlm.nih.gov/ pubmed/18029452.

[30] Park I-H, Arora N, Huo H, Maherali N, Ahfeldt T, Shimamura A, et al. Disease-specific induced pluri-potent stem cells. *Cell* [Internet]. 2008 Sep 5 [cited 2018 Aug 30];134(5):877–86. Available from: http://www. ncbi.nlm.nih.gov/pubmed/ 18691744.

[31] McKay R. Stem cells in the central nervous system. *Science* [Internet]. 1997 Apr 4 [cited 2018 Aug 30];276 (5309):66–71. Available from: http://www.ncbi.nlm.nih .gov/pubmed/ 9082987.

[32] Horner PJ, Gage FH. Regenerating the damaged central nervous system. *Nature* [Internet]. 2000 Oct 26 [cited 2018 Aug 30];407(6807):963–70. Available from: http://www. ncbi.nlm.nih.gov/pubmed/11069169.

[33] Victor FC, Gottlieb AB. TNF-alpha and apoptosis: implications for the pathogenesis and treatment of psoriasis. *J Drugs Dermatol* [Internet]. 2002 Dec [cited 2018 Aug 30];1(3):264–75. Available from: http://www. ncbi.nlm.nih.gov/ pubmed/12851985.

[34] Kim J, Heshka S, Gallagher D, Kotler DP, Mayer L, Albu J, et al. Intermuscular adipose tissue-free skeletal muscle mass: estimation by dual-energy X-ray absorptiometry in adults. *J Appl Physiol* [Internet]. 2004 Aug [cited 2018 Aug 30];97(2):655–60. Available from: http://www.ncbi.nlm.nih .gov/pubmed/ 15090482.

[35] Ross JJ, Verfaillie CM. Evaluation of neural plasticity in adult stem cells. *Philos Trans R Soc Lond B Biol Sci* [Internet]. 2008 Jan 12 [cited 2018 Jul 24];363(1489): 199–205. Available from: http://www.ncbi.nlm.nih.gov/ pub med/ 17282993.

[36] Taguchi A, Soma T, Tanaka H, Kanda T, Nishimura H, Yoshikawa H, et al. Administration of $CD34^+$ cells after stroke enhances neurogenesis via angiogenesisin a mouse model. *J Clin Invest* [Internet]. 2004 Aug 1 [cited 2018 Aug 16];114(3):330–8. Available from: http:// www.ncbi.nlm.nih .gov/pubmed/ 15286799.

[37] Shyu WC, Lin SZ, Yang HI, Tzeng YS, Pang CY, Yen PS, et al. Functional Recovery of Stroke Rats Induced by Granulocyte Colony-Stimulating Factor-Stimulated Stem Cells. *Circulation* [Internet]. 2004 Sep 20 [cited 2018 Aug 16];110(13):1847–54. Available from: .http://www.ncbi.nlm .nih.gov/pubmed/ 15381647

[38] Assmus B, Schächinger V, Teupe C, Britten M, Lehmann R, Döbert N, et al. Transplantation of Pro-genitor Cells and Regeneration Enhancement in Acute

Myocardial Infarction (TOPCARE-AMI). *Circulation* [Internet]. 2002 Dec 10 [cited 2018 Aug 16];106(24): 3009–17. Available from: http://www.ncbi.nlm. nih.gov/pubmed/12473544.

[39] Wollert KC, Meyer GP, Lotz J, Ringes Lichtenberg S, Lippolt P, Breidenbach C, et al. Intracoronary autol-ogous bone-marrow cell transfer after myocardial infarction: The BOOST randomised controlled clinical trial. *Lancet* [Internet]. 2004 Jul [cited 2018 Aug 16]; 364(9429):141–8. Available from: http://www.ncbi.nlm .nih.gov/ pubmed/1524 6726.

[40] Gnecchi M, Danieli P, Cervio E. Mesenchymal stem cell therapy for heart disease. *Vascul Pharmacol* [Internet]. 2012;57(1):48–55. Available from: http://dx.doi .org/10.1016/j.vph.2012.04.002.

[41] Lee VM, Louis SA, Reynolds BA. Neural Stem Cells M I N I-R E V I E W The Central Nervous System Identification of Neural Stem Cells. *Stem Cell Technologies* [Internet]. [cited 2018 Aug 10]. Available from: www.stemcell.com/NSC Webinar.

[42] Leung L. Cellular therapies for treating pain associated with spinal cord injury. *J Transl Med* [Internet]. 2012; 10(1):37. Available from: http://www.translational-med icine.com/content/10/1/37.

[43] Riemann L, Younsi A, Scherer M, Zheng G, Skutella T, Unterberg AW, et al. Transplantation of Neural Pre-cursor Cells Attenuates Chronic Immune Environment in Cervical Spinal Cord Injury. *Front Neurol* [Internet]. 2018 Jun 8 [cited 2018 Aug 10];9:428. Available from: http://www.ncb i.nlm.nih.gov/ pubmed/29951030.

[44] Raju T. Yoga Induced Brain Plasticity- Role of Neuro-trophic Factors. *Open Access J Neurol Neurosurg*. 2017; 6(1):10–2.

[45] Eric Domingos Mariano, Chary Marquez Batista, Breno José Alencar Pires Barbosa SK, Nagahashi Marie Manoel Jacobsen Teixeira, Matthias Morgalla, Marcos Tatagiba JL, Lepski G. Current perspectives in stem cell therapy for spinal cord repair in humans: A review of work from the past 10 years. *Views and Reviews*. 2014; 451–6.

[46] Monali Madhusmita, TMS, John Ebnezar, HR. Nagendra and PPM. Effect of Integrated Yoga as an Add-On to Physiotherapy on Walking Index, ESR, Pain, and Spasticity among Subjects with Traumatic Spinal Cord Injury: A Randomized Control Study. *J Stem Cells*. 2018;13(1):57–66.

[47] Marina Gazdic, Vladislav Volarevic, Randall Harrell, Crissy Fellabaum, Nemanja Jovicic NA and MS. Review: Stem Cells Therapy for Spinal Cord Injury. *Int J o f Mol Sci*. 2018;19:2–14.

[48] Berlowitz, DJ, Wadsworth, B, & Ross, J. (2016). Respiratory problems and management in people with spinal cord injury. *Breathe* (Sheffield, England), 12(4), 328–340. https://doi.org/10.1183/20734735.012616.

[49] Magia, F, Bhise, A, Prabhakar, M, & Shukla, Y. (2015). Special Interest Report Poster Presentation Number: SI-PO-21-12-Mon Monday 4 May 2015 13:00 Exhibit halls 401-403 Effect of Pranayama (Yogic Breathing) on Lung Function in Traumatic Thoracic Spinal Cord Injury Patients: An Interventional Study. *Physiotherapy*, 101, e927. https://doi.org/10.1016/j. physio.2015.03.1770.

[50] Schuldiner, M, Yanuka, O, Itskovitz-Eldor, J, Melton, DA, & Benvenisty, N. (2000). Effects of eight growth factors on the differentiation of cells derived from human embryonic stem cells. *Proceedings of the National Academy of Sciences of the United States of America*, 97(21), 11307–11312. https://doi.org/10.1073/ pnas. 97.21.1 1307.

[51] Zhang, N, Yin, Y, Xu, SJ, Wu, YP, & Chen, WS. (2012). Inflammation & apoptosis in spinal cord injury. *The Indian Journal of Medical Research*, 135(3), 287–296. Retrieved from http://www.ncbi.nlm.nih.gov/ pub med/22561613.

[52] Ahuja, CS, Nori, S, Tetreault, L, Wilson, J, Kwon, B, Harrop, J, Fehlings, MG. (2017). Traumatic Spinal Cord Injury—Repair and Regeneration. *Neurosurgery*, 80(3S), S9–S22. https://doi.org/10.1093/neuros/nyw080.

[53] Allison, D. J., & Ditor, D. S. (2015). Immune dysfunc-tion and chronic inflammation following spinal cord injury. *Spinal Cord*, 53(1), 14–18. https://doi.org/10.1038/sc.2014. 184.

[54] Lee, S, Zhao, X, Hatch, M, Chun, S, & Chang, E. (2013). Central Neuropathic Pain in Spinal Cord Injury. *Critical Reviews in Physical and Rehabilitation Medicine*, 25(3–4), 159–172. https://doi.org/10.1615/ CritRevPhysRehabilMed. 2013007944.

INDEX

C

D

E

F

G

H

I

K

L

M

N

Q

R

S

T

U

V

W

Y